W9-BYK-737

ADVANCES IN LIBRARY ADMINISTRATION AND ORGANIZATION

ADVANCES IN LIBRARY ADMINISTRATION AND ORGANIZATION

Series Editors: Edward D. Garten, Delmus E. Williams and James M. Nyce

Recent Volumes:

ADVANCES IN LIBRARY ADMINISTRATION AND
ORGANIZATION VOLUME 24

ADVANCES IN LIBRARY ADMINISTRATION AND ORGANIZATION

EDITED BY

EDWARD D. GARTEN
University of Dayton Libraries, Ohio, USA

DELMUS E. WILLIAMS
University of Akron Libraries, Ohio, USA

JAMES M. NYCE
Ball State University, Muncie, Indiana, USA

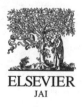

ELSEVIER
JAI

Amsterdam – Boston – Heidelberg – London – New York – Oxford
Paris – San Diego – San Francisco – Singapore – Sydney – Tokyo

JAI Press is an imprint of Elsevier

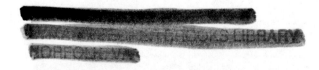

JAI Press is an imprint of Elsevier
The Boulevard, Langford Lane, Kidlington, Oxford OX5 1GB, UK
Radarweg 29, PO Box 211, 1000 AE Amsterdam, The Netherlands
525 B Street, Suite 1900, San Diego, CA 92101-4495, USA

First edition 2007

British Library Cataloguing in Publication Data
A catalogue record for this book is available from the British Library

ISBN-13: 978-0-7623-1410-2
ISBN-10: 0-7623-1410-9
ISSN: 0732-0671

For information on all JAI Press publications
visit our website at books.elsevier.com

Printed and bound in The Netherlands

07 08 09 10 11 10 9 8 7 6 5 4 3 2 1

CONTENTS

THE WORK PROCESS OF RESEARCH LIBRARIANS,
ELICITED VIA THE ABSTRACTION-
DECOMPOSITION SPACE

LIBRARY MANAGEMENT EDUCATION AND
REALITY: A CLEARER CONNECTION

INNOVATIVE LIBRARY PROGRAMS FOR THE
HISPANIC POPULATION: OPPORTUNITIES FOR THE
PUBLIC LIBRARY ADMINISTRATOR

LANDSCAPES OF INFORMATION AND
CONSUMPTION: A LOCATION ANALYSIS OF
PUBLIC LIBRARIES IN CALCUTTA

LIST OF CONTRIBUTORS

Dana W. R. Boden	University of Nebraska-Lincoln Libraries, Lincoln, NE, USA
Deonie Botha	Department of Information Science, University of Pretoria, Pretoria, South Africa
Zohra Calcuttawala	2224 Mountain Creek Trail, Hoover, AL, USA
Marvin J. Dainoff	Miami University, Cincinnati, OH, USA
Paula R. Dempsey	DePaul University Libraries, Chicago, IL, USA
K. Brock Enger	North Dakota State University, Moorhead, MN, USA
Rich Gazan	University of Denver Library & Information Program, Denver, CO, USA
Anna Maria Guerra	Boeing Aerospace Corporation, La Canada, CA, USA
Leonard S. Mark	Department of Psychology, Miami University, Oxford, OH, USA
Charles Osburn	School of Library & Information Science, University of Alabama, Tuscaloosa, AL, USA
Kevin J. Simons	Miami University, Cincinnati, OH, USA
Delmus E. Williams	University of Akron Libraries, OH, USA

INTRODUCTION

Over the years, *Advances in Library Administration and Organization* has worked to bring you research articles and well thought out essays on how we manage or ought to manage libraries and other information agencies. This volume is no exception. It brings together essays on an eclectic set of topics, many of which are based on research methodologies developed outside of librarianship and that are not often used in our field. We, the editors, feel that this is as consistently good a collection of pieces as we have ever offered readers and hope you will find that to be true.

The volume leads off with K. Brock Enger's essay on the development of our literature and that of higher education and her analysis of the ways in which the literature of the field defines the progress we and our education colleagues have made in establishing ourselves as full-fledged disciplines. Enger uses bibliometrics to understand how we look at ourselves and how we present data to our colleagues. She has come to interesting conclusions along the way. Her comparisons of the two disciplines are apt and provide guidance as to where we should go as we refine the study of libraries and their organizations.

Charles Osburn, whose work we have published before, follows with a fine essay on the library as a place. Much has been written on this topic over the last couple of years, but Osburn provides a thoughtful view of what it means to be a place rather than providing just one more view of how libraries use space. His consideration of place as a concept and a value draws on architectural literature and that of psychology, neurology, geography, and philosophy to add badly needed depth to our understanding of this issue.

Kevin Simons and his colleagues then discuss the work processes of research librarians based on a methodology imported from organizational psychology. The method chosen moves away from both normative (how we should do things) and descriptive (how we actually do our work) to a formative approach that can be particularly valuable in an information-dense environment. It is an interesting study that sheds new light to topics that have long been of interest to the Library and Information Sciences community.

Paula Dempsey, a sociologist, follows with an analysis of how interactive service workers collaborate with one another in conversations. The conversations studied are those that contribute to the construction of their professional identities in changing times.

Dana Boden uses a survey methodology to examine how chairs of library departments can support untenured librarians as they develop themselves professionally. In the same vein, Deonie Botha reexamines the role of mentoring as a tool for developing libraries. Her work is based on a case study developed in South Africa, but, even though it is set in the Third World, Botha's study does a good job of generalizing on unique situations so that they offer a strong analysis of librarianship's prevailing wisdom about mentoring, applies it to a specific situation, and then provides insights that can be easily generalized for use elsewhere.

Rich Gazan then uses a collaborative digital library development practice as an opportunity to analyze how we train library managers. He found a disconnect between what library schools now offer and the needs of the field and proposes a hybrid management course and practicum to address that disconnect.

Anna Maria Guerra's article brings together the available literature on services offered by public libraries in the United States to Hispanic populations, and to analyze both the work being done and the work libraries need to do to address the needs of this rapidly growing population. The work provides an exhaustive literature survey that can serve as a useful starting point for anyone trying to expand services in this area.

Finally, Zohra Calcuttawala offers us an empirical investigation of the spatial distribution, and changes in spatial patterns of Calcutta's public libraries. This study of a set of libraries in a non-western city talks about who benefits from these programs and combines an analysis of differences between south Asian and western experiences in library development. It offers methodologies that could be of value to any public library that wants to analyze how where it sits affects how it does its job.

In summary, we offer this volume to you as a strong yet varied analysis of some of the problems that we face in managing libraries and some of the methods we might use in analyzing those problems. Its strength is that the individual studies address timely and timeless problems using methods gleaned from a variety of disciplines. We hope you will find the volume informative and enjoy reading it as much as we have enjoyed assembling this group of authors.

Delmus E. Williams
Editor

UNDERSTANDING THE DEVELOPMENT OF DISCIPLINES AND THE WAYS THEY CONTRIBUTE TO KNOWLEDGE AND REFLECT PRACTICE: AN ANALYSIS OF ARTICLES PUBLISHED IN HIGHER EDUCATION AND LIBRARY AND INFORMATION SCIENCE

K. Brock Enger

ABSTRACT

Using bibliometrics to examine eight core journals in the year 2000 for the disciplines of higher education and library science, characteristics of the authors were determined, including gender or sex; Carnegie Classification or institutional affiliation; and position of the authors. Characteristics of the articles were also examined, including the research methods used such as descriptive statistics, inferential statistics, or qualitative analysis. A content analysis of each article was performed to determine the subjects

Advances in Library Administration and Organization, Volume 24, 1–51
Copyright © 2007 by Elsevier Ltd.
All rights of reproduction in any form reserved
ISSN: 0732-0671/doi:10.1016/S0732-0671(06)24001-X

discussed in each literature. For both disciplines, it was learned that males publish more, the highest Carnegie Classification, extensive research institutions, were represented the most, and authors came from academic departments other than their own disciplines. In higher education, inferential statistics were used frequently; in library and information descriptive statistics were used frequently; both disciplines failed to use research methodologies regularly. From these findings, it appears that both disciplines are still emerging and are in their early stages of development.

Does not wisdom call out? Does not understanding raise her voice? Proverbs 8:1

INTRODUCTION, BACKGROUND, AND LITERATURE REVIEW

The development of academic disciplines rests upon an evergrowing framework of ideas that is generated and tested over time through the collective research of scholars working toward the advancement of knowledge (Weber, Lassman, Velody, & Martins, 1989). The central purpose of the scholar, and the university, is to understand, create, and advance knowledge through research and instruction (Shils, 1984). Early scholars set the direction a field of study might take – consider Franklin's theory of electricity, or Bacon's history of heat, color, and wind (Kuhn, 1970). Scholarship contributes to human knowledge, confronts the unknown, and seeks understanding for its own sake (Boyer, 1990). Over time, with continued application, acceptance, and analysis, theories may become known as basic knowledge within a discipline (Cole, 1983). The underpinnings of specific theories eventually become widely accepted and passed along to students as primary tenets of understanding; knowing these tenets becomes necessary for progressing through a discipline and eventually discovering new theories and applications and further advancing knowledge.

Over the last century, one method of advancing knowledge has been through the publication of articles in academic journals (Kronick, 1962). Repeatedly, through articles published in academic journals, scholars point to areas of study that require further research and to previous studies calling for replication. Academic libraries serve as the conduits where researchers access this knowledge, "the academic library exits to make manifest and tangible the products of social processes aimed at putting us on the path to knowledge" (Budd, 2004, p. 364).

The progression of knowledge is central to the role of higher education in society, and the disciplines that move forward as a result of articles published in academic journals are central to the intellectual vitality and rigor of a nation:

> Knowledge has certainly never in history been so central to the conduct of an entire society. What the railroads did for the second half of the last century and the automobile for the first half of this century may be done for the second half of this century by the knowledge industry: That is to serve as the focal point for national growth. And the university is at the center of the knowledge process. (Kerr, 1963, p. 88)

The publication of articles in academic journals is a reflection of researchers and their work within a given field, and the study of the literature within any given discipline may reveal facets of its development and direction, as well as demographic features of those contributing to the discipline. The articles published in academic journals furnish a mechanism for establishing and formalizing branches of knowledge. Pierce (1990) suggested, "The boundaries of a discipline reflect the knowledge, interests, and practices of researchers actively working in the field" (p. 51).

An academic discipline is dependent on its literature for growth and development. Disciplines using research techniques to support findings in the literature deliver a framework for further study and development, and thereby encourage theoretical development. Wagenaar and Babbie (1989) point out:

> The scientific enterprise involves theory, research methods, and statistics. Research methods meet the scientific criterion of observation, theory meets the scientific criterion of logic or rationality by describing the logical relationships that exist among variables, and statistics help compare what is logically expected with what is actually observed. (p. 5)

Vigil (1991) defined an academic discipline as "a field of study with a unique theory base, research techniques, and body of knowledge" (p. 11). Academic disciplines have also been described by Ylijoki (2000) in this manner: "Disciplines have their own traditions and categories of thought which provide the members of the field with shared concepts of theories, methods, techniques and problems" (p. 339).

While some disciplines, such as biology, physics, and chemistry, are well-established and formalized, others, such as the disciplines of higher education and library and information science, are fairly young and in the process of formalization. The term higher education, as it is commonly used, refers to the practice and institutionalization of education in postsecondary institutions, namely colleges and universities. The discipline of higher education is a study of that practice. Higher education is considered a discipline that is still in the process of defining its own unique theoretical base and is defined as the study of the issues, problems, and opportunities associated with practice in institutions of higher learning (Burnett, 1973). Information science deals with the electronic technicalities associated with the organization, processing, and dissemination of knowledge created by humans, while library science is associated with linking humans to knowledge through service and access. Library science began as a discipline in the 1930s with the formalization of library education, while information science began in the 1950s with the computerization and mechanization of information, more openly recognized in the 1960s and 1970s with the organization of textual, tertiary computerized forms of organizing text through databases such as DIALOG and Science Citation Index. Saracevic (1999) determined that information science and library science were two distinct disciplines, with "strong interdisciplinary relations" (p. 1052). Bates (1999) noted that library science is more service-oriented than information science. Lack of research in the discipline of library science has been discussed for some time (Busha & Harter, 1980; Butler, 1933; Enger, Quirk, & Stewart, 1989; Ennis, 1967; Goldhor, 1972; Shera, 1964). Without substantial research, a discipline is yet in its formative stages. A further examination of the research methodologies employed in the literature of higher education and library and information science may show that the disciplines are still in the process of developing theories of their own.

Burnett identified the nature of the discipline of higher education as "the behavioral interaction of students, faculty, and administrators within the context of a college or university environment, and the interrelationship of this environment with the larger society" (p. 5). A study of the literature of higher education not only reflects the discipline's development, but the practices of those working within colleges and universities. The same is true for library and information science, or for any discipline. A study of its literature, and those publishing within that literature, reflects the work of the practitioners within that discipline.

This study follows a long-standing method of using literature to quantify written communication called bibliometrics. Bibliometrics is a method of analyzing communication among researchers, or "the application of mathematics and statistical methods to books and other media of communication as a research method" (Borgman, 1990, p. 11). As early as 1917, Cole and Eales analyzed the literature on comparative anatomy from 1550 to 1860 to discover the fluctuations of interest in the topic over time. Bibliometrics, or statistical bibliography as it was named then, was also discussed in two lectures delivered by Hulme (1923) at the University of Cambridge.

Much later, and more to the point, Pritchard (1969) suggested a standard and universal usage of the term bibliometrics to measure written communication in the development of a discipline as "the application of mathematics and statistical methods to books and other forms of written communication" (p. 349). In the early 1970s, Garfield (1972) established the Institute for Scientific Information, which used computerized databases to track citations, linking authors to journals and citations to authors. Through elaborate matches in *Social Science Citation Index* or *Science Citation Index*, searchers discovered which journals and authors were cited most frequently in specific disciplines, thus revealing the leaders of certain disciplines and their characteristics (Garfield, 1972). Through a bibliometric examination of the authors and articles of a discipline, characteristics, such as sex or institutional affiliation, may be determined, thereby revealing differences that may exist in publication within the discipline.

If the discipline of higher education reflects the development of American colleges and universities, a study of the articles published in higher education journals may reveal distinct characteristics regarding higher learning in this country. Likewise, the study of the literature of library and information science reveals characteristics of the practices of libraries and information processing, which, like higher education, is responsible for moving knowledge forward. In an early examination of the scientific literature in the *British International Catalogue* from 1901 to 1913, Hulme, who was librarian of the British Patent Office, predicted the pending decline of the industrial revolution through the waning publication of scientific patents (Hulme, 1923). His prediction, based on patterns revealed within the scientific literature, proved to be accurate.

This study will offer a reflection of the disciplines of higher education and library and information science through an examination of its literature for the year 2000 and present a profile of its contributors, a summary of its research methodologies, and a sense of its subject content. It will help clarify the current state of the disciplines that reflect the practices of those engaged in institutions of higher learning and in the dissemination of knowledge. The year 2000 was chosen as being as close to the current time period as possible, but not the most recent year (2005), because the literature was not available for examination. It was also chosen to reflect the nature of the two disciplines at the turn of a new century. *Journal Citation Reports*, the index that measures the citation rate of the most referenced journals, was not available in 2005 at the time of this publication.

Hefferlin (1969) recognized that academic reform may originate in forces external to the academy and change may reside in scholars' reactions to changing social conditions. Scholars themselves may actually mediate those wider forces through their scholarly interests (Gumport, 2002). A study of the literature of higher education and library and information science may indicate changes occurring in higher education and library science, overall; it may also indicate societal changes to which higher education and library and information science are adapting. Bibliometrics can provide useful perspectives on scholarly communication in emerging academic disciplines.

Summary of Early Written Scholarly Communication

Early scholarly communication provided the means for bringing the scholar out of seclusion and into a community where ideas and discoveries could more rapidly and universally be shared. Initially, this communication took the form of letters and other written correspondence, which was sometimes published, such as the *Epistolarum Medicinalm Centurea* (1663–67) in five volumes and the 400 letters of Thomas Bartholimus (Van Patten, 1932). The earliest written journal, the *Journal des Scavans*, a French weekly publication begun in 1665, played a major role in establishing the international scientific community (Gross, Harmon, & Reidy, 2000). In the *History of Scientific Periodicals*, Kronick (1962) identified the two primary functions of scientific periodicals: "that of serving as a vehicle for the communication of new discoveries and ideas, and that of acting as a repository of knowledge" (p. 8). These two measures accurately portray scholarly communication, as will be applied in this study.

Development and Growth of American Journals

The first American scientific journal, published by Johns Hopkins University in 1877, was *The American Journal of Mathematics* (Rudolph, 1962). A few years later, other universities published their own journals: *Astrophysical Journal* was first published at the University of Chicago in 1882; *Political Science Quarterly* began publication in 1886 at Columbia University; the *Quarterly Journal of Economics* was first published in 1886 at Harvard University; and the *Philosophical Review* appeared in 1892 from Cornell (Slosson, 1910). As time went on, scientific literature proliferated in the United States. In 1898, the University of Chicago printed 150,000 copies of their journals in 1 year (Goodspeed, 1916). Much later, by the 1950s, Price (1963) determined that the growth of scientific research doubled every 15 years, stating, "Scientists have always felt themselves to be awash in a sea of scientific literature that augments in each decade as much as in all times before" (p. 15). Chubin (1975) noted that the number of references per article in the sociological literature increased steadily from 1950 to 1970, indicating a burgeoning of the literature. Journal publication has grown at exponential rates since the inception of printed scientific communication. Between 1970 and 1990, the *Physics Abstracts* database grew from 624,000 to 2,852,000 records, doubling approximately every 10 years (Abel & Newlin, 2002). In part, this may be the result of the increased rate of spending money on research in the United States. The federal government spends $15 billion on university research, while industry and other sources spend $10 billion (Abel & Newlin, 2002).

The university plays a major role in supporting research and publication and in acquiring and promoting knowledge: "I view knowledge and its constituent bundles of fields as defining the work of universities and the people in them" (Stoner, 1966, p. 4). Looking at the origins of the modern university is useful in understanding its role in supporting research and publication and the proliferation of journal publication.

The Role of the University in Shaping and Supporting Research and Publication

The discussion of the modern university originated with Wilhelm von Humboldt in 1809 at the University of Berlin, which was sometimes referred to in the literature as the "Humboldt" University (Ash, 1997). Humboldt's summary of the German model:

> This much is agreed upon; it is easy to see that in the inner organization of higher institutions of learning everything depends on the preservation of the principle that knowledge is to be regarded as something not wholly found and never wholly findable, but as something ever to be searched out.

As soon as one stops searching for knowledge, or if one imagines that it need not be creatively sought in the depths of the human spirit but can be assembled extensively by collecting and classifying facts, everything is irrevocably and forever lost, lost for learning which soon vanishes so far out of the picture that it even leaves language behind like an empty pod, and lost for the state as well. For only that learning which comes from the inside and can be transplanted into the inside can transform character; and the state, like humanity in general, cares little about knowledge and talk but a great deal about character and actions (Humboldt, 1963, p. 134).

Humboldt (1963) recognized the importance of state support for higher learning but believed that the state should not play a role in dictating the

academic processes that occurred within the university. The German government provided funding for research universities and supported scientific
research extensively, allowing scholars to pursue their own research interests. The American research university was led by the German university in
its devotion to the advancement of science and the teaching of advanced
knowledge to students.

Prior to the development of the university in the United States, interested
scholars attended German universities to complete the Ph.D. and then returned to America to establish similar institutions (Cordesco, 1960). The
first Ph.D. awarded in the United States was from Yale in 1861, and it was
not until that time that the university began to take shape in the United
States (Jencks & Riesman, 1968). Daniel Coit Gilman, the first president of
Johns Hopkins University, was strongly influenced by the German model,
spending a winter at the University of Berlin where he absorbed the ideas
that he incorporated into the founding of Johns Hopkins in 1876 (French,
1946). The founding practices Gilman used from the German model included a focus on research, graduate education, and the hiring of German-
trained faculty (Hawkins, 1960). Gilman (1885) emphasized the importance
of the acquisition, conservation, refinement, and distribution of knowledge.
While Gilman emphasized research at Johns Hopkins, he continued to be
influenced by the early American college ideal:

> Let us hope that the American universities will cherish all branches of learning, giving
> precedence only to those that sound judgment indicates as most useful in our day...let
> neither novelty nor age prejudice us against that which will serve mankind. Let not our
> love of science diminish our love of letters. (Gilman, 1886, p. 211)

Harvard also played a role in establishing research as a model for American
higher education. Charles Eliot, president of Harvard from 1869 to 1909,
was influential in Harvard's development as a university. Eliot was a graduate of Harvard with a background and interest in chemistry and metal-
lurgy. He taught at Harvard's Lawrence Scientific School following his
graduation until he was dismissed in 1863. At the time he was dismissed
from the Lawrence Scientific School, he traveled in Europe, visiting German
universities and college preparatory schools in France. The concepts Eliot
learned from both the German and French models influenced his ideas in
establishing graduate and professional education at Harvard (Hawkins,
1972). When Eliot returned from Europe, he taught at the Massachusetts
Institute of Technology from 1865 to 1869. Once he had returned to
Harvard, Eliot was influential in developing graduate education. In 1890,

the Graduate Department at Harvard became the Graduate School, creating a new Faculty of Arts and Sciences (which combined the Harvard College and Lawrence Scientific School faculties), thus establishing the university at Harvard (Morison, 1946).

When the University of Chicago was formed in the late 1800s, colleges in the East took note. The primary focus of the University of Chicago was research, and most of its faculty acquired Ph.D.s from the research universities in Germany. While Chicago focused on becoming the best research university in the country, it was also devoted to the study of culture and the early classics (Veysey, 1965).

Founded for the explicit purpose of graduate research, Johns Hopkins emulated the German university model more than any other American institution and is regarded as the earliest dedicated primarily to research in the United States (Fye, 1991). Johns Hopkins retained funding to ensure that faculty could pursue research in advanced laboratory facilities, while teaching at the same time. The pursuit and furtherance of knowledge was the main goal of Johns Hopkins, a goal that became most evident with the opening of the medical school in 1893 (Harvey, Brieger, Abrams, & McKusick, 1989). Up to this point, medical education focused primarily on practice, with little regard to clinical research. By the end of the 19th century, other universities were forming their own research agendas, as well: "By 1910, if a research-oriented observer had been asked to name the leading American universities, he probably would have listed Harvard, Chicago, Columbia, and Johns Hopkins – in that order" (Veysey, 1965, p. 171). Charles Eliot at Harvard led the way in developing the elective system, which provided a basis for the division of the disciplines on university campuses (Hawkins, 1972). While disciplines stand on their own, universities give them status and legitimization (Geiger, 1986).

By the beginning of the First World War, about 25 major universities existed in the United States. Following the War, the American university shifted from the strict German ideal of pure research toward a uniquely American organization that combined both teaching and research (Worthington, 1997). Eventually, as the amalgamation of American colleges and universities evolved, even smaller, private institutions sought to emulate the larger institutions by adopting "university" into their titles or requiring faculty to publish to achieve tenure (Boyer, 1990; Jacobson, 1992; Morrow, 1993). A "scientific ethos" permeated American colleges and universities, creating among faculty a drive toward publication and research (Light, 1974). The concept of imitation of the larger institutions in higher education by smaller colleges and universities was recognized and articulated as the "academic procession" by critic Riesman (1956):

> What I do want to advocate, however, is that as long as institutions look to each other for models of what to accept and what to reject, they widen their awareness of the shifting contexts into which their communications fall. Thus, I hope that avant-garde professors can more often realize the way in which they are responsible for what happens in the large middle sections of the procession – how their kit of ideas, whether these are progressive education or the rejection of it, Freud or Jung, Bartok or Dave Brubeck, or the vogue of Kipling, spread through all the media which connect the centers of high culture with nationwide orbits and circuits. (p. 41)

Pace (1974) looked at the changes in academic programs and type of students from 1950 to 1970 and found that mission statements and specific programs had grown less distinctive over time. Montgomery (1994) argued that the increased emphasis on science as a model for graduate work had resulted in a race for institutions of higher education at all levels to pursue research. Fairweather (1994) noted the universal structural homogenization of faculty reward structures in higher education.

Throughout the late 1950s and 1960s, the government began increasing its allocation of dollars to universities for research, leading Eisenhower (1981) to surmise that government contracts had become substitutes for intellectual curiosity. Beginning in the late 1970s and throughout the 1980s, as student aid was decreasing and more students enrolled in higher education, the federal government increased research funding to major universities supporting defense and health initiatives as a result of the Cold War (Graham & Diamond, 1997). Hackett (1990) found that research had become more important as federal dollars to support it increased.

Research universities fuel the drive to perform research and publish, thereby giving structure to the furtherance and advancement of knowledge. Without the support of universities, very little would be done to provide the resources necessary for performing research and advancing knowledge. The meaning of university has generally "come to connote an educational institution of large size which affords instruction of an advanced nature in all the main branches of learning" (Brubacher & Rudy, 1996, pp. 143–144). The university provides infrastructure to advance knowledge, and the framework of what constitutes legitimate knowledge is built directly into the composition of the research university:

> Educational institutions have epistemologies. They hold conceptions of what counts as legitimate knowledge and how you know what you claim to know. These theories of knowledge need not be consciously espoused by individuals, for they are built into institutional structures and practices. (Schon, 1995, p. 27)

The mission and purpose of the university has been described in many treatises; this one, explicated by Ortega y Gasset (2001) in *Mission of the University*, identifies knowledge as its center:

> In its proper and authentic sense, science is exclusively investigation: The setting up of problems, working at them, and arriving at their solution to investigate is to discover truth, or inversely, to demonstrate an error. To know means to assimilate a truth into one's consciousness, to possess a fact after it has been attained and secured. (p. 50)

"The university *is* the intellect, it *is* science, erected into an institution" (p. 76). Veblen (1918/1954) also described the role of the university and its place among scholars:

> Yet, when all these sophistications of practical wisdom are duly allowed for, the fact remains that the university is, in usage, precedent, and commonsense preconception, an establishment for the conservation and advancement of the higher learning, devoted to a disinterested pursuit of knowledge. (p. 85)

Universities stand as a foundation for the performance of research and supply an avenue for representation and support of the disciplines. The research university gives shape to disciplines and the work expressed in disciplines through journal publications.

The Development of the Academic Library

Early American colleges developed library collections in a haphazard fashion, and the maintenance of those collections was not performed by full-time librarians until the introduction of research universities and professional schools at the end of the 19th and the beginning of the 20th century. In the early colonial years, the book collection consisted of donations and the keepers of the collection were either college presidents or faculty, leaving little time for access to the collection (Brubacher & Rudy, 1996, p. 27). In the early 1800s, literary societies formed on college campuses, and separate collections developed to support them. An example of the literary society at Harvard is reflected in Emerson's reading list during his Junior years. His required studies included the classical Harvard education. For his studies he read the following: In Greek, *The Iliad* and the *New Testament*; in Latin, Liby, Horace, Cicero, Persius; Geometry: plane, analytic, and spherical; Roman history; Science: physics, astronomy, and chemistry; Philosophy: Dugal Steward, Paley, and Lock's essays. Between December 1819 and February 1820, Emerson read the following material on his own:

Byron's *Don Juan*, Archibald Alison's *Essay on Taste*, Edward Channing's *Inaugrual Discourse*, Ben Jonson's *Life, Every Man in His Humour*, *and Every Man Out of His Humour*, a volume of Joanna Baillie's plays, Samuel Roger's poem *Human Life*, Thomas Campbell's *Essay on English Poetry*, and the new *North American Review* (which his father started), Thomas Blackwell's *Life and Writings of Homer*, Robert Lowth's *Lectures on the Sacred Poetry of the Hebrews*, Washington Irving's *Sketch Book*, Bacon's *Essays*, the first volume of Dacier's *Dialogues of Plato*, Scott's *Bridal of Triermain*, a volume of Crabbe, and H.H. Milman's *Samor, Lord of the Bright City* (Richardson, 1995).

From Emerson's reading list, it is obvious that he had access to an extensive collection and that it most likely did not come from the college library. At that time, literary societies had more extensive and wide-ranging collections than college libraries, and the literary society collections were vastly more accessible. "Not only did the literary societies often outstrip the college libraries in numbers of volumes, but the wide range of subject matter allowed far greater opportunity for the play of intellect than did the narrow religious fare of the usual college library" (Rudolph, 1990). Not much later, these same literary societies housed the essays of Emerson, such as *The American Scholar*, *Nature*, the *Over-Soul*, and others. Eventually, the literary society collections were folded into the college library collections.

In the decade before the Civil War, the popularity of literary societies dwindled. The extracurricular activity that replaced them was the fraternities. Students led the way in changing the focus of education throughout the historical development of American colleges. When the early focus was primarily religious, students enriched their education and access to literature by forming literary societies. As the nation approached Civil War, students formed fraternal societies, creating coalescence among groups and the development of strong alliances. The Civil War wreaked havoc on colleges, many of which were the sight of battles. Libraries burned to the ground, books and furniture were used as fuel. While the Civil War was tragic for academic libraries, the aftermath of the war spurred economic growth, catapulting libraries to the center of college life and making colleges a more central unit in the American experience.

The Morrill Federal Land Grant Act of 1862 was instrumental in bringing higher education to people who earlier did not have access to learning beyond primary school. The Morrill Act, in some ways, forced the formation of secondary schools, ensuring that students would come prepared to college life, and further lending the facility for educating future faculty. The Land Grant Act resulted in state funding for colleges, which included funding for academic libraries, and solidly placed the responsibility for the development and ongoing maintenance of colleges within the scope of state and federal government. Rudolph (1990) summarizes the land-grant movement most eloquently:

> The yeoman farmer and the self-made man are two versions of the same fundamental American myth: The myth of self-reliant free men achieving self-respect and security among equals. The land-grant college served both: It sustained the yeoman, it liberated the farm boy who would make his way in the city. And in doing so it kept its focus on the practical and allowed others to concern themselves with the theoretical. It made little effort to achieve a happy union between theory and practice; it became in America the temple of applied science, essentially institutionalizing the American's traditional respect for the immediately useful. In the end, the land-grant college incorporated in its rationale the Jacksonian temper; it became the common school on a higher level; it became one of the great forces of economic and social mobility in American society; it brought the government, both federal and state, firmly into the support of higher education. In the land-grant institutions the American people achieved popular higher education for the first time (p. 265).

At the time of the land-grant movement, colleges received government funding to develop the public institution of higher education. Some of the measures to bring education to the common citizen included funding for academic libraries. Colleges, for the first time, began to develop collections that moved beyond religious literature and included primary publications in the sciences and engineering. At the same time, some Americans continued to pursue doctoral studies in Europe and were introduced to the renowned research universities in Germany. German universities had libraries that supported a scientific education, and scholars returned to America expecting the same of the colleges here. Many of these returning scholars taught at private colleges and the new state colleges. Between 1861 and 1868, 134 Ph.D.s were awarded in the United States, so this country had its own means for developing a university curriculum (Atkins, 1991). Professional education developed at this time as well, and academic libraries responded by developing collections that could support medical and legal programs.

Johns Hopkins University was one of the first private schools to adapt a new approach to scientific and professional education; Harvard followed. A strong emphasis on the elective system took place, and along with it, increased investment in supporting library collections. As the curriculum changed from rote memorization to the elective system and scientific inquiry, the hours of the academic library increased as did the usage of the collection. In turn, as more and more students used the collections, attention was given to staffing, maintenance, and control. While formalized training in academic librarians did not yet exist, more campuses employed full-time library staff. While library collections were deemed more and more important, the skills needed to maintain them were not respected.

With the advent of public education in the 1850s, women were used as teacher candidates in the new pool of cheap labor needed in the teaching profession. At the same time, public libraries became instruments to educate the uneducated masses, and women were used in both public and academic libraries for cheap labor. As the 19th century came to a close, women were the primary library employees. This tradition has carried through to the present, along with the low salaries and status that accompanies librarianship.

By the 1920s several professional programs in library science opened, providing specific training in cataloging, reference and collection maintenance, and development (Smith, 1990). The period of 1912–1939 produced tremendous growth for college library collections. For example, in 1912, the collection at Harvard was just over one million volumes. By 1939, the collection consisted of slightly more than 4 million volumes. In comparison, both the University of California and the University of Illinois housed approximately 233,000 monographs in 1912, and both collections grew to over 1 million by 1939 (Gerould, 1945). After the Second World War, enrollments at colleges and universities boomed, and library collections continued to experience growth into the mid-1970s. The Higher Education Act of 1965 brought an infusion of funds into libraries, in some cases, academic libraries had so much money for the collection that librarians bought several copies of the same publication. From the 1970s to the present, except for the schools with large endowments (like Harvard), libraries have experienced a growing paucity of resources. Many external factors combine to contribute to this lack of funds.

Increasingly, libraries began to rely on automation and computerization for processing collections and making them available. In the early 1980s, most academic libraries automated their catalogs, and tossed their card catalogs. On many campuses, this raised controversy among those faculty and staff wishing to retain the card catalog. Indeed, the card catalog provides a snapshot of historical development of the library collection that cannot be found in the automated online catalog. The online catalog brought about many changes seen in the technical services departments of libraries. While the systems in place for providing access to materials were basically the same (the individual records in the online catalog look almost identical to the old 3 × 5 card in the card catalog), the change to computerization created an upheaval in the way things were traditionally done in academic libraries and on university campuses. Reliance on automation increased costs, which in turn, forced librarians to form consortia and share in the costs of development and maintenance of union online catalogs. The initial costs to automate the catalog and the yearly subscription fees for access to the online catalog were high, ongoing expenses. The replacement costs for hardware and software also added an additional burden to the financing of library automation. Once automation of the online catalog was completed at most academic libraries nationwide, the prices of journals and magazines sky-rocketed. In some years, inflation for journals reached 18–20%. In 1986, the average unit cost of serials in American Research Libraries was $87.09; by 1999, the same unit cost was $267.09 (Kyrillidou, 2000). Gone were the days of multiples copies of books. At this same time, the increase in publication of scientific literature multiplied exponentially. Most libraries can no longer keep pace with the publishing industry, and carefully select their collections to meet the curricular needs of their campuses.

Not only was the process of accessing books moving to electronic format, but traditional print indexes were also becoming electronic, and the variety of databases to choose from increased at a phenomenal rate. In 1975, DIALOG, a commercial vendor, allowed access to 300 online databases. By 1988, 3,893 online databases were available from 1,723 database producers and 576 online services (Meadow, 1988).

The most recent development in academic libraries is the advent of the electronic journal. In electronic publication, ownership no longer occurs, rather access to electronic collections is arranged through licensing agreements, which gives access, but does not necessarily allow for ownership of a collection. There is also a concern among academic librarians that the technology used now for the access to an electronic collection may not be available in the future.

The Development of a Discipline

The journal is quite distinct from the book in its periodicity, and in its publication at specific intervals of time. It is the collective achievement of thousands of individuals, and it imposes a process of critical review on professional work. Peers review one another's work and determine which articles are worthy of publication, attempting to ensure that the best work is published (Zuckerman & Merton, 1971). Through journals, scholars have the potential of influencing the direction of thought a discipline may take. Hagstrom (1965) noted that scholars writing in every discipline produce a "disciplinary ideology" that may come to serve as tradition within the discipline.

Kuhn (1970) created a conceptual framework for the development and emergence of scientific knowledge and introduced to popular understanding the concept of the paradigm – a unique way of viewing and thinking about particular models, problems, and ideas shared by a community of specialists. Kuhn observed the effect that personal experience and universal acceptance play in determining scientific discovery:

> Which of the many conceivable experiments relevant to the new field does he elect to perform first? And what aspects of the complex phenomenon that then results strike him as particularly relevant to an elucidation of the nature of chemical change or of electrical affinity? For the individual, at least, and sometimes for the scientific community as well, answers to questions like these are often essential determinants of scientific development. What differentiated these various schools was not one or another failure of method – they were all "scientific" – but what we shall come to call their incommensurable ways of seeing the world and of practicing science in it. Observation and experience can and must drastically restrict the range of admissible scientific belief else there would be no science. (p. 4)

Kuhn summarized what makes a field a discipline: a paradigm that "guides the whole group's research" (p. 22), where consensus determines reality. The level of consensus in a discipline determines the publication outcomes of its researchers and thereby influences the discipline's stratification system. Publication rates are higher in disciplines with highly developed theory and methodology, while publication rates in fields with less agreement among scholars tend to be lower (Zuckerman & Merton, 1971). In the natural sciences, it has been shown that rejection rates for publication average between 20 and 30%, while rejection rates in sociology and political science remain around 80%. Garvey, Lin, and Nelson (1970) showed that in the social sciences, rejection occurred as a result of an inappropriate match between the journal and the subject covered in the article; whereas, rejection in the physical sciences occurred as a result of weakness in theory or methodology. It has also been shown that longer dissertations are written in fields like the social sciences and humanities where low consensus occurs, while shorter dissertations are written in disciplines with high consensus, such as mathematics and the natural sciences (Hargens, 1975).

Biglan (1973) found similarities and differences between academic departments at a university in Illinois and a small private college in the State of Washington. He clustered academic areas into several dimensions by departmental task and practical application and showed that each academic area tests different sets of problems and methods, either hard/soft and/or pure/applied. Through his analysis of tasks, Biglan determined that educational administration and supervision was a soft/applied academic department, while departments such as astronomy and chemistry were hard/pure. Biglan assumed that classification by academic department represented the disciplines but was much easier than classification by discipline (Creswell & Roskens, 1981).

Biglan's model offered a systematic framework for exploring the role of cognitive processes in academic departments, linking his model to Kuhn's (1970) understanding of paradigm development, which is based on theoretical agreement among scholars within a field. Lodahl and Gordon (1972) surveyed 80 different university graduate departments in physics, chemistry, sociology, and political science to compare paradigmatic development of the disciplines in those departments. Four fields were chosen to represent two separate levels of paradigm development: physics and chemistry represented high levels of development, while sociology and political science represented lower levels of development. Through a variety of measures, Lodahl and Gordon found several distinctions between fields that were highly developed and those that were less developed. In the more developed fields, there was agreement among faculty regarding curriculum development; whereas, in the lesser developed fields, faculty could not easily agree on curriculum standards and offerings. In sociology and political science, for example, faculty were least willing to advise doctoral students, while faculty in more developed fields like chemistry solicited graduate advisees. Overall, the authors found that "university professors in a given scientific field must operate at the level of predictability permitted by the structure of knowledge within that field. Social scientists operate in a much less predictable and, therefore, a more anxious environment than physical scientists" (p. 70).

Kuhn (1970) speculated that paradigmatic development is still taking place in social sciences. If this is so, it may still be occurring in the field of higher education and library and information science. Development of a paradigm indicates maturity within a particular field or discipline; as defined by Lodahl and Gordon (1972), "the essence of the paradigm concept is the degree of consensus or sharing of beliefs within a scientific field about theory, methodology, techniques, and problems" (p. 58).

A more highly developed paradigm, or more clearly distinguished consensus among colleagues, facilitates increased communication among researchers and makes the process of teaching and research more amenable and defined. Hutchins (1949), in his report on *The State of the University, 1929–1949*, recognized that "the progress of scholarship varies directly with the freedom of communication among scholars" (p. 35). Collectively, a discipline is represented, shared, and developed through scientific communication, which is reflected through the publication of articles in the journal literature. Lodahl and Gordon (1972) noted:

> Our results seem to indicate that there are differences between disciplines that go to the heart of teaching, research, and student–faculty relationships. Any attempt to change the university must take into account the intimate relations between the structure of

knowledge in different fields and the vastly different styles with which university departments operate. (p. 71)

Research psychologist Jamie-Lynn Magnusson (1997) presented Kuhn's theory from a personal (constructivist) point of view:

> I assist in creating a social reality, develop hypotheses embedded within these realities, and then test these hypotheses against the data of social reality I myself have helped to create! But, unlike the students of literature described earlier, I have not been trained to read these activities like a text and to detect the sub-textual themes of my research practice. I have been indoctrinated, but have not been politicized in the critical sense of understanding my own indoctrination, and I have not been equipped with the skills to challenge my indoctrination. (p. 204)

The basic theoretical underpinnings of this study are sociological in nature, and the scholars referenced in this manuscript are primarily sociologists, rather than philosophers discussing epistemology, or social epistemology (Andersen, 2002; Budd, 2004; Egan & Shera, 1952). Study of knowledge development, or the theory of knowledge, may be philosophical or sociological in nature. Social epistemology primarily examines justified true shared belief and elaborates on how individual belief becomes collective belief (Fuller, 1988; Goldman, 1999). Since epistemology rests it arguments around belief, this author chooses a background nested in sociology, which explains the collective behavior of scientists at work. The collective nature of knowledge creation discussed in this manuscript assumes a basic understanding of theoretical development based on the scientific method, and on the method of qualitative analysis used in scientific discovery. The understanding of knowledge creation discussed in this study lies in the literature that follows accepted quantitative and qualitative procedures to determine collective accepted outcomes within disciplines. It does not presume to follow the social epistemological development of knowledge creation, which logically discusses how people come to know what they know through shared belief. There is an inherent distinction between an understanding derived from shared methodology and the construction based on justified true shared belief (Pahre, 1996). While social epistemology elaborates philosophically on the creation of knowledge, it does so within a system that would not find wide acceptance among scientists. Some of the sociologists referenced in this manuscript include Merton, Zuckerman, Cole, and others.

Bibliometrics and the Measurement of Scholarly Communication

Bibliometrics has been used primarily as an unobtrusive research process to examine the growth of scientific literature and "has clearly become established as a subdiscipline with applications in the history and sociology of knowledge, in communication, and in library and information science" (Lawani, 1981, p. 296). Bibliometrics reveals connections among scholars, such as citation patterns (citation analysis), the content of the material published (content analysis), or simple publication counts (King, 1987). It has been used in various disciplines, including communications (Reeves & Borgman, 1983), computer science (Subramanyam, 1976), economics (Coats, 1971), education (DeYoung, 1985), library and information science (Enger et al., 1989), psychology (Meyers, 1970), and sociology (Smalley, 1981), among many others.

Chemistry was the earliest discipline to utilize bibliometrics through citation analysis by ranking journals according to the number of times they were cited, and thereby producing a list of indispensable journals (Gross & Gross, 1927). Some bibliometric studies have shown a correlation between the research institutions where authors obtained their degrees and publication rates (Johnson, 1992). Using bibliometrics as a tool for examining the research within a discipline may indicate the maturity of the discipline itself, for without a body of extensive literature or research, bibliometrics cannot be performed. For example, citation analysis links references embodied within one article to the article of origin to determine the number of times a particular author or journal is cited a number of years after publication. Without an established literature over a period of time, citation analysis would not be possible.

The measurement of citations is based on the assumption that those articles, authors, or journals that are cited have an impact on the ongoing accumulation of scientific knowledge. Citations represent ideas and are symbolic in nature (Small, 1978). In one of the first-recognized articles using *Science Citation Index* to measure citation productivity, Bayer and Folger (1966) said, "What people cite in scientific writing is in general what they think is important; no other single measure gets at his contribution so directly" (p. 386). Citations symbolize ideas. The symbolic nature of citations gives scholar's ideas to discuss, systematizes them, and moves ideas forward. Essentially, with bibliometrics, the work performed and published by researchers is analyzed and examined:

> What is scientific about scientific research lies not in its execution but in its publication. Scientific research is recognizable as such not because of the conditions under which it is performed but because of the way it is presented and published. As researchers begin to question conventional wisdom regarding the workings of science, they turn to research papers as one directly observable scientific output available for analysis. (Pierce, 1990, p. 55)

The Theoretical Development of the Discipline of Higher Education and
Library and Information Science

It has been contested whether higher education itself is a discipline or field of study. Early in its development, as courses of study in higher education began to be taught more widely at colleges and universities, Burnett (1973) performed a review of the literature to determine whether or not higher education could be considered a specialized field and concluded that higher education still appeared to be "an emerging scholarly field of study but not considered a specialized field of study" (p. 13). In the same year, Hobbs and Francis (1973) sought to develop a taxonomy to distinguish among the publications produced by higher educationists, finding that "higher education is simply not a discipline" (p. 56), asserting two points: "Higher education needs theorists; it sorely lacks theory; [and] an absolute requisite for theoretical development in higher education is the active solicitation of theoretical material by the publication channels of the field, especially by the journals" (p. 59).

Theoretical development of the discipline of library and information science has long been contested by scholars who noted the lack of research methodologies employed in the literature (Busha & Harter, 1980; Butler, 1933; Goldhor, 1972; Shera, 1964). Information science in its own right is young and still in the process of developing a substantial body of research literature (Hawkins, 2001). Schmidt (1992) summarized what has long concerned scholars of library and information science:

> Whether librarianship is considered a profession or a discipline, there is general agreement that library research has major weaknesses, one of which is little theory or a unifying paradigm for research. It is also widely acknowledged that library research is primarily applied, rather than basic or pure, and that the focus of much research is related to solving local problems. (p. 357)

An example of theoretical development may be found through the research methodologies employed in the literature of a discipline (Enger et al., 1989). Kellams (1975) performed a content analysis of 1,130 abstracts to journals in higher education through the *Inventory of Current Research on Postsecondary Education 1972*. He discovered that "theoretical research, available in the disciplinary journals, is rare in the higher education journals" (p. 139), and that simple descriptive research techniques were most commonly employed. Of the field of higher education, Kellams stated:

> First, the field is immature and needs a descriptive knowledge base. Second, it is an applied professional field of study as reflected by about one-half of the studies falling into the policy research or developmental categories. Third, the relationship of the study of higher education to theory is a problematical one. (p. 152)

In their study of 25 core journals in library and information science, Enger et al. (1989) discovered that 68.2% of the 915 articles reviewed for 1985 contained no statistical measurement at all; 20.7% used some form of descriptive statistics, and 11.1% used inferential statistics. Years later, for 2,664 journal articles from 91 journals examined in 2001, Koufogiannakis, Slater, and Crumley (2004) found that descriptive research was published far more frequently than any other type. Many other studies have performed similar analyses and come to the same conclusion that to become a discipline, library and information science needs to conduct and publish more articles that contain statistical measures to develop a theoretical base.

Both higher education and library and information science are emerging fields, based on studies that show that each discipline is still determining a theoretical base and discovering how to perform effective research to develop theory. This study examined each field to determine the statistical measures used in performing research. It is assumed that an increased use of methodologies indicates maturation in the disciplines.

Bibliometrics and Social Stratification Publication

In his extensively cited work, *Little Science, Big Science*, Derek J. de Solla Price (1963) explained how many scientists may be working on the same idea or discovery at the same time in history, likening it to an apple tree that is ripe for picking (many apples ready to drop to the ground). Many scientists reach for the same fruit, or truth/reality at the same time, but not all of them are recognized for their work. Those who go unrecognized may well be making a significant contribution. Price (1963) observed that scientists publish their work in order to ensure that they receive recognition for their discoveries, much like inventors patent their ideas. In the literature, it can be seen that publishing operates as a collaborative process, bringing together in one place the work of certain areas of study, and giving opportunity for others to make progress. Price (1963) proposed a science to study science, by examining the exponential growth of publication in science. From the publication of the first journal, *Journal des Scavans*, science has "advanced steadily through more than five orders of magnitude in more than 250 years" (p. 16), and, therefore, moved from little science to big science. Through Price's (1963) analysis, he determined that few scholars publish many papers; numerous scientists publish a first or second paper and never go on to publish more, while other scientists exceed the first two, and go on to publish many. He likened the pooling of talent to population studies, where large number of people are located in cities, and few are located in rural areas. Likewise, in science, the most notable scientists congregate at the larger, more popular research universities.

Price (1975) used bibliometric analysis to show that "an author of many papers is more likely to publish again than one who has been less prolific" (p. 292). In this sense, a "Matthew Effect" is created: "Take therefore the talent from him, and give it unto him which hath ten talents. For unto every one that hath shall be given, and he shall have abundance: but from him that hath not shall be taken away even that which he hath" (Matthew 25:28, 29, KJV). This statement follows Jesus' parable of the talents, in which the person who buried his talents was chastised, and what he possessed was given to the person who had already taken his talents and increased them. Robert K. Merton introduced the "Matthew Effect" to the sociological literature in his notable publication in *Science* on January 5, 1968.

Lotka's (1926) law is a formulaic representation of how many times scholars are cited in literature. Examining *Chemical Abstracts* from 1907 to 1916 and Auerbach's *Geschichtstafeln der Physik*, which covers the range of history up to and including 1910, Lotka determined the frequency distribution of scientific productivity, using the inverse square law as a model and applying it to the number of times individual names were listed in the index. He discovered the following:

> In the cases examined it is found that the number of persons making 2 contributions is about one-fourth of those making one; the number making 3 contributions is about one-ninth, etc.; the number making n contributions is about $1:n^2$ of those making one; and the proportion, of all contributors, that make a single contribution is about 60 percent. (p. 323)

For instance, in the logarithmic frequency diagram plotted by Lotka, it was shown that of most of the articles published, say between 10 and 30% were published by 1% of the authors listed. In other studies, it has been shown that approximately 90% of the research literature is written by 10% of the scholars (Berelson, 1960; Ladd, 1979). Lotka's law has been used repeatedly throughout the literature utilizing this type of bibliometric analysis. Through this type of analysis, the social stratification of publications in science discussed by Merton (1968) and Cole and Cole (1973) may be made known.

Examples of Social Stratification

On the basis of Harriet Zuckerman's (1965) interviews with Nobel laureates, Merton (1968) postulated that renowned scientists publish more than scientists who are unknown, resulting "in the accruing of greater increments of recognition for particular scientific contributions to scientists of considerable repute and the withholding of such recognition from scientists who have not yet made their mark" (p. 58). Sociology is an example of a formal communication system that is stratified (Lin, Garvey, & Nelson, 1970; Lin & Nelson, 1969). Merton (1968) discussed whether universities with the most resources attracted the most talented scientists and published more than scientists from lesser endowed institutions:

> Without deliberate intent on the part of any group, the reward system thus influences the "class structure" of science by providing a stratified distribution of chances, among scientists, for enlarging their role as investigators. The process provides differential access to the means of scientific production. This becomes all the more important in the current historical shift from little science to big science, with its expensive and often centralized equipment needed for research. There is thus a continuing interplay between the status system, based on honor and esteem, and the class system, based on differential life-chances, which locates scientists in differing positions within the opportunity structure of science. (p. 57)

Social stratification in the structure of the disciplines is represented in the scholarly literature: "For the development of science, only work that is effectively perceived and utilized by other scientists matters" (Merton, 1968, p. 60).

The social stratification of science was clearly put forth by Cole and Cole (1967), who showed the inaccuracy of the assumption that many small contributions to science make way for the great contributions of science. In the same manner, with a different set of data, John R. Cole (1970) showed that the process of publication in the scientific literature is "highly stratified," so that "even the men who make these 'smaller' discoveries come principally from the top strata of the scientific community" (p. 379). Stephen Cole (1970) realized that authors with little or no recognition benefit from collaborating with authors who are well known. In accordance with Price's (1963) discoveries, John R. Cole (1970) found that 60% of all publications in physics came from a small group of physicists. Cole and Cole (1973) went on together to develop a typology of influences on scientific development that includes sources of influence both internal and external to the institution and types of influence that are intellectual and social. Cole and Cole, along with other science historians and sociologists of science, examined how science progresses, and how the various influences are played out in the academic sphere through publication, awards, and honors. They concluded that this communication process plays the most important role in what is advanced in a discipline and what is not:

Scientific advance is dependent on the efficient communication of ideas. Plainly, only those discoveries that come to be known can have an impact on the development of science. Only then do they become functionally relevant for the advance of science. Without efficient communication of ideas, rewards could not be allocated properly. Recognition is conditional upon the visibility of scientific work. Visibility is a function of effective communication. Only through an analysis of the scientific network of communication can we establish the "payoff " to scientists of being strategically located in that communication system. (p. 16)

Social Stratification and Females in Research and Publication in Higher Education and Library and Information Science

Cole and Cole (1973) performed a similar study to determine if there was sexual discrimination across institutions for females in science holding Ph.D.s and found that sex had only a minor effect on the prestige of the scientist's academic affiliation. However, there was a significant difference between the number of scientific papers published by males and females: males published more than females. It was also found that sex status had a significant independent effect on overall academic rank: females were not promoted as frequently to senior positions, especially at better universities. In a review of 50 studies of scientists from a variety of scientific disciplines and types of institutions during the mid-1970s to the early 1980s, Cole and Zuckerman (1984) learned that males publish 50–60% more than females. Cole and Zuckerman speculated that females might respond somewhat differently than males to positive and negative reinforcement of their work, resulting in lower production by females. In reviewing the progress of female scientists over the last 100 years, Harriet Zuckerman (1991) noted that careers "have changed considerably, but change has been slow and uneven" (p. 55). Price (1963) noted in *Little Science, Big Science* that a great deal of opportunity is lost when females do not enter scientific fields, and recognized in factoring the number of people who enter science and succeed is cut in half by the "wastage of scientific woman power" (p. 54). Many studies have shown that female Ph.D.s publish less than their male counterparts (Astin, 1969; Babchuk & Bates, 1962; Bernard, 1964; Centra, 1974; Long, 1990; Persell, 1983).

In recent studies in the literature of library and information science, it has been shown that males exceed females in publication. Hakanson (2005) examined references to female authors in three journals: *College & Research Libraries*, *The Journal of Academic Librarianship*, and *Library Quarterly* from 1980 to 2000. Hakanson learned that, while publications by females increased over the time period studied, references to male authors by both female and male authors exceeded those made to female authors by a range of 20–60% over 20 years, indicating that "gender bias has become more subtle and complex" (p. 321). Hakanson (2005) noted the following:

> The trends shown in the results are not to be considered a deliberate discrimination of female or male authors, but, rather, could be a part of the social stratification system of science that, in fact, contradicts central scientific principles such as objectivity. These particular tendencies might be called a "gendered Matthew effect." (pp. 321–322)

Through an overview of the journal *Knowledge Organization: An International Journal* from 1988 to 1999, Rekha and Parameswaran (2002) found that male authors published more articles than females with males at 105 articles (65.62%), while female authors published only 55 articles (34.8%).

Through an examination of the three major roles in a university, namely, research, teaching, and service, Park (1996) wondered why females are promoted to full professor less frequently than males, and pinpointed the emphasis at universities on research as the cause. Essentially, Park speculated that teaching and committee work is seen as "woman's work," while research, which is more quantifiable, is seen as "man's work." She wondered if the inherent structure of the university itself is biased against females since research and publication is necessary for promotion and tenure, while outstanding teaching and service, though necessary, will not by themselves ensure tenure.

These differences in "research productivity" can be explained by females' structural position in the university. Bordons, Morillo, Fernandex, and Gomez (2003) examined the productivity and impact of the Spanish Council for Scientific Research scientists in natural resources and chemistry by gender and professional category, and discovered the following:

> If professional category were to be taken into account, male scientists would show greater productivity than female scientists, a finding that has also been reported by other authors. However, productivity appears to be related to academic rank, and the lower productivity of women can be explained by the fact that they are working at lower professional ranks compared to men. (p. 169)

Females, as a group, carry heavier teaching loads, bear greater responsibility for undergraduate education, and have more service commitments. Females also have less access to graduate teaching assistants, travel funds, research monies, laboratory equipment, and release time for research. The net result is that utilizing research as the primary criterion for tenure and promotion while devaluing teaching and service, will not separate the men from the boys (or the women from the girls) so much as it will separate the men from the women. As Harding (1993) claims, women are in large part

> assigned responsibility for domestic and emotional labor in their workplaces as well as in their homes, whereas men are assigned the "head" work. And, as in the home, these two functions are causally related, hence inside the university, as outside it, we find a gendered division of labor wherein women assume primary responsibility for nurturing the young and serving men, but receive little credit for doing so. (p. 55)

In a considerable number of areas and across several measures, Valian (1998) found that in academia, females earned less than males and were overrepresented in low status and untenured positions. According to Valian, in 1996–1997, 96% of males at universities nationwide were in tenured or tenure-track appointments, compared with 85% of females, and females were also employed more often by low-prestige schools, and employed less often by high-prestige institutions. To summarize her extensive work compiling data to show the disparities between males and females in academe and other professional areas, Valian summarized:

> The data demonstrate that women in academia are substantially under-rewarded. They are paid less, promoted more slowly, and tenured more slowly. Except for the number of women in assistant and associate professor positions, progress from 1980 to 1996 was slow and slight in every area. Nor can women's slower advancement be accounted for by a lower standard of performance. Even when productivity is controlled for, women earn less and achieve tenure more slowly than men do. And, as chapter 12 shows, although women publish less than men (based on the 1984 work by Zuckerman and Cole), what they publish is of higher quality, as measured by the number of times their work is cited by other scholars in their field. (pp. 248–249)

In the July/August 1995 issue of *Academe*, an article entitled "Women Faculty Frozen in Time" by West (1995) noted:

> In 1920, when women won the right to vote, 26 percent of full-time faculty in American higher education were women. In 1995, 31 percent of full-time faculty in American higher education are women – an increase of 5 percent over seventy-five years. (p. 26)

In the same issue of *Academe* (July/August 1995) on a short overview of the contributions to higher education of M. Carey Thomas (second president of Bryn Mawr college in 1894), Horowitz (1995) discusses two lectures Thomas delivered to the Association of Collegiate Alumnae (subsequently renamed the American Association of University Women). In the lectures, Thomas posed a difficult question, "Why are there no women geniuses?" (p. 13). Horowitz points out, "Thomas argues that real scholarship is produced in social circumstances still denied to women" (p. 13). In later discussions, regarding graduate education for women, Thomas was noted as saying,

"The highest service which colleges can render to their time is to discover and foster imaginative and constructive genius" (p. 14).

Several studies have shown that females also publish less in higher education literature (Hunter, 1986; Hunter & Kuh, 1987). In a study of higher education journals regarding sex and publication, approximately 50% of the subjects studied by Hunter and Kuh held faculty appointments or institutional research appointments, while 30% were administrators. The prolific authors published an average of six books or monographs and 36 articles and chapters in their lifetimes. Seventy-six percent of the males were more likely than the females (50%) to describe their doctoral programs as research oriented. Hunter and Kuh summarized their work as follows:

> Members of the community of high producers are predominantly white males, a finding that underscores the importance of learning more about the existence and influence of cumulative advantages for men and cumulative disadvantages faced by women and minorities. (p. 458)

"It would be particularly helpful to know what might be done to increase the number of women and minority contributors to the higher education literature" (p. 459). Creamer (1994) found that between 1979 and 1983, only 8 females, compared to 25 males, accounted for four or more articles in seven journals over five years (most were found to be employed by doctoral-granting institutions). "The fact that women constitute a distinct minority on the faculty of most institutions, but especially at doctoral-granting research institutions, probably partly explains the lower rate of publication of women" (p. 38).

This study examined both literatures of higher education and library and information science to determine the sex of those publishing in these disciplines for the year 2000.

Position of the Authors Publishing in the Literature of Higher Education and Library and Information Science

In her doctoral thesis, *The Search for "Higher education" as an Academic Field of Study*, Vigil (1991) concluded that the discipline of higher education was still emerging. She based her conclusion on the fact that faculty mostly from outside the discipline of higher education did research or published in higher education. Vigil noted, "Higher education program faculty found themselves in the paradoxical position of trying to build a field of study, while what scholarship there was had been generated largely from outside higher education programs" (p. 71). In *Key Resources on Higher education Govern-ance, Management, and Leadership* (Peterson & Mets, 1987), a review of the literature about academic officers shows that "the literature on these posi-tions is uneven in quality and scattered throughout several fields" (p. 464).

John Henry Newman (1996) recognized that faculty advance knowledge through research and extend it through teaching. Full-time faculty are paid to perform research and publish, and rewarded through promotion and tenure when their work is published in the scholarly journals of their dis-ciplines (Hoyt, 1974). Sometimes, faculty may be more devoted to their discipline than the university. In other instances, faculty may be more ded-icated to teaching, and find that research limits the amount of time they can dedicate to teaching (Caplow & McGee, 1959). In any case, it is faculty who are responsible for the writing and lab work required to support the struc-tures in place that support research and carry on knowledge. Most faculty obtain their doctorates at major research universities where research is pro-moted. It is through training at the graduate level that faculty become scholars and pursue lifelong occupations of writing and research, regardless of the institution size and scope where they end up living out their careers (Braxton & Toombs, 1982; Daly, 1994).

Federal support of large research initiatives has also caught the attention of faculty who apply for and receive research funding. With the increase in enrollment and the increase in federal research dollars to major research institutions, faculty may be torn between a focus on teaching and attention to research (Braxton, 1983). Since funding for research has been allotted to specific areas, some of the smaller research institutions have not received funding comparable to the larger universities. It has been shown that the faculty at major research universities have performed more research and published more frequently than their counterparts at smaller institutions (Berelson, 1960; Ladd, 1979).

Studies indicate that faculty at all types of institutions are spending in-creasingly more time researching and publishing (Bentley & Blackburn, 1990; Milem, Berger, & Dey, 2000). Many studies have shown that faculty perform research and publish in order to achieve promotion and tenure (Babchuck & Bates, 1962; DeYoung, 1985; Fox, 1983; Holly, 1977; Kasten, 1984; Lewis, 1980; Ruscio, 1987; Tien & Blackburn, 1996) or to pursue their own curiosity and determination for discovering the unknown (McKeachie, 1979; Tien, 2000). Faculty and administrators at the research institutions surveyed by Pellino, Blackburn, and Boberg (1984) agree that "publishing is the essence of scholarship" (p. 114). In an extensive study of 494 deans and chairpersons, Suppa and Zirkel (1983) found that 89% regarded the publication of articles in refereed journals as an important factor in promotion and tenure decisions. In an article published in the March/April 2000 issue of *Change*, the National Center for Postsecondary Improvement shows the results of 378 interviews with faculty from a sample of 19 colleges and universities across the Carnegie Classifications from liberal arts colleges to research universities. It was found that 94% of the faculty consider tenure and promotion an important goal, while nearly 75% are motivated by salary and merit increases.

Faculty status for academic librarians plays an important role in research and publication in the literature of library and information science. It has been shown that faculty status and tenure for academic librarians ensures research and publication within the discipline because faculty status and tenure guarantees integration into the university's academic spheres (Welch & Mozenter, 2006). In a study of 12 library journals between 1973 and 1982, it was shown that the percentage of articles written by academic librarians increased from 28 to 42% (Krause & Sieburth, 1985). Watson (1985) analyzed the scholarly production of authors in 11 major library science journals from 1979 to 1983 and found that the requirements for academic librarians to publish affected publication productivity. Enger et al. (1989) examined 25 core journals in the literature of library and information science for 1985 and discovered that academic librarians published more than any other group, or 26.1% of the articles. In a study of collaborative efforts of authors in the library and information science literature Bahr and Zemon (2000) learned that university librarians published 69% of the literature in *College & Research Libraries* and the *Journal of Academic Librarianship* between 1986 and 1996. However, the most recent literature indicates that publication rates among academic librarians are reaching a plateau (Budd, 2006; Wiberley, Hurd, & Weller, 2006). In any case, faculty status among college and university librarians ensures the continuance of the literature.

This study examined the literature of higher education and library science to determine the position of the authors publishing in both disciplines for the year 2000.

Institutional Affiliation and Scholarly Productivity in Higher Education and Library and Information Science

Some studies have shown that the rank of the higher education institution influences publication and research activity (Bentley & Blackburn, 1990; Dey, Milem, & Berger, 1997; Milem et al., 2000). Milem et al. examined the influence of institutional setting on faculty time allocation by Carnegie

Classification and aggregating faculty data from three national surveys: (a) the American Council on Education 1972 Survey, with 53,034 respondents from 301 colleges and universities; (b) the 1989 Survey by the Higher Education Research Institute (HERI), with data from 51,574 respondents from 432 colleges and universities; (c) the 1992 Survey by the Higher Education Research Institute (HERI), with data from 43,940 respondents from 344 colleges and universities. All of the surveys were similar in design. The findings showed that faculty at research universities spent the greatest amount of time performing research; while faculty at other institutions also increased the time they spent on research. Specifically, Milem et al. noted that, even though the gap in time spent in research between the doctoral research institutions and other higher education institutions has narrowed, the greatest percentage of change involves faculty at doctoral and comprehensive institutions spending a greater amount of time doing research. It was shown that faculty at the institutions with the highest Carnegie Classification have a distinct advantage when it comes to faculty allotment of time for research. The researchers tested faculty rank across institutions and learned that there was no difference in the mean proportion of faculty who were tenured among the institutions. The study also showed that faculty across all institutional types spent an increased amount of time teaching and in preparation of teaching, as a whole.

Bentley and Blackburn (1990) analyzed data from four national surveys of college and university faculty between 1969 and 1988 and found that institutions at the top of the hierarchy retained their publication advantage over time, but that institutions at all levels were increasing their research activity. Hunter and Kuh (1987) identified prolific contributors to the literature of higher education, and interviewed them to determine their various characteristics, finding that over 75% of the respondents were employed at public Ph.D. granting institutions.

The fewest number of institutions represented by Carnegie Classification in the United States fall in the Intensive university category, which represents 110 institutions, or 2.8% of all institutions. The next smallest Carnegie category are institutions with research-extensive status, which is the highest ranking status (granting at least 50 doctoral degrees a year across 15 disciplines) representing 3.8% of the population of universities, or 151 institutions. The Baccalaureate classification contains 606 institutions, or 15.4% of the schools; the Master's institutions represent 15.5%, or 611 institutions; and all other categories, including Associate's colleges, represent the most institutions, or 62.4% of all institutions of higher education in the United States (Carnegie Foundation for the Advancement of Teaching, 2000).

Milem et al. (2000) observed that faculty at doctoral and comprehensive institutions spent a greater amount of time doing research, and that faculty at the institutions with the highest Carnegie Classification have a distinct advantage when it comes to faculty allotments of time for research. Bentley and Blackburn (1990) also found that institutions at the top of the hierarchy have retained their publication advantage over time.

Little research has been performed regarding the institutional affiliation of authors in library and information science publications. However, what research exists is pertinent and germane to the discipline. In a survey of 304 institutions for 1989, across Carnegie Classification type, research universities, doctorate-granting universities, comprehensive universities, and liberal arts colleges, it was found that 125 of the 304 institutions surveyed gave faculty status to librarians. Of the institutions that afforded faculty status to librarians, 20% of them were research universities; 50% were doctorate-granting universities; 56.8% were comprehensive universities, and 34.1% were liberal arts institutions. The study found that fewer research institutions were giving faculty status to librarians, while all the other institutions on the Carnegie Classification were noted for giving faculty status to librarians at a higher rate. The authors of this study ascertained that fewer research universities might be granting faculty status to librarians. In regard to scholarship, respondents in the survey acknowledged that scholarship was *considered* at 62.2% of all institutions, while it was *evaluated* at all 85% of the research, doctorate-granting, and comprehensive universities. However, only 17.8% of all surveyed *required* evidence of scholarship. Essentially, scholarship is *evaluated*, but not necessarily *required* for tenure among academic librarians at the top-tiered institutions.

In a paper using the 1994 Carnegie Classification for institutions, it was learned that university libraries, or librarians from a research university, doctoral university, or master's university or college constituted 69% of the articles published (out of 399 articles in *College & Research Libraries* and the *Journal of Academic Librarianship* between 1986 and 1996). In other words, nearly 70% of the articles published in these two journals were representing academic librarians from the top Carnegie institutions (Bahr & Zemon, 2000).

The journal articles tabulated for 2000 by institutional affiliation were categorized according to the Carnegie Classifications discussed and delineated in *The Carnegie Classification of Institutions of Higher Education*:

The 2000 Carnegie Classification includes all colleges and universities in the United States that are degree-granting and accredited by an agency recognized by the U.S. Secretary of Education. The 2000 edition classifies institutions based on their degree-granting activities from 1995–96 through 1997–98. (Carnegie Foundation for the Advancement of Teaching, 2000, p. 1)

At the time of this publication, the Carnegie Classification system was under revision. Since the articles examined for this study were from the year 2000, the Carnegie Classification during the year 2000 was chosen. Park and Riggs (1993) note:

> Although a number of schemes are used to categorize colleges and universities, the Carnegie Classification (first developed by Clark Kerr in 1973) is generally recognized as the most credible. The Carnegie Classification groups colleges and universities according to their missions and educational functions. Among the factors used to distinguish institutions are numbers and types of degrees awarded, priority given to research and graduate education, and selectivity of admission. (p. 72)

Core journal articles in higher education and library and information science were examined for the year 2000 to determine the institutional affiliation of the authors, or more specifically, the Carnegie Classification of the institutions where the authors worked. In this manner, it will be determined if social stratification is occurring in the two disciplines in regard to publication.

Content Analysis of the Disciplines of Higher Education and Library and Information Science

Little has been done in the literature of higher education to determine the subject content of the literature published. Hood et al. (1979) examined the *Journal of College Student Development* for the years 1959–1974 and found that a large portion of the articles dealt with orientation, housing, discipline, student activities, and a small portion related to admissions and placement. Kuh and Bursky (1980) examined 1,268 articles in four student affairs journals between 1970 and 1978 and categorized the articles by type of article, such as Philosophical/Theoretical, Research/Evaluation, Review of the Literature, and Program Description, finding that approximately 50% fell within the Research/Evaluation category. Kellams (1975) performed a content analysis on the literature of higher education to determine the research orientation of the literature and found that "theoretical research was rare among the abstracts analyzed" (p. 152). While Kellams performed a content analysis, he did not examine the subject content of the abstracts studied. Overall, very little research exists discussing the subject content of the literature of higher education.

In the literature of library and information science, there is a fair amount of research on content analysis. Using *College & Research Libraries* and the *Journal of Academic Libraries* for articles published from 1990 to 1999,

Xue-Min Bao (2000) found that the majority of articles discussed library collections and services. An analysis of 517 professional and 127 research articles in *Turk Kutuphaneciligi* from 1952 to 1994 showed that the most popular category in Turkey, in both the professional and research articles, was "Library and Information Science Service Activities." Koufogiannakis et al. (2004) examined 91 library and information science journals (2,664 journal articles) for 2001 and found that the following subjects were discussed, in order of discussion: (1) Information Access & Retrieval, (2) Collections, (3) Management, (4) Education, and (5) Reference. In a survey of subject trends discussed in conferences, seminars, and meetings from 1957 to 1986 in Denmark, it was reported that the three areas discussed the most, other than "Unclassified/Miscellaneous," were Administration and Management, Materials/Collections, and Automation of Library Processes (Kajberg, 1995). In an overview of research productivity among library professionals in Iran from 1966 to 1998 (2,490 titles), the areas of highest priority were Information Storage and Retrieval and Information Technology (Horri, 2004). Overall, it appears that there is an eclectic mix of subjects discussed in the library and information science literature worldwide. It must be noted that of all the subjects discussed in the literature, these particular subjects "rose to the top," so as to speak. Collectively, there were many topics that were discussed in the literature, but those noted as the top areas of content are the ones that took priority over others, thereby reflecting the orientation and focus, overall, of the discipline. As discipline reflects practice, these areas are most reflective of practice in library and information science for the titles and years covered. Of the topics discussed, the following took precedence over others:

- Information retrieval/technology/automation
- Collections
- Service
- Management/Administration
- Education

This study examined journals in higher education and library and information science to determine the subject content of the journal for the year 2000. It is assumed that the discussion of topics reflects the direction of the disciplines at the turn of the new millennium, and also reflects what is important in the practice of the two disciplines at that point of time.

METHODOLOGY

Bibliometrics was used to tabulate the research methodologies used and the subject content contained in eight core journals in higher education and eight core journals in library and information science for the year 2000. Bibliometrics was also used to determine the gender, Carnegie Classification, and academic position of the authors in the journals. The statistical package SAS, created one-way frequency and percentage (descriptive) tables and two-way (inferential) chi-square tables to determine, first of all, the frequencies and percentages of the variables tested for higher education and library and information science. Once the frequencies and percentages were performed, a chi-square test was performed on the variables tested to infer whether or not two categorical variables were associated with each other. The variables include research methodologies, gender, Carnegie Classification, position, and content analysis. Definitions of the variables and other units measured in this study, such as journal article and subject headings, are seven pages long and are not included in this publication. For definitions, please contact the author. The hypotheses were the following:

- There is no significant difference in the research methodologies employed between the discipline of higher education and the discipline of library and information science in the eight core journals examined for each discipline in the year 2000.
- There is no significant difference in the sex of the authors in higher education and library and information science core journals.
- There is no significant difference in the Carnegie Classification the authors were affiliated in higher education and library and information science core journals.

The position of the authors and the content of the articles were also examined. A simple descriptive analysis occurred for each. It was assumed that higher educationist published the most in higher education, and that librarians published the most in library and information science.

DATA COLLECTION

The eight selected journals in higher education were taken from Budd's (1990) study, which ranked education journals according to the number of times they were cited in the education literature. No other examination of the literature represents this number of a ranking of higher education journals. In another study, Burnett (1973) listed several of the same journals used in Budd's (1990) study as the best-known journals reporting the study of higher education, including the *Journal of Higher education, College and University,* and *Journal of College Student Development.* Silverman (1982) employed three of the journals used in this current study for his analysis: *Research in Higher education, Journal of Higher education,* and *Higher education.* Smart (1983) found that citation measures could be utilized to discover those journals discussed the most often in education literature and learned that, of the journals to be used in this study, the *Journal of College Student Development* ranked among the highest. Bayer (1983) sought to identify the journals in higher education based on three criteria: (a) journals most frequently publishing article titles with a higher education focus, 1977–1979; (b) journals most frequently referencing Carnegie Commission and Jossey-Bass volumes; (c) reputation ranking of journals by the American Society for Higher Education (ASHE) members. While the result was a cross-disciplinary representation, several of the higher education journals – *Journal of Higher Education, Higher Education, College and University* – met all the three criteria, and one other journal – *Journal of College Student Development* – met two of the three criteria. Other education studies used to rank order journals include Luce and Johnson (1978). By examining previously developed lists and querying respondents affiliated with the American Educational Research Association (AERA), Luce and Johnson developed a list of the highest ranking journals by specific education categories to include journal rankings for administration, for learning and instruction, and for journals relating to the social context of education. Luce and Johnson found the *Journal of Higher Education* was ranked as one of the highest journals for administrators. Two of the top 10 publications in Budd's (1990) list, *Change* and *The Chronicle of Higher Education,* do not directly represent research and are omitted from this study. *The Chronicle of Higher Education* is primarily a newspaper in higher education, reporting on the results of research, and *Change* is primarily a magazine, not a research journal. The journal articles in the eight most cited journals were examined for 2000.

The eight core journals in higher education were:

- Research in Higher Education
- Journal of Higher Education
- Review of Higher Education
- Journal of College Student Development
- Academe

- College and University
- New Directions for Institutional Research
- Higher Education

The eight selected journals for library and information science were taken from the journals that were cited the most in Journal Citation Reports (JCR) in the category "Information and Library Science" for the years 2001, 2002, 2003, and 2004. The journals from 2000 are calculated for the 2001 JCR list. The eight core journals in library and information science were:

- Journal of the American Society of Information Science and Technology
- MIS Quarterly
- Information & Management (Amsterdam)
- Information Processing & Management
- Journal of Management Information Systems
- International Journal of the Geographical Information Society
- College & Research Libraries
- Journal of Academic Librarianship

The following information was recorded: Journal Title; Year; Volume; Pages; Article Title; Up to Three Authors listed in the article, including Last Name, First Name or Initials, and Sex; Research Methodology, including Qualitative Research: Biography, Phenomenology, Grounded Theory, Ethnography, Case Study, Miscellaneous, and Quantitative Research: Descriptive, Inferential, and Miscellaneous, as well as No Research Methodology; Subject Topics of the Articles, listing the first four subject headings assigned to the articles in the Education Resources Information Center (ERIC) database, using the ERIC thesaurus as a guide for the journals in higher education, while keyword descriptions were compiled to determine the subject of the articles in library and information science. In order to ensure integrity of the data, each element listed above was recorded. The investigator recorded all of the information needed for this study alone so that no misunderstanding regarding the definitions of the variables would occur. Two separate files were created, an author file and a journal file, and the two files were linked by a number assigned to each journal article. For instance, in the Excel database, the first article in *Academe* (January/February 1995, vol. 81, pp. 7–11) was given the code of 1 and so on for each article. No distinction was made regarding the ranking of first, second, or third author.

The two variables were tabulated for Gender. Sometimes, with the names given in the article, the sex of the author could not be determined. For instance, one author's name was Yinong Chong. Upon searching the

Internet, several articles were found about Yinong Chong; one article was located from a newsletter published by the Cedar Valley Medical Specialists at this site: http://www.cedarvalleymedical.com/centers/osteoporosis/recent-headlines/newtesturged.htm. Dr. Yinong Chong, an epidemiologist with the National Center for Health Statistics, Hyattsville, Maryland, told Reuters Health, "This test, *she said* (emphasis added), provides women and their doctors a solid piece of information on which to decide." From the article, it is clear that Chong's sex is female. In other cases, when the sex could not be determined from the article, such as the article by G.L. Donhardt, the author was located at a university through a search on the Internet, and sent an e-mail. When the sex still could not be determined, the field was left blank.

The Carnegie Classification was a variable with the levels of: Extensive, Intensive, Master's, Baccalaureate (including Associate's), and Miscellaneous (including International). To find information regarding the Carnegie Classification of the institutional affiliation of the authors publishing, each institution was recorded. *The Carnegie Classification of Institutions of Higher education* (Carnegie Foundation for the Advancement of Teaching, 2000) was consulted to determine the Carnegie Classification of each institution and was recorded on the data collection instrument. In the initial data collection, all of the Carnegie Classifications were recorded and tabulated; but each level recorded did not meet the criteria of five tabulations in each category, so the following categories were collapsed into the Miscellaneous category: Master's I and II categories were collapsed into Master's; Baccalaureate Colleges – Liberal Arts, Baccalaureate Colleges – General, and Baccalaureate/Associate's Colleges; Specialized Institutions and Tribal Colleges.

The variable "position" contained the following levels: Faculty, Administrators, and Miscellaneous (including Students). All of the people in the study who teach at the college level were recorded as Faculty, including Lecturers, Visiting Professors, Professor Emeriti, Assistant Professors, Associate Professors, and Full Professors. Positions that were recorded as administrator are included in, but not limited to, the following categories: Chancellor, Vice Chancellor, Provost, Vice President, Associate Vice President, Dean of Graduate School, Assistant Dean, Assistant Dean of Students, Director, Associate Director, Registrar, etc. The Miscellaneous category included Students and Staff and other areas. The position variables for library and information science included Academic Librarians, Faculty, Researcher, and Student.

The categories representing faculty departments in higher education were Education (other than higher education), Higher Education, and

Miscellaneous. The categories representing departments of authors of library and information science journals included Business, Computer Science, Geography, Institute, Library and Information Science, and Management.

The Research Methodologies used in this study were Descriptive (quantitative), Inferential (quantitative), Qualitative, or No Research Methodology. Each article in the journals for 2,000 was examined for the research methodologies employed. Initially, the qualitative category specified the particular type of qualitative analysis in each article, such as Biography, Phenomenology, Grounded Theory, Ethnography, and Case Study. When there was not enough data for individual categories for qualitative analysis, the individual categories for qualitative analysis were collapsed into one category, qualitative analysis. The other three quantitative research categories tabulated included descriptive and inferential and were not collapsed into one category.

DATA ANALYSIS AND DISCUSSION

Research Methodologies

The research methods tested in the eight core journals for higher education and for library and information science included Descriptive, Inferential, Qualitative, and No Research Methodology. Other measures, such as formulas or models, were tabulated as No Research Methodology.

Research Methodologies Used in Eight Higher Education Core Journals for 2000

Frequency tables were created for each discipline with the following results: of the 235 articles examined for higher education, 37 (15.74%) were Descriptive; 109 (30.64%) were Inferential; 41 (17.45%) were Qualitative; and 194 (36.17%) contained No Research Methodology. Quantitative measures (Descriptive and Inferential) combined for a total of 46.36%, or nearly half of all the articles examined for 2000. It should be noted that 17.45% of the articles were qualitative. Of the authors publishing in the eight core journals in higher education chosen for this study, 375 authors were represented.

A chi-square test was given for gender and research methodologies for higher education, resulting in a significant difference in the proportions of males using each different research methodology compared to females, with a p value equal to .0037, at the alpha value of .001, showing a significance and rejection of the null hypothesis. 62.5% of the articles using inferential statistics had male authors and 37.5% of the inferential articles had female authors.

Research Methodologies Used in Eight Library and Information Science Core Journals for 2000

In a frequency tabulation for the eight core journals in library and information, it was discovered that a total of 34.69% of the journals contained both Descriptive and Inferential statistics; while 60.63% of the journals contained No Research Methodologies (or statistical measures). Six of the eight journals in the Information and Library Science list were information science journals. Few of the studies published in information science employed traditional statistical measures, but used models and formulas to discover methods of information management and retrieval to develop web-based interfaces. Primarily, these studies are doing research, but not of the type measured in this study.

For a cross tabulation using research methodologies and gender, it was discovered that of the publications employing inferential statistics, 81.05% of them were published by males; while 18.95% were published by females. Males did not use any statistical analysis 63.66% of the time, while females did not use any analysis 49.69% of the time.

Overall, only 34.69% of the eight library and information science journals published in 2000 contained some form of descriptive and inferential statistics, assuming that over 60% of the journals lacked any form of quantifiable statistics. Without continued statistical analysis in a literature, it is difficult to develop a theoretical base. In contrast, given the fact that the journals cited the most in library and information science are information science journals, one must seriously examine why information science journals are being cited more than library science journals.

Has library science become a subdiscipline of information science, or are they now becoming more distinct, separate disciplines? A more accurate portrayal of the two disciplines may warrant separate categories in tabulating citation ranks, one for information science and the other for library science. A change has occurred from this author's research in 1989 of twenty-five core journals in library and information science for 1985 (Enger et al., 1989) to the present 2000 study. The most cited journals were primarily library science journals, and reflected the discipline of library science. In this study, a distinction between the two has become apparent, questioning whether they are becoming two distinct, separate disciplines.

Gender of the Authors

Comparing males publishing in higher education to library and information science, 56.2% in higher education were male; while 70.73% of the authors were male in library and information science. The total female authors for both disciplines were 327, while the total male authors for both disciplines were 602. When counting (or describing) only the number of authors by discipline, 29.27% of the authors in library and information were female while 70.73% were male. It appears that males publish a much higher percentage of the articles in library science than in higher education.

Carnegie Classification of the Authors

There were a total of 930 authors between the two disciplines represented in this study. Of the 930 authors, 489 (or 53%) worked at Carnegie Extensive institutions for the year 2000, representing more than half of all the institutions in the Carnegie list. In addition, 245 authors were from institutions outside of the United States, or international authors. Of the 489 authors from Carnegie Extensive institutions, 220 were published in the higher education literature and 281 were published in the library and information science literature. In other words, for higher education, 57.94% of all Carnegie Categories were represented in the Extensive category and 15.60 in the International category. For library and information science, 49.21% represented the Extensive category, while 33.10% represented the International category (the two largest representations in both disciplines) All other Carnegie areas represented the remaining categories. In performing the chi-square test on higher education and library and information science, there was a significant difference in representation of authors by Carnegie Classification with a probability of $p = .0095$. The difference may be explained that when cross tabulation occurred, the distribution between both Extensive and Other classifications appeared to be similar, or nearly equal.

When cross tabulating for gender and Carnegie Classification for higher education, 40.58% of the authors from Extensive institutions were female while 59.42% were male. In library and information science, 34.30% of the authors from Carnegie Extensive institutions were female while 65.70% representing Carnegie Extensive institutions were male. A disparity exists in each discipline among sexes regarding who is represented by the highest tiered institutions. It also exists in authors represented by the highest tiered institutions, overall.

Position of the Authors

On a frequency rating, faculty published the most articles in higher education, with 61.71% of authorship; administrators published 22%, while students published 10.57% of the articles. For library and information science, the findings were similar. Faculty published 64.34% of the articles, academic librarians 12.94%, Researchers 10.49%, and Students 5.24% of the articles. The departments represented in higher education were Other (48.80%) (meaning departments other than those listed here), Higher Education (20.64%) (meaning people representing departments of higher education), Education (17.86%) and Psychology (12.80%). The departments represented in the library and information literature were very diverse, with 97 departments represented and listed in order with the highest first: Computer Science (10.70%), Business (10.08%), Institutes (10.08%), Geography (6.58%), Library and Information Science (7%), Management (4.73%), Management Information Systems (2.88%). All of the other percentages were too low to discuss here.

In regard to gender of the authors, the most significant difference was noted in the library and information science literature where Academic Librarians who were female represented authorship in 63.01% of the publications, while male academic librarians represented 36.99%. The reverse is true for faculty – 75.99% of the faculty publishing in library and information are male, while 24.01% of the faculty are female.

In both areas, faculty publish the most and are widely represented from areas other than higher education and library and information science.

Content Analysis

The area discussed the most in the higher education literature was College Students (34.21%), College Administration (16.67%), College Faculty (16.23%), and Institutional Evaluation and Research (10.96%). In library and information science, 210 content areas were tabulated on the basis of keywords. The following topics were discussed, with the highest listed first: Geographical Information Systems (4.39%); the World Wide Web (2.82%); Relevance (1.88%); a tie ensued for the following (1.57%): Collection Development, End User Searching, Information Retrieval Systems, Librarians, Service, Online Searching. The literature of higher education is tied to the operation of the academy, while it appears that the literature of library and information science is tied to information/technological access and service.

SUMMARY

In both disciplines, the use of research methodologies in developing the literature, and subsequently the disciplines, requires further progress, since both disciplines used quantifiable statistics less than 50% of the time. There was a contrast by gender in the library and information science literature, with males publishing at a much higher rate than females. In future studies, a distinction between the library science and information science literature must be made and compared. It appears that information science has come to dominate the literature, since the highest ranking journals for 1999–2003 were information science journals. Males dominated the literature of information science. This may suggest something meaningful in regard to practice. Are the practitioners in information science mostly male? Are females primarily practicing library science? If so, what implications does this have for the future of the discipline of library and information science? In a 1997 article in *Wired Magazine*, Caulfield notes that for too long, "librarians got too narrow by defining themselves in terms of a particular social institution – they were organized around libraries rather than information in general" (p. 64). From 1976 to 1996 enrollment in library schools dropped from 8,037 to 4,845. As a new literature begins to emerge around information science, what will become of the literature of library science? If literatures define disciplines, and disciplines reflect practice, what is the future practice of library and information science? In addition, it is clear that a social stratification is occurring in the literature at this time in regard to a disparity between males and females and publication.

Social stratification as discussed in this manuscript also exists in both literatures in regard to Carnegie Classification of the authors. There is no disputing that most of the authors publishing in both higher education and library and information science are from the highest tiered research institutions for the year 2000, the Carnegie Extensive institutions. It was also shown that a large number of authors came from institutions outside the United States. Omotayo (2004) found in studying *Lfe Psychologia* from 1993 to 2002 that foreign authorship rose from 21.7% in the first six years to 52% in the last four years.

In both disciplines, faculty published the most. It is interesting to note that faculty in disciplines other than higher education and library and information science published more than higher educationists and librarians and information scientists. This, too, may indicate something about the maturation of the discipline. If authors outside the discipline represent it the most, who takes ownership for the development of the discipline? How is scholarship defined? Then again, it simply may indicate the interdisciplinary nature of the disciplines, which should be recognized and considered by educators developing curricula.

Finally, the content of the literatures indicated what may be central to practice. In higher education, college students were the most frequent subjects of study, and this is reassuring, particularly when the study also indicates that the authors come primarily from Carnegie Extensive institutions. While it is assumed that research institutions focus on research, there is a generous discussion of students in this literature. The discussion of students in the higher education literature was over twice as high as the other two subjects discussed. From this literature, it became apparent that students are important among practitioners.

In the library and information science literature, the discussion focused on matters of libraries, and on information science – both library science and information science issues were discussed. Both library science and information science represent access – access to knowledge in either physical or virtual form. Organization and access was at the core of the library and information science literature, while passing knowledge on to students was the axis of the higher education literature. Both disciplines advance knowledge through practice. At the heart of each is the human endeavor to move forward, to make sense of the world, and to make life better for one another.

ACKNOWLEDGMENTS

The author would like to acknowledge Curt Doetkott, Statistician at North Dakota State University, for his ongoing support and expertise.

REFERENCES

Abel, R. E., & Newlin, L. W. (Eds) (2002). *Scholarly publishing: Books, journals, publishers, and libraries in the twentieth century.* New York: John Wiley & Sons.

Andersen, J. (2002). The role of subject literature in scholarly communication: An interpretation based on social epistemology. *Journal of Documentation, 58,* 463–481.

Ash, M. G. (1997). *German universities, past and future: Crisis or renewal?* Providence, RI: Berghahn Books.

Astin, H. S. (1969). *The woman doctorate in America.* New York: Sage.

Atkins, S. E. (1991). *The academic library in the American university.* Chicago: American Library Association.

Babchuck, N., & Bates, A. (1962). Professor or producer: The two faces of academic man. *Social Forces, 40*, 341–344.

Bahr, A. H., & Zemon, M. (2000). Collaborative authorship in the journal literature: Perspectives for academic librarians who publish. *College & Research Libraries, 61*, 410–419.

Bates, M. J. (1999). The invisible substrate of information science. *Journal of the American Society for Information Science, 50*, 1043–1050.

Bayer, A. E. (1983). Multi-method strategies for defining higher education journals. *The Review of Higher Education, 6*, 103–113.

Bayer, A. E., & Folger, J. (1966). Some correlates of a citation measure of productivity in science. *Sociology of Education, 39*, 381–390.

Bentley, R., & Blackburn, R. T. (1990). Changes in academic research performance over time: A study of institutional accumulative advantage. *Research in Higher Education, 31*, 327–344.

Berelson, B. (1960). *Graduate education in the United States.* New York: McGraw-Hill.

Bernard, J. (1964). *Academic women.* University Park: Pennsylvania State University Press.

Biglan, A. (1973). Relationships between subject matter characteristics and the structure and output of university departments. *Journal of Applied Psychology, 57*, 204–213.

Bordons, M., Morillo, F., Fernandex, M. T., & Gomez, I. (2003). On step further in the production of bibliometric indicators at the micro level: Differences by gender and professional category of scientists. *Scientometrics, 57*, 159–173.

Borgman, C. L. (1990). *Scholarly communication and bibliometrics.* Newbury Park, CA: Sage Publications.

Boyer, E. L. (1990). *Scholarship reconsidered: Priorities of the professoriate.* Princeton, NJ: Carnegie Foundation for the Advancement of Teaching.

Braxton, J. M. (1983). Teaching as performance of scholarly-based course activities: A perspective on the relationship between teaching and research. *Review of Higher Education, 7*, 21–33.

Braxton, J. M., & Toombs, W. (1982). Faculty uses of doctoral training: Considerations of a technique for the differentiation of scholarly effort from research activity. *Research in Higher Education, 16*, 265–282.

Brubacher, J. S., & Rudy, R. (1996). *Higher education in transition: A history of American colleges and universities, 1636–1976.* New York: Harper & Row.

Budd, J. M. (1990). Higher education literature: Characteristics of citation patterns. *Journal of Higher Education, 61*, 84–97.

Budd, J. M. (2004). Academic libraries and knowledge: A social epistemology framework. *The Journal of Academic Librarianship, 30*, 361–367.

Budd, J. M. (2006). Faculty publishing productivity: Comparisons over time. *College & Research Libraries, 67*, 230–239.

Burnett, C. W. (1973). Higher education as a specialized field of study. *Journal of Research and Development in Education, 6*, 4–15.

Busha, C. H., & Harter, S. P. (1980). *Research methods in librarianship: Techniques and interpretation.* San Diego: Academic Press.

Butler, P. (1933). *An introduction to library science.* Chicago: The University of Chicago Press.

Caplow, T., & McGee, R. J. (1959). *The academic marketplace.* New York: Basic Books.

Carnegie Foundation for the Advancement of Teaching. (2000). *The Carnegie classification of institutions of higher education* (5th ed.). Menlo Park, CA: Carnegie Publications.

Centra, J. A. (1974). *Women, men, and the doctorate.* Princeton, NJ: Educational Testing Service.

Chubin, D. (1975). The journal as a primary data source in the sociology of science: With some observations from sociology. *Social Science Information, 14,* 157–168.

Coats, A. W. (1971). The role of scholarly journals in the history of economics: An essay. *Journal of Economic Literature, 9,* 29–44.

Cole, J. R. (1970). Patterns of intellectual influence in scientific research. *Sociology of Education, 43,* 377–403.

Cole, J. R., & Cole, S. (1973). *Social stratification in science.* Chicago: University of Chicago Press.

Cole, J. R., & Zuckerman, H. (1984). The productivity puzzle: Persistence and change in patterns of publication on men and women scientists. In: P. Maehr & M. W. Steinkamp (Eds), *Advances in motivation and achievement* (pp. 217–256). Greenwich, CT: JAI Press.

Cole, S. (1970). Professional standing and the reception of scientific discoveries. *American Journal of Sociology, 76,* 286–306.

Cole, S. (1983). The hierarchy of the sciences? *American Journal of Sociology, 89,* 111–139.

Cole, S., & Cole, J. R. (1967). Scientific output and recognition: A study in the operation of the reward system in science. *American Sociological Review, 32,* 377–390.

Cordesco, F. (1960). *The shaping of American graduate education: Daniel Coit Gilman and the protean Ph.D.* Totowa, NJ: Rowman and Littlefield.

Creamer, E. G. (1994). Gender and publication in higher education journals. *Journal of College Student Development, 35,* 35–39.

Creswell, J. W., & Roskens, R. W. (1981). The Biglan studies of differences among academic areas. *The Review of Higher Education, 4,* 1–16.

Daly, W. T. (1994). Teaching and scholarship: Adapting American higher education to hard times. *Journal of Higher Education, 65,* 45–58.

Dey, E. L., Milem, J. F., & Berger, J. B. (1997). Changing patterns of publication productivity: Accumulative advantage or institutional isomorphism? *Sociology of Education, 70,* 308–323.

DeYoung, A. (1985). Assessing "faculty productivity" in colleges of education: Penetration of the technical thesis into the status system of academe. *Educational Theory, 35,* 411–412.

Egan, M. E., & Shera, J. H. (1952). Foundations of a theory of bibliography. *Library Quarterly, 22,* 125–137.

Eisenhower, D. D. (1981). *Farewell radio and television address to the American people, January 17, 1961.* Boston: Council for a Livable World Education Fund.

Enger, K. B., Quirk, G., & Stewart, J. A. (1989). Statistical methods used by authors of library and information science journal articles. *Library and Information Science Research: An International Journal, 11,* 37–46.

Fairweather, J. S. (1994). Faculty rewards: The comprehensive college and university story. *Metropolitan Universities: An International Forum, 51,* 54–61.

Fox, M. F. (1983). Publication productivity among scientists: A critical review. *Social Studies of Science, 13,* 285–305.

French, J. C. (1946). *A history of the university founded by Johns Hopkins.* Baltimore: The Johns Hopkins Press.

Fuller, S. (1988). *Social epistemology.* Bloomington: Indiana University Press.

Fye, W. B. (1991). The origin of the full-time faculty system: Implications for clinical research. *Journal of the American Medical Association, 265,* 1555–1573.

Garfield, E. (1972). Citation analysis as a tool in journal evaluation. *Science, 78,* 471–479.

Garvey, W. D., Lin, N., & Nelson, C. E. (1970). Some comparisons of communication activities in the physical and social sciences. In: C. E. Nelson & D. K. Pollock (Eds), *Communication among scientists and engineers* (pp. 61–84). Lexington, MA: D. C. Heath.

Geiger, R. L. (1986). *To advance knowledge: The growth of American research universities, 1900–1940*. New York: Oxford.

Gerould, J. T. (1945). *Statistics of university libraries, 1913-1940*. Princeton, NJ: Princeton University.

Gilman, D. C. (1885). *The benefits which society derives from universities*. Baltimore: Johns Hopkins University.

Gilman, D. C. (1886). *The relation of universities to the progress of civilization*. New York: State University of New York.

Goldhor, H. (1972). *An introduction to scientific research in librarianship*. Urbana: The University of Illinois Press.

Goldman, A. I. (1999). *Knowledge in a social world*. Oxford: Oxford University Press.

Goodspeed, T. W. (1916). *A history of the University of Chicago*. Chicago: The University of Chicago.

Graham, H. D., & Diamond, N. (1997). *The rise of American research universities: Elites and challengers in the postwar era*. Baltimore: Johns Hopkins University Press.

Gross, A. G., Harmon, J. E., & Reidy, M. S. (2000). Argument and 17th-century science: A rhetorical analysis with sociological implications. *Social Science Information, 30*, 371–389.

Gross, P. K., & Gross, E. M. (1927). College libraries and chemical education. *Science, 66*, 1229–1234.

Gumport, P. J. (2002). *Academic pathfinders: Knowledge creation and feminist scholarship*. Westport, CT: Greenwood Press.

Hackett, E. J. (1990). Science as a vocation in the 1990's: The changing organizational culture of academic science. *Journal of Higher Education, 61*, 241–279.

Hagstrom, W. O. (1965). *The scientific community*. New York: Basic Books.

Hakanson, M. (2005). The impact of gender on citations: An analysis of College & research Libraries, Journal of Academic Librarianship, and Library Quarterly. *College & Research Libraries, 66*, 312–323.

Harding, S. (1993). Rethinking standpoint epistemology: What is "strong objectivity?". In: L. Alcoff & E. Potter (Eds), *Feminist epistemologies* (pp. 49–82). New York: Routledge.

Hargens, L. L. (1975). *Patterns of scientific research: A comparative analysis of research in three fields*. Washington, DC: American Sociological Association.

Harvey, A. M., Brieger, G. H., Abrams, S. L., & McKusick, V. A. (1989). A model of its kind: A century of medicine at Johns Hopkins. *Journal of the American Medical Association, 261*, 3136–3143.

Hawkins, D. T. (2001). Information science abstracts: Tracking the literature of information science. Part 1: Definition and map. *Journal of the American Society for Information Science and Technology, 52*, 44–53.

Hawkins, H. (1960). *Pioneer: A history of the Johns Hopkins University, 1874–1889*. Ithaca, NY: Cornell University Press.

Hawkins, H. (1972). *Between Harvard and America: The educational leadership of Charles W. Eliot*. New York: Oxford University Press.

Hefferlin, J. B. Lon. (1969). *Dynamics of academic reform*. San Francisco: Jossey-Bass.

Hobbs, W. C., & Francis, J. B. (1973). On the scholarly activity of higher educationists. *Journal of Higher Education, 44*, 51–60.

Holly, J. W. (1977). Tenure and research productivity. *Research in Higher Education, 6*, 181–192.

Hood, A. B., Hull, S. B., & Mines, R. A. (1979). The role of the *Journal of College Student Personnel* in the literature of various student services. *Journal of College Student Personnel, 20*, 469–475.

Horowitz, H. L. (1995, July/August). A man's and a woman's world. *Academe*, 81, 10–14.

Horri, A. (2004). Bibliometric overview of library and information science research productivity in Iran. *Journal of Education for Library and Information Science, 45*, 15–25.

Hoyt, D. P. (1974). Interrelationships among instructional effectiveness, publication record, and monetary reward. *Research in Higher Education, 2*, 81–88.

Hulme, E. W. (1923). Statistical bibliography in relation to the growth of modern civilization: Two lectures delivered in the University of Cambridge in May, 1922, by E. Wyndham Hulme, B. A, Sandars reader in bibliography, some time librarian of the patent office. London: Grafton & Co.

Humboldt, W. F. (1963). *Humanist without portfolio: An anthology of the writings of Wilhelm von Humboldt*. Detroit: Wayne State University Press.

Hunter, D. E. (1986). Women who write: Prolific female scholars in higher education and student affairs administration. *Journal of the National Association for Women Deans, Administrators, and Counselors, 50*, 33–39.

Hunter, D. E., & Kuh, G. D. (1987). The "write wing": Characteristics of prolific contributors to the higher education literature. *Journal of Higher Education, 58*, 443–462.

Hutchins, R. M. (1949). The state of the university, 1929-1949: A report by Robert M. Hutchins covering the twenty years of his administration. Chicago: The University of Chicago Press.

Jacobson, R. L. (1992, November 11). Public-college officials struggle to respond to growing concern over faculty productivity. *The Chronicle of Higher Education*, pp. A17–A18.

Jencks, C., & Riesman, D. (1968). *The academic revolution*. New York: Doubleday.

Johnson, V. R. (1992). Utilizing prolific writers and their interconnections when expanding on the histories of a discipline: American geography as a case study (Doctoral dissertation, University of Kentucky, 1992). *Dissertation Abstracts International, 53*, 0732.

Kajberg, L. (1995). A content analysis of formalized interpersonal communications in the library-information field in Denmark, 1957–1986. *The New Review of Information and Library Research, 1*, 85–112.

Kasten, K. L. (1984). Tenure and merit pay as rewards for research, teaching, and service at a research university. *Journal of Higher Education, 55*, 500–514.

Kellams, S. E. (1975). Research studies on higher education: A content analysis. *Research in Higher Education, 3*, 139–154.

Kerr, C. (1963). *The uses of the university*. Cambridge, MA: Harvard University Press.

King, J. (1987). A review of bibliometric and other science indicators and their role in research evaluation. *Journal of Information Science, 13*, 261–276.

Koufogiannakis, D., Slater, L., & Crumley, E. (2004). A content analysis of librarianship research. *Journal of Information Science, 30*, 227–239.

Krause, S. C., & Sieburth, J. F. (1985). Patterns of authorship in library journals by academic librarians. *Serials Librarian, 9*, 127–138.

Kronick, D. A. (1962). *A history of scientific and technical periodicals: The origins and development of the scientific and technological press, 1665–1790*. New York: Scarecrow Press.

Kuh, G. D., & Bursky, M. (1980). Knowledge dissemination by publication in student affairs: Who publishes what where? *Journal of College Student Personnel, 21*, 387–393.

Kuhn, T. S. (1970). *The structure of scientific revolutions*. Chicago: The University of Chicago Press.

Kyrillidou, M. (2000). Perspectives on research library trends: ARL statistics. *Journal of Academic Librarianship, 26*, 427–436.

Ladd, E. C., Jr. (1979). The work experience of American college professors: Some data and an argument. In: R. Edgerton (Ed.), *Current issues in higher education* (pp. 3–12). Washington, DC: American Association for Higher education.

Lawani, S. M. (1981). Bibliometrics: Its theoretical foundations, methods, and applications. *Libri, 31*, 294–315.

Lewis, L. S. (1980). Academic tenure: Its recipients and effects. *Annals of the American Academy of Political and Social Science, 448*, 86–101.

Light, D. (1974). Introduction: The structure of the academic professions. *Sociology of Education, 47*, 2–28.

Lin, N., Garvey, W. D., & Nelson, C. E. (1970). Publication fate of material presented at an annual ASA meeting: Two years after the meeting. *American Sociologist, 5*, 22–25.

Lin, N., & Nelson, C. E. (1969). Bibliographic reference patterns in sociological journals, 1965–1966. *American Sociologist, 4*, 47–50.

Lodahl, J. B., & Gordon, G. (1972). The structure of scientific fields and the functioning of university graduate departments. *American Sociological Review, 37*, 57–72.

Long, J. S. (1990). The origins of sex differences in science. *Social Forces, 68*, 1297–1315.

Lotka, A. J. (1926). The frequency distribution of scientific productivity. *The Journal of the Washington Academy of Sciences, 16*(317), 320–323.

Luce, T. S., & Johnson, C. M. (1978). *Rating of educational and psychological journals* (ERIC Document Reproduction Service No. ED155209).

Magnusson, J. L. (1997). Higher education research and psychological inquiry. *Journal of Higher Education, 68*, 191–211.

McKeachie, W. J. (1979). Perspectives from psychology: Financial incentives are ineffective for faculty. In: D. R. Lewis & W. E. Becker (Eds), *Academic rewards in higher education* (pp. 3–20). Cambridge: Ballinger Publishing.

Meadow, C. T. (1988). Back to the future: Making and interpreting the database industry timeline and online database industry timeline. *Database, 11*, 14–16, 119–132.

Merton, R. K. (1968). The Matthew effect in science: The reward and communication systems of science are considered. *Science, 159*, 56–63.

Meyers, C. R. (1970). Journal citations and scientific evidence in contemporary psychology. *American Psychologist, 25*, 1041–1048.

Milem, J. F., Berger, J. B., & Dey, E. L. (2000). Faculty time allocation: A study of change over twenty years. *Journal of Higher Education, 71*, 454–475.

Montgomery, S. L. (1994). *Minds for the making: The role of science in American education, 1750–1990*. New York: Guilford Press.

Morison, S. E. (1946). *Three centuries of Harvard, 1636–1936*. Cambridge, MA: Harvard University Press.

Morrow, L. E. (1993). The roles of the education professoriate in private institutions (faculty productivity) (Doctoral dissertation, Ohio State University, 1993). *Dissertation Abstracts International, 54*, 4410.

Newman, J. H. (1996). *The idea of a university*. New Haven, CT: Yale University Press.

Omotayo, B. (2004). A content analysis of life Psychologia, 1993–2002. *International Information & Library Review, 36*, 95–103.

Ortega y Gasset, J. (2001). *Mission of the university.* New Brunswick, NJ: Transaction Publishers.

Pace, C. R. (1974). *The demise of diversity: A comparative profile of eight types of institutions.* Berkeley, CA: Carnegie Foundation for the Advancement of Teaching.

Pahre, R. (1996). Patterns of knowledge communities in the social sciences. *Library Trends, 45*, 204–225.

Park, B., & Riggs, R. (1993). Tenure and promotion: A study of practices by institutional Type. *The Journal of Academic Librarianship, 19*, 72–77.

Park, S. M. (1996). Research, teaching, and service: Why shouldn't women's work count? *The Journal of Higher Education, 67*, 46–84.

Pellino, G. R., Blackburn, R. T., & Boberg, A. L. (1984). The dimensions of academic scholarship: Faculty and administrator views. *Research in Higher Education, 20*, 103–115.

Persell, C. H. (1983). Gender, rewards, and research in education. *Psychology of Women Quarterly, 8*, 33–47.

Peterson, M. W., & Mets, L. A. (1987). *Key resources on higher education governance, management, and leadership: A guide to the literature.* San Francisco: Jossey-Bass.

Pierce, S. J. (1990). Disciplinary work and interdisciplinary areas: Sociology and bibliometrics. In: C. L. Borgman (Ed.), *Scholarly communication and bibliometrics* (pp. 46–58). Newbury Park, CA: Sage Publications.

Price, D. J. de Solla. (1963). *Little science, big science.* New York: Columbia University Press.

Price, D. J. de Solla. (1975). *Science since Babylon.* New Haven, CT: Yale University Press.

Pritchard, A. (1969). Statistical bibliography or bibliometrics? *Journal of Documentation, 25*, 348–349.

Reeves, B., & Borgman, C. L. (1983). A bibliometric evaluation of journals in communication research. *Human Communication Research, 10*, 119–136.

Rekha, G., & Parameswaran, W. (2002). Knowledge organization, 1988–1999: A bibliometric analysis. *Journal of Information management, 39*, 355–362.

Richardson, R. D., Jr. (1995). *Emerson: The mind on fire.* Berkeley: University of California Press.

Riesman, D. (1956). *Constraint and variety in American education.* Lincoln: University of Nebraska Press.

Rudolph, F. (1962). *The American college and university: A history.* Athens: The University of Georgia Press.

Ruscio, K. P. (1987). The distinctive scholarship of the selective liberal arts college. *Journal of Higher Education, 58*, 205–222.

Saracevic, T. (1999). Information science. *Journal of the American Society for Information Science, 50*, 1051–1063.

Schon, D. A. (1995, November/December). The new scholarship requires a new epistemology (theory of knowledge). *Change, 27*, 26–34.

Schmidt, N. J. (1992). Research without theory: Data collection as an end in itself. *Journal of Academic Librarianship, 17*, 357–358.

Shera, J. (1964). Darwin, Bacon, and research in librarianship. *Library Trends, 13*, 141–149.

Shils, E. (1984). *The academic ethic.* Chicago: The University of Chicago Press.

Silverman, R. J. (1982). Journal manuscripts in higher education: A framework. *The Review of Higher Education, 5*, 181–196.

Slosson, E. E. (1910). *Great American universities.* New York: Macmillan.

Small, H. G. (1978). Cited documents as concept symbols. *Social Studies of Science, 8*, 327–340.

Smalley, T. N. (1981). Trends in sociology literature and research: A comparison of characteristics of journal articles, 1968 and 1978. *Behavioral & Social Sciences Librarian, 2*, 1–19.

Smart, J. C. (1983). Perceived quality and citation rates of education journals. *Research in Higher Education, 19*, 175–182.

Smith, E. (1990). *The librarian, the scholar, and the future of the research library.* New York: Greenwood Press.

Stoner, N. W. (1966). *The social system of science.* New York: Rinehart & Winston.

Subramanyam, K. (1976). Journals in computer science. *IEEE Transactions on Professional Communication, 19*, 2–25.

Suppa, R. J., & Zirkel, P. A. (1983). The importance of refereed publications: A national survey. *Phi Delta Kappan, 64*, 739–740.

Tien, F. F. (2000). To what degree does the desire for promotion motivate faculty to perform research: Testing the expectancy theory. *Research in Higher Education, 41*, 723–752.

Tien, F. F., & Blackburn, R. T. (1996). Faculty rank system, research motivation, and faculty research productivity: Measure refinement and theory testing. *Journal of Higher Education, 67*, 2–11.

Van Patten, N. (1932). Obstetrics in Mexico prior to 1600. *Annals of Medical History, 4*, 203–212.

Valian, V. (1998). *Why so slow? The advancement of women.* Cambridge, MA: The MIT Press.

Veblen, T. (1954). The higher learning in America: A memorandum on the conduct of universities by business men. Stanford, CA: Academic Reprints. (Original work published 1918).

Veysey, L. R. (1965). *The emergence of the American university.* Chicago: The University of Chicago Press.

Vigil, T. A. (1991). The search for "higher education" as an academic field of study. *Dissertation Abstracts International, 52*, 06A. (UMI No. 9132927)

Wagenaar, T. C., & Babbie, E. (1989). *Practicing social research.* Belmont, CA: Wadsworth Publishing.

Watson, P. D. (1985). Production of scholarly articles by academic librarians and library school faculty. *College & Research Libraries, 46*, 334–342.

Weber, M., Lassman, P., Velody, I., & Martins, H. (1989). *Max Weber's science as a vocation.* London: Unwin Hyman.

Welch, J. M., & Mozenter, F. L. (2006). *College & Research Libraries, 67*, 164–176.

West, M. S. (1995). Women faculty frozen in time. *Academe, 81*, 26–29.

Wiberley, S. E., Hurd, J. M., & Weller, A. C. (2006). Publication patterns of U.S. academic librarians from 1998 to 2002. *College & Research Libraries, 67*, 205–216.

Worthington, D. E. (1997). Advancing scholarship in wartime: World War I research experience and its impact on American higher education, 1900–1925 (Doctoral dissertation, University of Illinois at Urbana-Champaign, 1997). *Dissertation Abstracts International, 58*, 2366.

Xue-Ming Bao (2000). An analysis of the research areas of the articles published in C & RL and JAL between 1990 and 1999. *College & Research Libraries, 61*, 536–544.

Ylijoki, O. H. (2000). Disciplinary cultures and the moral order of studying: A case study of four Finnish university departments. *Higher Education, 39*, 339–362.

Zuckerman, H. (1965). Nobel laureates in the United States: A sociological study of scientific collaboration (Doctoral dissertation, University of Illinois at Urbana, Champaign, 1965). *Dissertation Abstracts international, 54*, 4294.

Zuckerman, H. (1991). The careers of men and women scientists: A review of current research. In: H. Zuckerman, J. R. Cole & J. T. Bruer (Eds), *The outer circle: Women in the scientific community* (pp. 27–56). New York: W. W. Norton.

Zuckerman, H., & Merton, R. K. (1971). Patterns of evaluation in science: Institutionalization, structure, and functions of the referee system. *Minerva, 9*, 66–101.

REGAINING PLACE

Charles B. Osburn

ABSTRACT

This paper situates the concept of library as place in its broader context of relevant theory and research in a number of fields, primarily psychology, neurology, geography, philosophy, and architecture. The term "place" is defined, its powers described, and its role in library administration and design thus revealed to be one of very considerable significance at the highest levels of library mission in any setting.

INTRODUCTION

Recently, there has been a decided surge of interest registered in our professional literature about "the library as place." And this is true even of the popular press, where questions of both the library as a physical place and the place of the library as a social institution are raised for the consideration of the general public. Inspiring these questions of such a fundamental nature are the closely intertwined thoughts of related phenomena, among which figure the infusion of information technologies throughout most of society, the heightened awareness of the ubiquity of information sources and of the simultaneity of access to them, the unknown potential of the Internet, the equally unknown implications of the vast digitization projects in progress, the proper blending of paper and electronic sources in the hybrid library,

Advances in Library Administration and Organization, Volume 24, 53–90
Copyright © 2007 by Elsevier Ltd.
ISSN: 0732-0671/doi:10.1016/S0732-0671(06)24002-1

and, not least among the issues raised for consideration, projections about the demise of the book in a supposed paperless society.

When the library as place is discussed in this context, often the outcome is couched in two polarized conceptualizations of the future. One is the model represented by no free-standing physical structure at all called library because in this model, individuals are connected directly from anywhere to the sources of whatever type of information interests them. At the opposite end of the pole is the model suggested by the great library in ancient Alexandria, Egypt, which is invoked now more than it has been before in modern times. It is a proven model and one that commentators find lends its spirit quite readily to the possibilities offered by the communication technologies at our disposal.

Slowly emerging in the context of these opposed futures of the library, however, is the attention to intrinsic attributes of the library that would make it considerably more than a physical space for books, computers, and related transactions. Discussion is turning to the library as a space of a very special kind, a location wherein the individual can sense and benefit from a unique and valued spirit. Moving into focus is the library as a conceptualized place in a philosophical and psychological sense, which is defined more fully below. This essay is about enriching the library experience through the conscious nurturing of a sense of place. Its purpose is to set this concept in the broader context of germane research and thought within several disciplines, so that place can be understood as an essential dimension of human life and, accordingly, be incorporated into the profession's thinking about library service.

This paper does not purport to be a review of the literature on the concept of place. But, it may have some of the appearances of such, because, except for brief parts of it, the essay leans very heavily on the published work of others in half a dozen or more fields. This multi-perspective approach affords rewarding insight into a concept of human interest, generally, and of heightened interest to librarianship, specifically, at this time. Within that framework, and due to both the approach adopted and the elusive nature of the concept under examination, this essay employs an unusual number of extended quotations. Discussion of place is not constructed on simple, hard facts, for by all accounts, place is a humanistic concept.

As employed across disciplines, there is no single definition for the word "concept," although certain aspects of its meaning and use are commonly agreed upon. It is widely understood as a principal part of classification and a construct of knowledge and thought. A concept often is considered to function in thought the way a word functions in a sentence. From a different perspective, according to Paul Thagard, researchers in psychology and artificial intelligence view concepts "as mental structures analogous to data structures in computers" (Thagard, 1992, p. 21). A principal role of concepts[1] is the explanation of phenomena in a way that is memorable and relatively efficient to communicate. "To say that concepts have a categorization function is to acknowledge that concepts are essentially pattern-recognition devices, which means that concepts are used to classify novel entities and to draw inferences about such entities" (Smith & Medin, 1981, p. 8). H.H. Price concludes his classic work on thinking and experience with the assessment that "The most remarkable function which concepts have is that they make cognition in absence possible. If we possess concepts, or to the extent that we possess them, we are able somehow to think of objects, events or situations which we do not at the moment see or feel" (Price, 1953, p. 325). Finally, neurologist C. Judson Herrick summarizes the function of concepts in his observation that conceptual knowledge "provides the mental tools of all rational thinking at higher levels" (Herrick, 1956, p. 301).

The sense of place constitutes a very rich concept, the potential influence of which clearly indicates it to be a genuine entity endowed with much power from which the community can benefit, if we choose to give it appropriate attention. Therefore, place is worthy of the most serious consideration, especially at a time when so many fundamental options present themselves for the future of the library. This essay proceeds from the general to the specific: from analysis of the generic sense of place to an attempt at an embracing definition of place and discussion of its power and, from that foundation, on to consideration of the library as place. It is primarily about an understanding of the specific sense called place, which could well be adopted as a vision in the planning of library facilities and services, tailored to local situations.

Throughout at least two decades during the second half of the 20th century, the library profession seems to have lost track of the deeper, more human, values of the library experience that had evolved over preceding centuries. A large segment of librarianship, and perhaps also of the public, seems almost to have judged itself too sophisticated to be influenced by insubstantial notions, such as the "feel" of the library and the inspirational qualities of the library as part of an experience. Certainly, these are unquantifiable attributes and, therefore, lend themselves to the intellectualization of description, analysis, and explanation only with the greatest of difficulty. Consequently, the importance of this aspect of librarianship has in large measure eluded recognition in library management. Although the coeditors of the de facto manual for library space planning did allude to something like the concept of place two decades ago, they did not attempt to define it, to identify it in any specific way with the purposes of the library, or to assess its importance. "The desired 'feel' of a space," they write, "is at best difficult to establish in words. Words such as *inviting, stimulating, low key, quiet, durable, pleasant, easy to maintain, vandal resistant, student proof, conducive to research or reading,* and *comfortable* are common descriptions of the desired effect" (Metcalf, 1986, p. 115). But these simple qualifiers could just as well be applied to any number of architectural and design projects.

Now, however, the apparently wide-spread aversion to the slippery concept of place is slowly beginning to be addressed in librarianship. This is demonstrated not only by the recent flurry of publication about the library as place, as is reflected in the list of references appended to this essay, but also by more formalized means: The 2005–2006 American Library Association president's six-point recommendation for libraries to become more competitive in securing their resources includes the objective of "promoting the cultural and social value of the library as place" (Gorman, 2006, p. 4).[2]

The history of the concept of place throughout the past four decades or so raises several provocative questions, the consideration of which should cast light on the concept's value to the planning and presentation of library services over the long term. For example: Why did place experience a decline in attention, generally, and with regard to the library as place, specifically. Why are these positions turning around? What, indeed, does the concept of place signify, and what does it mean for the library? What is the role or fit of the concept in library management? Consideration of these issues is essential to answering the question that ultimately is so timely at this moment, which is why, in a society whose thirst for information is quenched so effortlessly by the push-button transaction, would the place matter if appropriate information can be retrieved from virtually any place?

PLACE STUDIES

Librarianship is not alone in its apparent neglect of the significance of place, for there is a fairly long history behind the devaluation of that concept in many other fields. For example, geographer John A. Agnew examines two causative trends within the broader context of the social sciences, the first having to do with national and world developments. He argues that the expansion of nationalism in the 19th century supported a place-transcending ideology, while the Cold War of the 20th set the ideologies of East and West in an apparent life-and-death conflict. Thus, "at the root of the intellectual devaluation of place in orthodox social science is the oppositional dichotomy of community and society and its image of total temporal discontinuity between two totally different forms of human association" (Agnew, 1989, p. 16). Accordingly, the theory of social change incorporated a specific transformation of life, whereby its emphasis moved from the concept of community to the concept of society; and in this process, Agnew argues, "as society displaces community, place loses its significance since it is closely intertwined with community" (p. 16).

The other development Agnew interprets as a force for the devaluation of the concept of place is the powerful influence of the natural sciences, especially theories of evolution, on late 19th-century social thought. There were various motivations for the adoption of these ideas by the social sciences, but one of the more forceful attractions, according to Agnew, was the thought that natural explanations "would be free of the tinge of religion, ideology, and 'free opinion' that had previously characterized social thought" (Agnew, 1989, p. 17). Thus, objectification, functional relationships between individuals and things, and exclusion of exception or idiosyncrasy became the dominant considerations of social theory, crowding out the more subjective – some might well have said foggy – notions inspired by perceiving and feeling. J. Nicholas Entrikin explains the stance of those who write about the significance of place but have avoided justifying their concepts in terms of prevailing standards of scientific concept formation. They have done so, he reasons, because they find that scientific concept formations are misleading through their limitations. He argues further that, from an academic perspective, place is a poorly understood concept because it does not fit into standard methodological and epistemological categories and does not lend itself to the conventional thinking that separates objective and subjective approaches (Entrikin, 1991, p. 57).

Within the social sciences, the field of psychology had long relegated place to an inferior position even though it had been known through published research since the 1930s that the environment exerts an influence on human behavior. In her review of the early research in environmental psychology, Claude Lévy-Leboyer finds that field work emphasized relationships between the individual's psychological traits and behavior, while laboratory techniques investigated environmental/behavior relations "at the micro- rather than macrolevel, thus having little relevance to real life" (Lévy-Leboyer, 1982, p. 11).

Philosopher Edward Casey observes that even the philosophical underpinnings of the concept of place have just recently become the object of analysis. "It is only with extreme belatedness in the history of philosophy that ... place is considered with regard to living organisms and, in particular, the lived human body" (Casey, 1997, p. 332). Casey traces the vagaries of place in philosophical thoughts from its prime position with Aristotle through a long period of decline in importance, leading to its present resurgence as an enlightening area for exploration. More pointedly, the geographer Entrikin would support this observation with his own that the term "placelessness" (more about which is discussed below) signifies "one aspect of the loss of meaning in the modern world" (Entrikin, 1991, p. 57). If place is powerful in its absence, it must be doubly so in its presence.

More cogent to the library profession, place also was submerged in thought partly owing to the influence of contemporary research and theory in the social sciences, and even more simply because of the increasing press of daily business. The latter phenomenon was experienced most forcefully during the last two decades of the 20th century due to the competition of professional principles, such as ownership and access, and concepts, such as patron and client, as the practice underwent far-reaching transformation. Sam Demas captures the spirit of that time, which he characterizes as euphoric in the midst of this unsettling experience of innovation:

> A kind of siege mentality developed in the library profession, reinforcing a narrow view of libraries as being solely about access to information ... Discussion about library as place and about the larger cultural and educational role of academic libraries was marginalized by many librarians' determination to 'get with the digital program'. (Demas, 2005, p. 27)

The spiritual sense of the library experience thus lost whatever priority it may have held previously. It was set aside as priority was assigned to the expediency of labor-saving devices, questions of access and ownership, insecurities of personal and professional status, and issues of technological ambiguity. To some extent, it was a brief era of convenience over substance and of operations over service. Image became paramount in a very new way, as the need to appear ultra "21st century" in rejection of the 20th guided response to change. "We have come to believe," writes Theodore Roszak, "that mankind is never so essentially human as when it is cast in the role of *homo faber*" (Roszak, 1972, p. 14). Some librarians seemed to become fearful even that the library was no longer a legitimate place in the new age. Innovation of function was privileged over significance of form. And in that regard, art philosopher Susanne Langer's admonition about the role of art seems highly applicable, even if paradoxical: "Indifference to art is the most serious sign of decay in any institution; nothing bespeaks its old age more eloquently than that art, under its patronage, becomes literal and self-imitating" (Langer, 1953, p. 403). Librarianship may be a science, but the best librarianship combines it with art.

CURRENT SCOPE OF PLACE STUDIES

The expression "sense of place" refers to an infinite number of possible settings that range, for example, from a rocking chair to a nation or beyond. The location and type of place vary, as does the quality of the sense they invoke. And, for reasons that will become evident, each instance is unique. As a concept, place is of increasing interest to theorists in many fields, among them are architecture, art, interior design, psychology, psychiatry, sociology, music, geography, politics, literature, philosophy, environmental studies, neurology, and economics. But the great preponderance of contribution to the present understanding of the concept called place comes from the disciplines of psychology (environmental psychology) and geography (humanistic geography). Place may always have been of interest to all the above and other fields, but noticeable growth in publication about it is fairly recent, belonging largely to the past 40 years.

A number of theories have been advanced about the apparent upswing in attention to the concept of place. One draws on the observation that the record of publication on this topic "synchronizes fairly well with periods of relatively abrupt change either within the social or physical environment or in the world of ideas" (Buttimer, 1980, p. 166). Another postulates that "As developments in science and technology allowed people to dominate and even dispense with environment and terrestrial space, it appeared that human beings could escape from place; that they were infinitely adaptable and could mold their relationship to place and space as they saw fit" (Seamon, 1980, p. 194). Yet another theory sets forth four capitalist influences since about 1970: restructured space relations related to global patterning of capital accumulation; diminished transport costs; competition among locales for mobile capital; and speculative space development (Harvey, 1992, pp. 7–8). We are reminded elsewhere that preservationists seek to stabilize the meanings associated with places, and that "They do so in a self-conscious manner, as responses to a perceived human need for attachment and identity" (Entrikin, 1991, p. 58). Still another theory traces the stimulus in study of place to the more recent findings of science, noting that "New modern science is confirming that our actions, thoughts, and feelings are indeed shaped not just by our genes and neurochemistry, history and relationships, but also by our surroundings" (Gallagher, 1993, p. 12).[3] This science writer continues in the same vein, seeing the trend as a direct reversal of one of the effects of the industrial revolution, which "drew the West indoors. Turning away from the natural world, huge populations gravitated toward a very different one made up of homes and workplaces that were warm and illuminated regardless of season or time of the day" (Gallagher, p. 13). A literary scholar points out that during the 20th century place became an important element in literature, but also that it became a much more important issue in general, citing the role of concern over the global environment: "There is a growing conviction that man's use of the earth's resources, his alteration of places in every corner of the globe, must proceed now with a view not only to present profit and pleasure but to the survival of the very next generation. The great question is whether man can change his perception of himself in relation to his surroundings in such a way as to achieve this end" (Lutwack, 1984, p. 2). But more recent influences have diverted the trend that had directed the concept of place into obscurity. J. Nicholas Entrikin describes a movement that led away from the strict rationality of social science. He sees a reaction by those who have sought to redirect geographical research away from the scientific mode toward a concern for the richness of human experience and an understanding of human action. Their skepticism of the interpretative powers of science in matters of place, he says, "stems in part from the fact that they are taking seriously the cultural significance of everyday life" (Entrikin, p. 40).

Against this background, the field of environmental psychology was developed in the late 1950s, primarily in the United States, and most recognizably with the establishment in 1958 of a research group by William Ittelson[4] and Harold Proshansky. The field's initial interest in the physical characteristics of the environment soon developed into the larger issue of the interface between human behavior and the sociophysical environment (Bonnes & Secchiaroli, 1995, p. 1). In a conference paper he presented in 1975, Kenneth H. Craik suggested that to the two traditional questions of personality research, a third should be added to address how a person behaves in relation to the physical environment; this, he said, relates ultimately to the prediction of behavior in specific situations. He observed that "Environmental psychology is extending the scope of personality research by contributing new techniques for assessing environmental dispositions, a heretofore neglected array of personal attributes" (Craik, 1976, p. 60), and that "In the case of the personality research paradigm, the field of man-environment relations not only engages its most technically refined components but also affords a milieu for its conceptual growing edge"

(p. 75). Thus, the sense of place has come to be understood and analyzed as something more than a kind of vague nostalgia bearing negligible significance.

Even the language of everyday life, according to a geographer, "conceptually fuses experience and its geographical context" (Entrikin, 1991, p. 41). During roughly the same era that produced environmental psychology, humanistic geography also emerged. The term "humanistic geography" was first used in English by Yi-fu Tuan in the title of a paper he presented in 1975 (Tuan, 1976), and was given prominence in 1978 with the publication of a collection of essays edited by David Ley and Marwyn S. Samuels (Ley & Samuels, 1978). The roots of humanistic geography are traced to the French geographer Paul Vidal de la Blache (Bird, 1993, p. 65) and his early-20th-century school of human geography. The tenets of this school of thought are set forth in his book, *Principes de géographie humaine*, which was published posthumously (Vidal de la Blache, 1922). Humanistic geography emphasizes ontology and is directed more toward the understanding sought by humanism than the explanation demanded by science.

DEFINING PLACE

Study of the history of ideas can lead quickly to the conclusion that humanity does not really change, at least not over relatively short periods of time as measured in global history. Human concerns and interests and the questions they pose are in most instances the same now as centuries past, only expressed with greater elaboration. Technologies and social structures do change, to be sure, but the basic fears, aspirations, and intellectual quests of human beings seem not to. Thought is refined and made more complex with the increasing production of information, but the fundamentals remain.[5] Consequently, the concept of place is at least as old as the written word and surely very much older. There are "many dimensions to meanings ascribed to place: symbolic, emotional, cultural, political, and biological. People have not only intellectual, imaginary, and symbolic conceptions of place, but also personal and social associations with place-based networks of interaction and affiliation" (Buttimer, 1980, p. 167). In fact, the word "place" is so rich in variant meanings that it occupies 12 long columns of extremely fine print in the second edition of the *Oxford English Dictionary*. Therefore, the following selection of definitions that apply to the meaning understood in this essay is intended as the first step in an attempt to cut through that dense field of significance by providing a context for further refinement of the more specific concept of place at issue throughout this essay.

Place is a special kind of object. It is a concretion of value, though not a valued thing that can be handled or carried about easily; it is an object in which one can dwell. (Tuan, 1977, p. 12)

We call locations of experience 'places'. Experience means perceiving, doing, thinking, and feeling. Every event happens some *where*, but we don't often locate an experience by its latitude and longitude ... A place has a name and a history, which is an account of the experience located in that position. (Walter, 1988, p. 117)

Places are not just presences in some 'nature' abstracted from human being; places are *presences in that nature* raised to some sort of human significance or, perhaps more broadly, raised to significance for some sentient being. (Flay, 1989, p. 6)

The concept of place provides an organizing concept for what is termed to be immersion in, or interpenetration with, the world. With its experiential perspective and varied scale, place relates to an area which is abounded and has distinctive internal structure, to which meaning is attributed and which evokes an affective response .... (Pocock, 1981, p. 17)

Place is a center of meaning constructed by experience ... Place is known not only through the eyes and mind but also through the more passive and direct modes of experience, which resist objectification ... To know a place fully means both to understand it in an abstract way and to know it as one person knows another. (Tuan, 1975, p. 152)

Place has two aspects: The *sense of place*, which is the particular experience of a person in a particular setting, (feeling stimulated, excited, joyous, expansive, and so forth); and the *spirit of place*, which is the combination of characteristics that gives some locations a special 'feel' or personality (such as a spirit of mystery or of identity with a person or group ... A sense of place is the pattern of reactions that a setting stimulates for a person. (Steele, 1981, pp. 11–12)

Place, at all scales from the armchair to the nation, is a construct of experience; it is sustained not only by timber, concrete, and highways, but also by the quality of human awareness. (Tuan, 1975, p. 165)

To get into the spirit of a place is to enter into what makes that place such a special spot, into what is concentrated there like a fully saturated color. (Casey, 1993, p. 314)

Personal place depends on and influences actions. Virtually anything can help constitute this place, and virtually anything can change it ... Personal place does not simply exist— it requires constant (though often preconscious) effort to support and is connected to the more physically visible and stable places in the landscape. (Sack, 1992, p. 31)

Place is, in other words, the place of freedom from the contingent impositions – and crises – of what we have come to know as history [meaning politics, society, and economy]. It is the transcendental value – hence its 'verticality' – that defines humankind in its authentic essence, and defines a community in its organic identity. (Dainotto, 2000, p. 33)

Drawing upon these and other explanations of the concept of place and related phenomena, the following definition is constructed for use in the present essay: "Place" is a setting of any dimension and type in which an individual perceives a special spirit (genius loci) that is generated by the quality of experience related to the values and associations it recalls, and whose significance to the individual captures an extraordinary order and heightens related awareness that becomes an inspiration for imagination and behavior. More will be said about the important role of perception in understanding the concept of place, but it may be useful to note here a neurologist's finding that "Perception is at a level of psychological integration intermediate between sensation and conception" (Herrick, 1956, p. 352).

This definition of place logically raises the question of its relation to space. Both explicitly and implicitly, the relevant literature makes the distinction that space is the physical container, while place is the metaphysical content. "It is not spaces which ground identifications, but places ... Place is space to which meaning has been ascribed" (Carter, Donald, & Squires, 1993, p. xii). This distinction is not a recent fabrication, but extends at least as far back as ancient Greece, where two separate words for place, *chora*, which is the older word, and *topos* were used to represent different features, much the same as space and place are used for purposes of distinguishing the special features understood in the phrase *a sense of place*. According to psychiatrist Eric V. Walter:

> In antiquity, a writer could say *chorophilia* for love of place, but never *topophilia*. In the classical language, *topos* tended to suggest mere location or the objective features of a place ... The older word, *chora* – or sometimes *choros* – retained subjective meanings in the classical period. It appeared in emotional statements about places, and writers were inclined to call a sacred place a *chora* instead of a *topos*. (Walter, 1988, p. 120)

The concept of place, then, has long signified a set of unusual, perceived human properties that are worthy of closer consideration.

But place does not possess these powerful and unusual properties through inherence, although some spaces are more conducive than others; it is endowed with them only by the beholder whose awareness of the experience generates it. Thus, "these personal views are the most elementary and accessible ways of being in geographical space and place, for it is the way we constantly experience the world and act upon it" (Sack, 1992, p. 11). This differentiation of the many physical spaces in one's life has been called "indexing," which is accomplished both explicitly and implicitly. "I submit that one will always be at a loss to define place without taking into account this human indexing" (Flay, 1989, p. 5). Nor, of course, can place even be identified without it.

Although there probably are as many manifestations of the sense of place as there are individuals and physical spaces, most often they convey emotional and moral qualities. As interpreted by the individual, "The 'soul' of a place is the pure, expressive meaning of a location, a concrete image that represents its quality of expressive space" (Walter, 1988, p. 145). Indexing spaces so that they consequently become places requires that such a space be "lived in" in the sense that the individual fully experiences it[6] and is "aware of it in the bones as well as with the head" (Tuan, 1975, p. 165). Thus, places have "soul." Something that we take so for granted within ourselves is nonetheless a highly complex phenomenon[7] for reasons that are brought together quite poignantly in the analysis by philosopher J.E. Malpas:

> Place ... possesses a complex and differentiated structure made up of a set of interconnected and interdependent components – subject and object, space and time, self and other ... The fact that place possesses such a variously complex structure, and is capable of presenting itself in such differentiated and multiple ways, leads to an inevitable multiplicity in the ways in which place can be grasped and understood; place may be viewed in terms that emphasise the concrete features of the natural landscape; that give priority to certain social or cultural features; or that emphasise place purely as experienced. (Malpas, 1999, p. 173)

Ultimately, a geographer asserts, physical place "is 're-placed' in the mind and through our sensibilities by an image of place." (Pocock, 1981, p. 17). These images can have much or little to do with reality, for they are partial and may be either exaggerated or understated. Collectively, a set of place images shared by segments of society forms a place myth (Shields, 1991, pp. 60–61). The myth can be identified – as it has been at least since antiquity – with hierarchical levels of value, usually in three positions: upper, middle, and lower. "The high place inspires feelings of elation, domination, transcendence; it is the traditional home of poetry." (Lutwack, 1984, pp. 39–40). This is the level of place sense, or the image, to which many regular users of the library place assign it.

POWER OF PLACE

Although the identification of place varies with the variety of experience, it also exerts several extraordinary powers. Foremost among them are the power to help define self-identity, the power to stimulate imagination, and the power to enhance or otherwise alter one's world view.[8] They are examined below, following which is a consideration of the processes involved in arousing the sense of place.

The capacity of a sense of place to encourage self-discovery and self-identity is the most widely agreed upon attribute of a sense of place, and arguably is its single greatest power, while self-identity also has assumed increasing importance in contemporary society. In his survey of the concept of global identity crisis, Wilbur Zelinsky finds use of the term "identity" in the social sciences to have increased about 30-fold from 1965 to 1998 (Zelinsky, 2001, p. 130), and even concludes that "The scholarly literature treating questions of contemporary personal and group identity has been growing at an alarming rate in recent years" (p. 147).[12] Following are some assessments of the powers of place as they relate to the discovery and formation of self-identity.

> Since places carry out a relevant role in the satisfaction of biological, psychological, social and cultural needs of the person in the many situations faced in his/her lifetime, they assume the function of meaningful reference points in the processes of identity definition. (Bonnes & Secchiaroli, 1995, p. 186)

> The concept of self, then, that system of thoughts and experiences which enables each one of us to regard ourselves as unique and to distinguish ourselves from others, is an integral aspect of the psychology of place. (Canter, 1977, p. 179)

> The specific dependence of self-identity on particular places is an obvious consequence of the way in which self-conceptualisation and the conceptualisation of place are both interdependent elements within the same structure. Our identities are thus bound up with particular places or localities through the very structuring of subjectivity and of mental life within the overarching structure of place. (Malpas, 1999, p. 177)

> Whatever its sources of explanation, this literature on the sense of place reveals several consistently recurring themes. It appears that people's sense of both personal and cultural identity is intimately bound up with place identity. Loss of home or 'losing one's place' may often trigger an identity crisis. (Buttimer, 1980, p. 167)

> Place identity "is anchored to the particular possibility individuals have of perceiving and/or knowing that specific component of the self defined through interaction with the physical environment." (Bonnes & Secchiaroli, p. 187)

> ... the subjective sense of the self is defined and expressed not simply by one's relationships to other people, but also by one's relationships to the various physical settings that define and structure day-to-day life. (Proshansky, Fabian, & Kaminoff, 1983, p. 58)

From these statements, one can infer a composite description of the sense of place as a key element in the defining of self, as follows: The conceptualization of place and the conceptualization of self are interdependent functions, both being forms of differentiation to which the sense of place provides reference points for the process of identity definition.

The second of these unusual powers of place is the triggering of imagination, which instills meaning and value in the conceptualized place. Imagination identifies or differentiates the place and builds the image,[9] which then reflects in the image of self. According to psychologist David Canter, "it has been argued that interactions with our surroundings are a major base for the *development* of conceptual systems in the first place" (Canter, 1977, p. 153). And psychologist Joachim Wohlwill observes that "Individuals give evidence of more or less strongly defined attitudes, values, beliefs, and affective responses relating to their environment" (Wohlwill, 1970, p. 304). Imagination seems to be boundless. "A marvel of economy," notes a literary scholar, "the imagination may thrive on the most meager materials to make a place meaningful" (Lutwack, 1984, p. 33). And he explains that "Places lend themselves readily to symbolical extension because there is so little that is inherently affective in their physical properties" (p. 35). In his inaugural address as president of the American Geographical Society several decades ago, John K. Wright chose as his subject the role of imagination in geography, and concluded with the thought that "the most fascinating *terrae incognitae* of all are those that lie within the minds and hearts of men" (Wright, 1947, p. 15).

Although some of what is created or captured in the imagination as an idea or a concept can be described verbally, not all of it lends itself to communication, not even internal communication. Some of it eludes the logic and clarity required of verbalization, but it is no less an entity to be reckoned with. In his work on philosophical universals, R.I. Aaron discusses the situation of having a thought or idea or concept in mind but, even so, failing to put the thoughts into words. He contends that "these thoughts or concepts must be other than the words; they are objects in the mind which can be there even if we fail to express them in words" (Aaron, 1952, p. 200). Similarly, a neurologist notes that "The perceptual experience has a past and a future reference; it is selective, directive, and purpose-like, though most of these processes go on below the level of awareness" (Herrick, 1956, p. 349). Even when articulation can be achieved, frequently it is the case, whether inadvertent or intended, that the concept or the experience being described leads in more than one direction; it is ambiguous. A psychiatrist reminds us that "The highest form of ambiguous language we call 'poetry.' An ambiguous place or object leads the mind somewhere else" (Walter, 1988, p. 72). For a mind that is led somewhere else, there are few spaces more conducive to the free association of thoughts than the library place.

Sense of place is an excellent venue for introspection, but it also contains a strong social dimension. In their analysis of research on the social dimension of place, a team of environmental psychologists reports that "the socio-cultural meanings associated with a setting are viewed as the 'glue' that binds groups to particular places" (Bonnes & Secchiaroli, 1995, p. 177). How a physical location becomes a place in the sense that it gains the psychological power to become the kind of place examined in this essay can be explained with reference to the degree of differentiation afforded it in the individual cognitive system, as James Campbell explains. "We become ourselves," he says, "in large part, by a process of differentiation from various groups of others. In addition, we find the examination and fostering of this social place to be a source of self-understanding and stability" (Campbell, 1989, p. 68). The links between place and activity, David Canter adds, and "the expectation of finding certain people in certain places,[10] all indicate how a particular physical location can have its psychological power; indeed, how it becomes a 'place' rather than simply a location" (Canter, 1977, p. 123). And more explicitly, according to Bobby Wilson, "the self can be characterized as an ontological structure which manifests itself in social space. A place-based social space is essential for some groups' development and maintenance of self" (Wilson, 1980, p. 145).

Because place has a very strong social dimension, it follows that the term "placelessness,"[11] which refers to the spread of standardized landscapes and designs that diminish differentiation among spaces, "signifies one aspect of the loss of meaning in the modern world" (Entrikin, 1991, p. 57). The spirit of reaction to the rapid standardization of space around the globe was captured several decades ago by Theodore Roszak in the phrase "Almost every place is becoming Anyplace" (attributed to Roszak by Lutwack, 1984, p. 183).

But all individuals do not see spaces the same way, much less understand and interpret them the same way.[12] Some see the library experience very positively, others negatively. They do not form the same images because the quality of spaces is determined by the subjective response of people (Lutwack, 1984, p. 35). For example, some are far more dependent on the stabilizing influence of behavior settings than others (Gallagher, 1993, p. 130). A long-time scholar in the field of humanistic geography tells us that "One person may know a place intimately after a five-year sojourn; another has lived there all his life and it is to him as unreal as the unread books on his shelf" (Tuan, 1975, p. 164). And a philosopher reminds us of the simple basis for these differences: that "values alter facts" (Bachelard, 1994, p. 100). To some extent, differing perspectives on a physical space can be understood to relate to differences that result not only from the way society is structured, but also from the very fact of its structuring. "In demonstrating that there are differences in conceptions of places ... we are highlighting an inevitable potential for confusion and disagreement built into our existing social structure" (Canter, 1977, p. 138). Place differentiation is highly social and deeply rooted.

Places are neither good nor bad nor of any other quality without their human valuation. The identification of individually held values with a particular location constitutes an especially significant consideration in matters of place. A neurologist notes that "The desires of men and the needs of all other creatures arise as expressions of their own inner natures, however much they may be inflected by social and other environmental conditions. This sets the most significant criteria of value within the organism" (Herrick, 1956, p. 142). Value, therefore, is generated biologically. "There are impersonal standards of value, but there are no impersonal values," he adds (p. 138). The impressions and memories they create correspond to the values assigned by the individual, and in turn inspire a mood, which prompts either good or bad behavior, often in the most subtle ways.[13] "We needn't even be consciously aware of a pleasant or unpleasant environmental stimulus for it to shape our states" (Gallagher, 1993, p. 132). This lack of awareness of the nature and content of place differentiation stems in part from the fact that these perceptions begin in the earliest processes of socialization when the child is not consciously participating in the process or even aware of such perceptions (Proshansky et al., 1983, p. 63).

These revelations notwithstanding, philosopher and social and political theorist Charles Taylor observes that "The search for the self in order to come to terms with oneself ... has become one of the fundamental themes of our modern culture" (Taylor, 1988, p. 316).[14] In that context, the power of place to define one's own identity and to influence the imagination takes on even greater significance. This is accomplished through means that are complex, most often elusive, and not necessarily recognized by the individual, as place recognition engages a process that is at once psychological (which has been addressed), physiological (which is addressed below), and metaphysical. Robert D. Sack summarizes the range of metaphysical experience.

> Being in the world is being in, and constructing, this personal sense of place, with ourselves at the center. Personal place expands and contracts as our interests and actions wax and wane. And personal place moves as we move through space. In a closely knit and geographically isolated community, the contents of our personal place can be shared by others and can coincide with (or develop into) a place fixed in space and publicly recognized. But in a fragmented and dynamic society, personal place is less likely to be shared and so can appear private, idiosyncratic, and subjective. (Sack, 1992, pp. 11–12)

The social context of place is the collection of forces that operate on an individual as a result of relationships to other people and social institutions. The context also "helps to determine the impact of the physical setting" (Steele, 1981, p. 15), while conversely "The physical setting also affects the impact of the social setting, rendering certain forces more or less potent" (p. 17). As indicated earlier, this interactive quality is among the defining characteristics of place.

Sir Russell Brain addresses in terms of knowledge the physiology of place sensing in a lecture series on "The Nature of Experience." This neurologist notes that the human brain is the product of millions of years of evolutionary selection to achieve the capacity to react commensurately with an ever more complex physical environment.[15] More specifically, he states that "the receptive function of the cerebral cortex is to provide us with a symbolical representation of the whole of the external world ... at the same time giving us similar symbolical information about our own bodies and their relationship with the external world" (Brain, 1959, p. 32). There is a connection between the environment and the human capacity to react to it that is real in a physical sense. A team of psychologists describes this phenomenon as a function of the cognitive system:

> Like any other cognitive system, place-identity influences what each of us sees, thinks, and feels in our situation-to-situation transactions with the physical world. It serves as a cognitive backdrop, or perhaps better said, as a physical environment 'data base' against which every physical setting experience can be 'experienced' and responded to in some way. Broadly speaking, what is at stake is the well-being of the person. (Proshansky et al., 1983, p. 66)

LIBRARY AS PLACE

As described above, individuals are far from unanimous in the sense they ascribe to the same locations, and we know that, as well, from our own personal experience with people. Response to environment varies from person to person, sometimes in ways that may be imperceptible, sometimes in ways that put them at the extreme ends of a continuum. One could make a long list of settings that might generate such opposed, even antagonistic, feelings one way or the other. For example, among them might figure a primeval forest, a busy city street, a dimly lit tavern, home, a church, a football stadium on game day, and a library on any day. Some individuals view the library in a positive sense, others in a negative sense, while still others may register no response at all. And, anytime we talk about the library as place, we need to bear in mind that, throughout history, the library has been labeled with an elitist connotation,[16] only part of which is owed to the normal use requirement of literacy.

Unfortunately, unlike the hard sciences, librarianship would be hard pressed to record for purposes of replication any particular experience, least of all one as subjective as the sensing of place. However, a composite perception can be extracted from a combination of one's own personal experience and those experiences heard and read about over the years. Accordingly, the library presents a commingling of culture, nature, and human nature through a range of virtually all subjects, tastes, and points of view. And, of particular importance, it does so in a manner that situates the potential of this intellectual experience immediately in evidence to those who may be receptive. It offers the possibility of easy immersion in a vast, complex, and layered network of knowledge, understanding, and expression, whose connections are created only by the individual contemplating them, when and as the individual chooses.

For the individual, this setting invites communication with the thoughts, creations, and discoveries of many others, both past and present. These conditions lead to the pursuit of insight and the continuous construction of completeness, raising further questions and, in turn, rekindling the quest for answers. Such pursuits are undirected by anyone else, but the library does provide just enough fundamental order by which to find one's own way to one's own destination even if that destination is imprecise or unknown. One's guiding thoughts and methods during this intellectual voyage are protected to the extent that the individual determines them to be. The library does not create this free style process, but enables and encourages it. The library sets the stage then steps back to allow us to construct, create, and clarify exactly as we may wish, and to take whatever deviations from what might at first seem to be the logical course toward what we may originally have thought to be the objective, which changes without warning. The library is not demanding and not judgmental about reasons and motivation. A unique social institution, the library also creates the locus for a sense of special community among the apparently like-minded. The visitor knows that in large measure, he/she is communing with others of similar world view, with kindred spirits undeclared, even though their exact interests almost surely differ. It is the experience of library that they share, albeit in quite different ways. One feels like a privileged guest in the library place, but at the same time like its steward.

The library is dependable in this regard, despite operational problems that do, on occasion, give rise to frustration. But even in the face of them, the library remains an anchor of reliability and stability for the spirit and the intellectual experience it contains just for the taking. We know that it will help us put our thoughts and feelings into a broader context for better understanding. So we return to the library. It is often a sense of context we lack and seek in the confidence that we can discover it in that place and in ways not necessarily clear even to us. Context makes possible the kind of distancing that provides new perspective and discovery.[17] Contemplation and informed serendipity are the tools that are crafted in the library to achieve this through the stimulation of imagination, curiosity, and creativity.[18] Whether or not we find the specific piece of information we have been seeking, we will have had a fulfilling experience because of other discoveries made along the way and within ourselves.

So the library is, indeed, an outstanding place for self-discovery, for energizing the imagination, and for seeing the world anew. The inner self can be revealed continuously through the process of identification with the intellectual intersections of one's chosen paths of inquiry leading toward a higher level of understanding. This process of discovering the inner self also encourages self-expression. The library can thus be a place of great intellectual comfort, even if not always physical comfort.

Comfort is a recurring theme in any description of place and, again, there must be as many connotations of that sense as there are individuals to experience it. Moreover, "At various times and in response to various outside forces – social, economic, and technological, the idea of comfort has changed, sometimes drastically" (Rybczynski, 1986, pp. 230–231).[19] It is particularly useful in the examination of library as place to note that the Latin root of the present-day English noun "comfort" is the verb *confortare*, which conveyed the meanings "to strengthen" and "to console." These concepts aptly describe the positive experience of the kind of intellectual comfort afforded by the library. And, Fritz Steele points out that "One of the most consistently important contributions of place has been to provide a sense of security to individuals and groups: a feeling that they are at home or have a home that they can go back to, which provides a sense of control over their own fate" (Steele, 1981, p. 7). Indeed, Robert David Sack states categorically that "control is a defining quality of home" (Sack, 1997, p. 263, note 31), and that while home provides security and comfort, it also stimulates "a sense of responsibility for that place" (p. 14). Like the sense of home, the library connotes both a physical place and a state of being. The library is an intellectual home.

Another recurring theme in place description is that of the production of a world view, which provides both the context for self-definition and its product. To discover one's self is to rediscover the world. Robert David Sack makes this relationship quite clear.

> As a locus of experience, personal place provides a holistic sense, interweaving elements from the realms of nature, meaning, and social relations. From its other side, it sets in motion the potential to see the world from somewhere else, and then unravel the threads and trace them back to the particular realms. The key to understanding the relation between these moments lies in the connection of place to awareness. (Sack, 1992, p. 30)

As we learn about ourselves through the introspection that is stimulated by heightened awareness, we interpret the world around us differently and gain a more advantageous perspective on life, thereby achieving a greater understanding of our situation in the world. So, it is logical that "The more we experience a behavior setting, the greater its power to alter our perception of the 'real world'" (Gallagher, 1993, p. 129).[20] Synesthetic experience is commonly associated with the identification of place, as can readily be judged from references to the literary work of Marcel Proust, which figure prominently among examples offered by scholars who are representative of diverse fields. In the novel's most famous scene, the protagonist of *Remembrance of Things Past* dips a Madeleine cookie into a cup of lime blossom tea, the resulting combination of whose flavor and aroma unleashes his involuntary memory and thus helps him better understand the present. The experience is not just literary, of course, but more broadly human and physiological. The neurologist Sir Russell Brain notes that "an object seen is seen endowed with those qualities which experience has shown it to have for other sensory modalities, tactile shape, texture, temperature, weight, &c" (Brain, 1959, p. 33). Yi-fu Tuan advances this information: "An object or place achieves concrete reality when our experience of it is total, that is, through all the senses as well as with the active and reflective mind" (Tuan, 1977, p. 18). The library is about providing information; but it is more, or more profoundly, about understanding. At its best, the library experience is about both understanding of self and understanding of world.

LIBRARY EXPERIENCE AT THE CROSSROADS

An understanding of the qualities and powers produced by a sense of place suggests that it would be greatly to the benefit of those who use the library to present them the fullest sense of the potential library experience possible. This means drawing out the sense of place that may to a greater or lesser extent be intrinsic in the institution, but which needs to be made more perceptible in a given location. The first and single-most important step in that direction is recognition of the full range of the values of place and the power it possesses. Action that is oriented to the future of the library as place means sustaining, enhancing, or re-creating the space to permit, to encourage or to facilitate the natural bonding process that is innate, even if dormant, in most humans. It should now be evident that "the perception of the environment is a great deal more than the sum of the perceptions of those objects which make up that environment" (Lévy-Leboyer, 1982, p. 46). Perception of place invokes and gives further definition to a world view, it provides a special comfort by enabling the continued definition of self, and it stirs the imagination. Place is an essential and inspiring sense, but one that sometimes needs to be aroused and sustained through the right kinds of nurturing. It arguably is among the responsibilities of librarianship to work toward that vision.

Fortunately, creating library place does not require us to start from a blank slate, but rather makes us identify and strengthen those elements in the library setting that have tended naturally toward the most likely effect to be achieved. Whatever positive connotations are best emphasized, it is a matter of thoughtfully blending the design of the digital environment commensurately with the concept of place. Perception, image, cognitive systems, and feelings are not simple considerations to integrate into library management. But the most challenging aspect of this undertaking stems from what seems to be the mixture of conflicting temperaments that it entails today. We cannot afford to ignore or gloss over the likelihood that the temperament that drives the speed and precision of the library's technological dimension, which is integral to most library services, is at odds with the temperament that encourages the contemplation and exploration that are expected of place. This must be dealt with directly. But the raw materials are there to be shaped; the potential is there to be realized. "I would suggest," says David Canter, "that the real significance of environmental change and the concomitant change in conceptual systems, is the change in the interaction we have with our surroundings" (Canter, 1977, p. 156). We do not need an entirely new library. But we do need to take stock of the essence, or the latent essences, of the library as place and of the full potential of the library as experience, and to set them, figuratively, in bold relief. First, we need to understand these influences ourselves; then we need to bring that understanding to bear on the fashioning of space that will be conducive to the very subtle experiential essence that can be valued by those many individuals who are most susceptible to its influence.

We have arrived at a fortuitous moment in that regard, for, as observed earlier, what now appears to be the beginning of a gradual displacement of print text by digital[21] is accompanied by an unprecedented intensity of attention to the library as place. The ubiquity of points of access to information and, therefore, the convenience of information at fingertip, argues loudly the possibility that the physical library can be bypassed, and consequently raises logical questions about the function of its space. Surely, we do not really believe that convenience of access to the world's information is either the sole function or the ultimate goal of the library in the long term. Study of the concept of place indicates that the library's function should and can be considerably more than that.

A proposition advanced decades ago by environmental psychologist Harold Proshansky and his colleagues provokes circumspective thought about the current library situation; they concluded that "When a change in a physical setting is not conducive to a pattern of behavior that has been characteristic of the setting, that behavior will express itself at a new time or locus" (Proshansky, Ittelson, & Rivlin, 1970, p. 33). Of course, the library profession would prefer that the chosen locus for library-type activity be the institution that the library has become or can become. But the profession is not alone in that preference, because the logic of it is so compelling and so well supported by the established positive senses of place already associated with the library, even if they have been taken largely for granted in the recent whirlwind of technological innovation.

Because the image an individual generates about the qualities perceived in surrounding space prompts action, the manner in which change is introduced assumes even greater significance as "It is these changing environmental roles which mediate the changes in conceptual systems" (Canter, 1977, p. 156). David Canter speculates further that "increasing differentiation is an aspect of certain types of cultural development, especially those involving the importation of new technologies or modes of space use" (p. 118). None of this means that place is ignored or is rendered less significant as the culture evolves but, rather to the contrary, that it can be defined more distinctly.

Speaking at a national conference on the library as place, an architect reminds us of what we already know about an academic library, but of which we do not always seem fully convinced and confident.

The library is the only centralized location where new and emerging information technologies can be combined with traditional knowledge resources in a user-focused,

service-rich environment that supports today's social and educational patterns of learning, teaching, and research. Whereas the Internet has tended to isolate people,
the library, as a physical place, has done just the opposite. Within the institution, as
a reinvigorated, dynamic learning resource, the library can once again become the cen-
terpiece for establishing the intellectual community and scholarly enterprise. (Freeman,
2005, p. 3)

Among the many other similarities between academic and most other types
of libraries, the fact that the library is a unique institution within its community remains clear. Not to seize the opportunity presented by this
uniqueness in the interests of the users of the library would be a most
unfortunate mistake.

In contrast to creating physical space, the subject of creating or sustaining
place as an identifiable experience has begun to receive a level of attention in
the library press that is unprecedented. Meanwhile, as much professional
and scholarly writing outside librarianship addresses the more general aspects of place, most of which are highly applicable to the library, the few
theories advanced for the creation or design of place also share in their
fundamentals. Yi-fu Tuan observes that successful architecture most evidently generates a strong sense of place simply by housing the accumulated
experiences of work or worship or whatever is the regular activity of the
space, but that "a great building is also an image of communal life and
values: it is communal experience made into a tangible and commanding
presence" (Tuan, 1975, pp. 161–162). Elsewhere he states that while human
beings not only discern geometric patterns in nature and create abstract
spaces in the mind, "they also try to embody their feelings, images, and
thoughts in tangible material" (Tuan, 1977, p. 17).[22] Psychiatrist Eugene V.
Walter summarizes the special place created by experience:

The totality of what people do, think, and feel in a specific location gives identity to a
place, and through its physique and morale it shapes a reality which is unique to places –
different from the reality of an object or a person. Human experience makes a place, but
a place lives in its own way. Its form of experience occupies persons – the place locates
experience in people. A place is a matrix of energies, generating representations and
causing changes in awareness. (Walter, 1988, p. 131)

These are the most fundamental of guidelines, to which informed imagination must give shape. For centuries, the library has presented a unique
experience for those who sought it or discovered it by chance. As place, it
has encouraged, in the most subtle and passive ways, the reflection and
introspection that arouse the individual subconscious. If the library profession recognizes this value and chooses to adopt it as a fact with the same
degree of certainty as the undeniable fact that library services incur a cost,

then the challenge is to maintain the quality of that unique experience, but with such accommodations as may be necessary in a hybrid environment that emphasizes its digital dimension. It is a matter of more purposefully applying the theories of the concept of place to the physical library through a merger of the developing technologies into the perception of one holistic library experience. This will require much thought, but it will be a fascinating intellectual venture.

As suggested earlier, it is not the purpose of this paper to recommend specific library operations or services, logistics or mechanics, but to consider the much subtler and more qualitative dimensions of human experience that can interact to create the library as place. First among them is the single most significant characteristic of the library, and therefore its foundation for further refining, which Betsy Baker aptly describes as convergence:

> For the library to be a true convergent point in the information landscape, we need to develop an environment from which users can intuit that they are in a hub where an abundance of intellectual and informational resources, from a wide variety of disciplines, schools of thought, times, geographic locations, ethnic voices, production formats, and so on, are coming together. It is in this desire to be a place of convergence that we set ourselves apart from other information providers. (Baker, 2000, p. 87)

How this vision can be realized is a matter to be determined within each library and its community, but there are many other considerations, as well, that would build upon Baker's suggested foundation for the library as place.

By abstracting the concepts advanced in the works of a number of mostly recent writers,[23] they can be brought together into a coherent vision, such that they are applicable in principle to all types of libraries. Thus, among the perceptions to be encouraged are those of sanctuary and solitude required to engage in the refinement of analytical and critical thinking, yet with the awareness of ready support systems; available collaborative learning processes and varied learning environments; and the drama of community that makes one feel a greater sense of self and higher purpose; the sense of a contemplative oasis for the spirit and intellect, both in reaction against conformism and to provide a sense of control over individual fate; the perception of comfort, including the olfactory and tactile experiences, which is important to endowing the library with the sense of a special kind of familiarity that befits an intellectual home; the perception of the library as an iconic symbol, as a presence that recalls historical experience and tradition in the midst of a world of constant change and innovation. J. Nicholas Entrikin makes a special point of noting that some places are given significance as symbols of a shared past or in recognition of their cultural distinctiveness, and that it is the job of preservationists "to stabilize the meanings associated with places. They do so in a self-conscious manner, as responses to a perceived human need for attachment and identity" (Entrikin, 1991, p. 58). It is that human need that we should strive to meet in planning the future of the physical library and the library as place. Our responsibility is to preserve what can reasonably be preserved of the library as place and to accommodate current and emerging service potentials accordingly.

When the stage is set to invite the appropriate perceptions, they will then be conducive to the three great achievements that the library as place can offer: the nurturing of imagination,[24] the refinement of self-identity, and the extension of thought into invention and the rediscovery of the surrounding world. Arguably, these potentials embrace the core of the mission of any library, the differences being how and to what extent they are intended to be achieved. It is not uncommon that settings provide a level of predictability that guides toward an accepted and expected behavior, and even that "We unconsciously rely on ... behavior settings to supply much of the stability of our social institutions" (Gallagher, 1993, p. 128).

This essay attempts to reference the generic physical library, although my bias that whatever else we may be, we are also and always students, may show through more than necessary. But the learning dimension of the library surely is highly worthy of emphasis when contemplating the power of place. Whoever is the user of the library, our primary purpose in managing it is to help the users do what they do better as a result of their library experience. It is precisely because of the possibility of the fathoming experience it offers that the library is a social institution, not a public utility. Understood in its fullest sense, for example, the concept of learning occupies a particularly significant segment of the voyage from the library as utility to the library as place in the way place has been described here. To be sure, the library is a tool. But in its fullest sense the library is that and much more. The fundamental purposes of the "learning library" are described succinctly:

> The central idea of the learning library is that of integration ... Rather than an external 'add on' to the educational experience, the library, as information resource and gateway, is a primary catalyst for cognitive, behavioral, and affective changes in students – as they interact with information resources as directed by faculty, as they complete assignments and study with peers, as they extend their knowledge at multiple levels, seeking connections and making meaning in more self-directed ways. The learning library, rather than a repository of materials or a study hall, is therefore an agency of change in students' lives. (Simons, Young, & Gibson, 2000, p. 124)

More than a belief, an unwritten theory has long held that the library can be an agency of individual and societal improvement: Students become better students, workers become better workers, citizens better citizens, and all of humanity benefits. Taken to their limits, notions of the library as place are attempts to more nearly realize the potential portrayed in this theory.

CONCLUSIONS

Consideration of the high ideals incorporated in this generalized theory brings us to the purpose of the library and the role of place as its ultimate mission. Based on his two decades of experience in the design and production of theme park attractions for the Walt Disney Corporation, Barry Braverman reminds us that "it is usually advantageous to define your mission at the deepest and most profound level possible" (Braverman, 2000, p. 100), which is a thought so essential to planning that we should not have needed reminding. But we did and we do. Librarianship is a highly pragmatic profession which, at the same time and as noted above, also is guided by lofty ideals. The influence of these ideals, however, has been limited since the last quarter of the 20th century almost exclusively to transactions carried out within the library, then between and among libraries, then between library consortia and conglomerations of information producers and vendors. Due in some measure to this increasingly outward look, with its focus on transactions, the reach of our ideals has fallen short in terms of the architecture, the interior design, the ambiance of the library building and, in summary, the experiential place for the community and its individuals that is the heart of library activity. There are exceptions to this sweeping declaration, of course,[25] but like any recognizable exception, they do not represent the mainstream of thinking. Yi-fu Tuan, who is the most prolific writer and, judging from informal bibliometric comparison, one of the most influential thinkers about the concept of place,[26] emphasizes the value of cultural representation in extending that reach:

> Culture makes people truly human and distinguishes them from other animals. This is a widely held view. Common sense suggests that if this is true of culture, then *high* culture in complex societies enables people to explore the further reaches of human potential in both an intellectual and a moral-spiritual sense. (Tuan, 1989, p. 69)

But in recent years, it has begun to look as though the connection between the ideals and the house in which they are to be realized through service either has become severely frayed or is at least seriously weakened. Joshua Meyrowitz has examined aspects of the so-called placelessness of America that were created solely by the rapid adoption of communication technologies prevalent in the early 1980s (Meyrowitz, 1985). A quarter century later, the situation he described has changed only to be intensified, especially within the microcosm of the library as it begins to assume the features of many other business settings. Scott Bennett surely is correct in his assertion that "in designing library space we attend too exclusively to library operations and pay too little attention to student learning" (Bennett, 2005, p. 21), but the disconnect goes well beyond the academic setting and purpose he describes.

Part of the problem resides in the fact that planning place is a much more complex enterprise than planning operations, for place is a much more elusive kind of entity. It is unlike most other things we do for place, after all, is a perception drawn from individual experience, a perception that may then be transformed into a concept that informs the design of space. Place identity "is a complex cognitive structure which is characterized by a host of attitudes, values, thoughts, beliefs, meanings and behavior tendencies that go well beyond just emotional attachments and belonging to particular places" (Proshansky et al., 1983, p. 62).

But, regardless of its complex, even ethereal, nature, the sense of place is real.[27] Political philosopher Hannah Arendt reasons that, in addition to the conditions of life presented to humankind, humans create their own conditions, which "possess the same conditioning power as natural things. Whatever touches or enters into a sustained relationship with human life immediately assumes the character of a condition of human existence" (Arendt, 1958, p. 9). Stated otherwise, place creation is about feelings, but about feelings that can be conveyed to the understanding of others; it is about connecting feelings to the intellect.[28] Because this perception or "conditioning power," as Arendt calls it, is so well rooted, so intimately embedded in being, it should be no surprise that when it is disturbed, threatened, or lost, that disruption, threat or loss carries a weighty negative impact,[29] even if subconsciously. Whatever is done with the space called library, surely we do not want it to become a space that offers so inconsequential an experience that it conveys insufficient essence even to evoke a sense of threat at the thought of it being taken away. Marc Augé, anthropologist and president of the Ecole des Hautes Etudes en Sciences Sociales, issues the sobering admonition that "The possibility of non-place is never absent from any place" (Augé, 1995, p. 107).

Much as librarianship tries to design its services according to the inferred predilections and motivations of both the individual and society, trying to create place for both presents an even greater ambiguity for the designers. But failure to address this challenge conscientiously would be no less an abdication of responsibility than failure to deliver any other fundamental library service.[30] "To design a place is therefore to try to design meaning and value" (Relf, 1996, p. 919). And in the end it must be a design whose presence is sufficiently strong that it can readily be sensed (grasped) by those for whom it is intended.

Values both inspirational and practical merge in the library place. "Memory and imagination, crucial elements in the quality of a place ... shape what is called the spirit of a place" (Walter, 1988, p. 118). It is largely a question of knowing the most essential characteristics of likely users, and selecting the values to determine the "experiences that 'should' happen there" (Steele, 1981, p. 18). This is not a simple assignment. Occasionally throughout this paper, there has been allusion to art, while science always is more overtly implied in the melding of art into functional design. But there is more to making place than the combining of art and science. What remains is a third dimension made up of values and, still more subjectively, feelings. A librarian–architect team describes the process as follows:

> Place-making involves the art and science of crafting spaces in ways that transcend their physical attributes. The successful library building, with its programs and its staff, creates a sense of connection to the values, traditions, and intellectual life of the community, and helps the patron participate in building its future. (Demas & Scherer, p. 65)

They elaborate on this explanation by describing a transcendent/transportive coexistence that distinguishes the library as place[31] and recalls the description of place articulated by Yi-fu Tuan, that place "is the past and the present, stability and achievement ... It is the human home in the cosmic scheme of things ... Place is created by human beings for human purposes" (Tuan, 1975, p. 165), meaning purposes peculiar to the condition of being human. David M. Levy speculates on the reasons behind the recent boom in new library construction in the midst of emphasis that concurrently is being placed on the virtual nature of cyberspace. He suggests that it may be because

> people want the advantages of the online world, but not at the expense of the physical, the material side of life. People recognize the value of shared, communal spaces where they can meet and greet or where they can work by themselves while surrounded by others. Libraries may be the only institution currently capable of creating and maintaining trusted, nonpartisan spaces of this kind. It may also be that physical libraries serve as symbols of certain shared, sacred values.(Levy, 2006, p. 250)

This still leaves the goal of establishing and sustaining the library as place a rather less clear goal than normally is employed in planning. But the concept of place is not unique in that regard. The concept of corporate culture,[32] which in recent decades has claimed a significant position in the literature of library management, also has in common with "place" a high degree of intangibility to which we are becoming rather accustomed in library management. In fact, occupying a key point between the services offered in the library and the place in which we wish the clientele to experience them is the experience that is generated daily by the library employees. Through the application of a predetermined quality of interpersonal and interdepartmental communication, they have much to do with the environment; they have the potential to make or break the perceptions we may try to bring about through architecture and interior design. Library employees can be either thoughtful interpreters of the intended sense of place or they can be impediments to the communication of that experience. The culture and the physical space as place function symbiotically in creating the library experience.[33]

As asserted earlier, this essay is not about the functions that should or should not take place in the library or even about how they should be laid out. Nor is it about furnishings or lighting or acoustics or staffing responsibilities or whether the library should be digital or print or even the proper proportions thereof. It has nothing specific to do with the architecture or interior design of the library. All these considerations will vary from one type of library to another and are dependent on institutional mission and other local matters. There is no "how to""manual for library place creation, for it is neither a simple mechanism nor a step-by-step process. Yet, on another plane, place does have everything to do with all of the aforementioned: "If places are indeed a fundamental aspect of man's existence in the world, if they are sources of security and identity for individuals and for groups of people, then it is important that the means of experiencing, creating, and maintaining significant places are not lost" (Relph, 1976, p. 6).

Though the differentiation of place is highly individualized, there evidently is something about the values assigned by the perceiving individual to the library that is widely shared. These are the qualities that are essential to being human. Because of the great range of conditions surrounding the life of each individual, these values have been cultivated in some individuals more than in others; their residence is buried deeper in the self of some than in the self of others, but they are there to be aroused. Creating or sustaining the library place does not mean maintaining the tradition in toto and with no further accommodation any more than it means replacing whatever may be considered the traditional experience with something entirely new or opposite. It does mean, above all, achieving an understanding of the total library essence and ultimately employing that understanding as a context to inform local planning and management decisions, just as do other environmental considerations and anything else that influences the quality of library service. Toward the close of his penetrating study of the place concept, psychologist David Canter states that "If the reader is looking for a key to unlock the practical, day-to-day implications of the research with which I have been dealing, then I would suggest the slogan: *The Goal of Environmental Design is the Creation of Places*" (Canter, 1977, p. 157). If spaces can be designed for political and commercial purposes, surely they can be designed specifically for purposes of the library. Because the library is a place with a latent essence that is rich in potential for experience, there may not be a right way or wrong way to accomplish this. But there may be better ways of strengthening, emphasizing, and drawing upon the potential. However subtle and complex they may be, concepts of place have an essential function in making the library successful in its community.

NOTES

1. Thagard (1992, p. 22) presents a list of 10 basic functions of concepts, including examples.

2. Gorman also contributes a chapter on the significance of the library as place in his book *Our Enduring Values* (Gorman, 2000).

3. This had been understood for at least several decades. Describing the role of environment in providing stability, naturalist Alexander Petrunkevitch was quite clear about this in his conclusion that "Normal development and normal; morphological structure can not be therefore attributed to the structure of the germ plasm alone. To be sure, there must be a certain chemo-physical structure to start with; and this structure must be very much alike in the case of all animals belonging to the same species. Nevertheless, its further fate, its mode of development and its ultimate characters, whatever their hereditary value, are dependent upon, and in a way are a function of, the environment" (Petrunkevitch, 1924, pp. 76–77).

4. Ittelson introduced the term "environmental psychology" in New York in 1964, using the term in the title of his paper. The group's first volume of research was published in 1970, using the term in its title. The leading American journal in the field, *Environment and Behavior*, was begun in 1969 (Bonnes & Secchiaroli, 1995, pp. 1–11). Claude Lévy-Leboyer claims that the German philosopher of science and subsequently psychologist Kurt Lewin "was the first psychologist to propose a coherent theoretical structure corresponding to the needs of environmental psychology" (Lévy-Leboyer, 1982, p. 23).

5. Arthur O. Lovejoy, philosopher and founder of the history of ideas movement, recalls "a celebrated remark of Professor [Alfred North] Whitehead's that 'the safest general characterization of the European philosophical tradition is that it consists in a series of footnotes to Plato'" (Lovejoy, 1936, p. 24).

6. Tuan elaborates: "Experience takes time. Sense of place is rarely acquired in passing. To know a place well requires long residence and deep involvement. It is

possible to appreciate the visual qualities of a place with one short visit, but not how it smells on a frosty morning ... To know a place is also to know the past ... If it takes time to know a place, the passage of time itself does not guarantee a sense of place. If experience takes time, passage of time itself does not ensure experience" (Tuan, 1975, p. 164). A neurologist confirms that "The perceptual experience has a past and a future reference; it is selective, directive, and purpose-like, though most of these processes go on below the level of awareness" (Herrick, 1956, p. 349).

7. Another description of the process, a bit more detailed, is that cited by David Canter, a psychologist, who finds a statement published in 1920 by the neurologist Henry Head to contain "the seeds of almost every major development in the psychology of place"(Canter, 1977, p. 16). Head wrote that "the sensory cortex is also the storehouse of past impressions. These may rise into consciousness as images, but more often, as in the case of spacial impressions, remain outside central consciousness. Here, they form organised models of ourselves, which may be termed 'schemata.' Such schemata modify the impressions produced by incoming sensory impulses in such a way that the final sensations of position, or of locality, rise into consciousness charged with a relation to something that has happened before. Destruction of such 'schemata' by a lesion of the cortex renders impossible all recognition of posture or of the locality of a stimulated spot in the affected part of the body" (Head, 1920, pp. 607–608). Employing terms less technical, art psychologist Rudolf Arnheim writes that "My contention is that the cognitive operations called thinking are not the privilege of mental processes above and beyond perception but the essential ingredients of perception itself" (Arnheim, 1969, p. 13), and that "What we need to acknowledge is that perceptual and pictorial shapes are not only translations of thought products but the very flesh and blood of thinking itself" (p. 134). C. Judson Herrick argues that "perception may be regarded as a behavior because we know by experiment that the polarization of the perceiving self against the objects perceived must be learned by actual experience gained through the motor responses made to the setup of sensory stimuli received" (Herrick, 1956, p. 339).

8. The definition of world view is summarized by W.T. Jones: "The world view of any individual is a set of very wide-range vectors [which he explains] in that individual's belief space (a) that he learned early in life and that are not readily changed and (b) that have a determinate influence on much of his observable behavior, to the verbal and nonverbal, but (c) that he seldom or never verbalizes in the referential mode, though (d) they are constantly conveyed by him in the expressive mode and latent meanings" (Jones, 1972, p. 83).

9. David Canter claims that "It is to [Kenneth E.] Boulding that we owe the notion of an overall, all-pervading cognitive system: an image which embraces all our interactions with our surroundings" (Canter, 1977, p. 26).

10. He goes on to state that "A further important implication of place differentiation is that it leads to the identification of places within a wider network of reactions. In recognizing a place as having a specific set of behaviours associated with it, it is also possible to anticipate that particular people will be found in those places" (Canter, 1977, p. 119). Another psychologist is even more emphatic on this point. She notes that "... the perception of the physical features of the environment is inseparable

from affective, aesthetic, and normative assessments, that is to say, from a social evaluation. This evaluation depends upon the perception of objects, but exceeds that perception in complexity and significance" (Lévy-Leboyer, 1982, p. 46).

11. For a full discussion of this concept, see Chapter 6, "Placelessness," of Relph (1976, pp. 79–121).

12. Thus, the terms topophilia and topophobia are used to distinguish these basic reactions to place. On the topophobic side, for example, Yi-fu Tuan has written a book about places that are likely to cause fear (Tuan, 1979). A review of environmental psychology research shows that, like every other cognitive system, place identity is meant to accomplish the cognitive backdrop function that enables people to recognize what they see, think, and feel in locations. Place identity primarily allows for discrimination between what is familiar and what is not in different environments (Bonnes & Secchiaroli, 1995, p. 188).

13. Psychologist Joachim Wohlwill asserts that "... the physical environment does not only arouse strong affective reactions in the individual, but is frequently an object of approach and avoidance behavior, in a literal sense and on a large scale" (Wohlwill, 1970, p. 306). Art philosopher Susanne Langer explains the subtleties: "What we call a person's 'inner life' is the inside story of his own history; the way living in the world feels to him. This kind of experience is usually but vaguely known, because most of its components are nameless, and no matter how keen our experience may be, it is hard to form an idea of anything that has no name. It has no handle for the mind" (Langer, 1957, p. 7).

14. Taylor explains that "No one ever doubted that there were individual differences, that one person differed from another. What is new in the modern era is that these have a specific kind of moral relevance. Although differences of endowment and temperament were thought to define relevant conditions for moral action ... nowhere before the modern era was the notion entertained that what was essential to us might be found in our particular being. But this is the assumption underlying the identity question" (Taylor, 1988, p. 316).

15. He concludes that "All knowledge is both subjective and objective, or it would not be knowledge. The objective features are the information which it gives about the external object; the subjective features those which make it *my* knowledge, namely, its relationship to my other past and present experiences, and any contribution which my brain may make to the representation of the object" (Brain, 1959, p. 33). Yi-fu Tuan finds a paradox in the thought process: "Here is a seeming paradox: thought creates distance and destroys the immediacy of direct experience, yet it is by thoughtful reflection that the elusive moments of the past draw near to us in present reality and gain a measure of permanence" (Tuan, 1977, p. 148). About the purpose of turning our thought inward, Charles Taylor says that "... we go to discover or impart some order, or some meaning or justification to our lives ... To the extent that this form of self-exploration becomes central to our culture, another stance of radical reflexivity becomes of crucial importance to us alongside that of disengagement. It is different from and in some ways antithetical to disengagement. Rather than objectifying our own nature, and hence classing it as irrelevant to our identity, it consists of exploring what we are in order to establish this identity because the assumption behind modern self-exploration is that we do not already know who we are" (Taylor, 1988, pp. 314–315).

16. An especially thought-provoking perspective on the social paradigm that has structured and maintained this assessment of the library is advanced most forcefully by Harris (1986).

17. Neurologist C. Judson Herrick observes that "An essential feature of perceptual integration is the polarization of the perceiving subject against the things perceived, of the self against the not-self. This implies the presence of self-consciousness at a higher level of mentation than primitive undifferentiated 'feeling,' and this in turn is a prerequisite for that sharp contrast between perceptual knowledge and conceptual knowledge" (Herrick, 1956, pp. 349–350). Hannah Arendt explains that "It is in the nature of the human surveying capacity that it can function only if man disentangles himself from all involvement in and concern with the close at hand and withdraws himself to a distance from everything near him. The greater the distance between himself and his surroundings, world or earth, the more he will be able to survey and to measure and the less will worldly, earth-bound space be left to him" (Arendt, 1958, p. 251). Charles Taylor is more specific in terms of establishing and being guided by moral direction: "I want to defend the strong thesis that doing without frameworks is utterly impossible for us; otherwise put, that the horizons within which we live our lives and which make sense of them have to include these strong qualitative discriminations ... living within such strongly qualified horizons is constitutive of human agency" (Taylor, 1989, p. 27).

18. In the estimation of John K. Wright, "Much of the world's accumulated wisdom has thus been acquired, not from the rigorous application of scientific research, but through the skillful intuitive imagining – or insight – of philosophers, prophets, statesmen, artists, and scientists" (Wright, 1947, p. 6).

19. He explains that "the idea of comfort has developed historically. It is an idea that has meant different things at different times. In the seventeenth century, comfort meant privacy, which lead [sic] to intimacy and, in turn, to domesticity. The eighteenth century shifted the emphasis to leisure and ease, the nineteenth to mechanically aided comforts – light, heat, and ventilation. The twentieth-century domestic engineers stressed efficiency and convenience" (Rybczynski, 1986, p. 231).

20. Sharing this understanding, Susanne Langer extends it: "It is perception molded by imagination that gives us the outward world we know. And it is the continuity of thought that systematizes our emotional reactions into attitudes with distinct feeling tones, and sets a certain scope for an individual's passions" (Langer, 1953, p. 372).

21. Nicholas C. Burckel sets this issue in a larger context in his sanguine conclusion that "Technology enhances the library's capability to extend its services and collections, but it does not replace the physical library. Digital technology in particular has dramatically increased the synergy of content and technology" (Burckel, 2006, p. 229). More specifically, Donald Lindberg, Director of the U.S. National Library of Medicine, summarized a two-day symposium held in November 2004 on "The Library as Place: Building and Revitalizing Health Sciences Libraries in the Digital Age," with his moderate, final comment that "the future is both print *and electronic*" (Klose, 2005, p. 19).

22. Susanne Langer describes the work of architecture: "The architect creates a culture's image: a physically present human environment expresses the characteristic rhythmic functional patterns which constitute a culture ... Architecture creates the

semblance of that World which is the counterpart of a Self. It is a total environment made visible" (Langer, 1953, p. 98). From a different perspective we are told by neurologist Sir Russell Brain that "... our awareness of the spatial relations of objects is never limited to perceptions of the objects themselves: it is imbued with past experiences of movement and time" (Brain, 1959, p. 33).

23. These perceptions of place are treated by the following writers: Arendt (1958), Baker (2000), Bennett (2005), Braverman (2000), Freeman (2005), Frischer (2005), Ludwig and Starr (2005), Rybczynski (1986), Simons, Young & Gibson (2000), Steele (1981), Tuan (1975), Walter (1988), Wright (2006).

24. Yi-fu Tuan analyzes the relevant values of symbolic space, which he says "offers good examples of how the human imagination works. Space becomes symbolic when it intimately conjoins human and social facts with those of nature. Symbolic space is a mental artifact, necessary to the ordering of life, and so in this sense it is a practical venture; and yet it is also infused throughout with the aesthetic values of balance, rhythm, and affect. Symbolic spaces have different foundations and exist at different scales" (Tuan, 1993, p. 172).

25. Not the sole example, but a fine one, is the new Seattle Public Library (Marshall, 2004).

26. See the tribute to Tuan by J. Nicholas Entrikin (2001).

27. Psychiatrist E.V. Walter follows Plato in clarifying this otherwise blurry idea: "Plato tells us that to grasp the nature of place, 'we must try to express and make manifest a form obscure and dim.' It lies outside both reason and sensation, to be apprehended by a kind of sensuous reasoning. 'Some sort of bastard reasoning, which is hardly trustworthy,' Plato writes, gives us the knowledge of place. It is not a legitimate kind of knowledge in his view, being neither within the rules of rational thought nor even a product of sensory experience, but something else – a curious, spurious mode of grasping reality. It is a knowledge that must be 'grasped,' because it cannot be conceived and it cannot be perceived. Yet it is not less real than the objects of reason and perception" (Walter, 1988, pp. 121–122).

28. Susanne Langer writes that "Artistic form is congruent with the dynamic forms of our direct sensuous, mental, and emotional life; works of art are projections of 'felt life' ... into spatial, temporal and poetic structures. They are images of feeling that formulate it for our cognition. What is artistically good is whatever articulates and presents feeling to our understanding" (Langer, 1957, p. 25).

29. Following is a selection of concurring views: "The sentiment [of place] is there, and we learn how strong it is when these small foci of our world are disturbed or threatened" (Tuan, 1975, p. 154); "... perception helps us organize external information so that we can feel that we 'know' something about what surrounds us and what is likely to happen to us. Having this information provides us with some control over our own fate, so that we are not always at the whim of unpredictable events. The importance of this sense of control is brought home to us when we lose it, as in the experience of diving into murky water where sights and sounds are suddenly cut off" (Steele, 1981, p. 22); "Consequently simply asking questions about the future of libraries, let alone working to transform them for the digital age, almost inevitably evokes anguished, poignant, and even hostile responses filled with nostalgia for a near-mythical institution" (Campbell, 2006, p. 28).

30. A serious attempt to understand the reasons behind both aversion to and ignorance of the library place could prove useful in the creation of perceptions of library as place and of the library experience. This understanding could possibly even lead to an extension of the library's horizons.

31. They define their terms: "*transcendent*, in the sense of buildings that delimit physicality through imaginative understanding and application of virtues; and *transportive*, in design that uplifts the patron and enhances the unique experience of sensing past, present, and future simultaneously. It is this *transcendent/transportive* coexistence, with particular reference to its local, place-specific manifestations, that distinguishes a library with what we are calling *esprit de place*, or spirit of place" (Demas & Scherer, 2002, p. 65).

32. For further discussion of the influence of corporate or organizational culture, see Osburn (2007).

33. "Organizational climate has also been used to describe social contributions to a spirit of place. Many organizations impart a distinct feel or atmosphere to those who work in them ... Physical features help to create this climate, but a good portion of it is maintained by the ways that the social system impacts on people with its norms, rules policies, expectations, and management style" (Steele, 1981, p. 71). Kenneth H. Craik made a similar observation early in the history of environmental psychology: "Unlike other attributes of places, institutional characteristics also relate to a social system which may extend beyond the spatial-physical setting itself" (Craik, 1971, p. 60).

REFERENCES

Aaron, R. I. (1952). Concepts. In: *The theory of universals* (pp. 190–215). Oxford: Clarendon Press.

Agnew, J. A. (1989). The devaluation of place in social science. In: J. A. Agnew & J. S. Duncan (Eds), *The power of place. Bringing together geographical and sociological imaginations* (pp. 9–29). Boston: Unwin Hyman.

Arendt, H. (1958). *The human condition*. Chicago: University of Chicago Press.

Arnheim, R. (1969). *Visual thinking*. Berkeley: University of California Press.

Augé, M. (1995). *Non-places. Introduction to an anthropology of supermodernity*. London: Verso (Original French edition 1992).

Bachelard, G. (1994). *The poetics of space*. Boston: Beacon Press (Original French edition 1958).

Baker, B. (2000). Values for the learning library. *Research Strategies, 17*, 85–91.

Bennett, S. (2005). Righting the balance. In: K. Smith (Ed.), *Library as place: Rethinking roles, rethinking space* (pp. 10–24). Washington, DC: Council on Library and Information Resources.

Bird, J. (1993). *The changing worlds of geography. A critical guide to concepts and methods* (2nd ed.). Oxford: Clarendon Press.

Bonnes, M., & Secchiaroli, G. (1995). *Environmental psychology. A psycho-social introduction*. Thousand Oaks: Sage.

Brain, R. (1959). *The nature of experience*. London: Oxford University Press.

Braverman, B. (2000). Libraries and theme parks: Strange bedfellows. *Research Strategies, 17*, 99–105.

Burckel, N. C. (2006). Library space in the digital age. In: D. B. Marcum & G. George (Eds), *Digital library development* (pp. 225–241). Westport: Libraries Unlimited.

Buttimer, A. (1980). Home, reach, and the sense of place. In: A. Buttimer & D. Seamon (Eds), *The human experience of space and place* (pp. 166–187). New York: St. Martin's Press.

Campbell, J. (1989). Place as social and geographical. In: D. W. Black, D. Kunze & J. Pickles (Eds), *Commonplaces. Essays on the nature of place* (pp. 67–79). Lanham: University Press of America.

Campbell, J. D. (2006). Changing a cultural icon: The academic library as a virtual destination. *EDUCAUSE Review*, *41*, 16–30.

Canter, D. (1977). *The psychology of place*. London: Architectural Press.

Carter, E., Donald, J., & Squires, J. (Eds) (1993). *Space and place. Theories of identity and location*. London: Lawrence & Wishart.

Casey, D. S. (1993). *Getting back into place. Toward renewed understanding of the place-world*. Bloomington: Indiana University Press.

Casey, E. S. (1997). *The fate of place. A philosophical history*. Berkeley: University of California Press.

Craik, K. H. (1971). The Assessment of places. *Advances in Psychological Assessment*, *2*, 40–62.

Craik, K. H. (1976). The personality research paradigm in environmental psychology. In: S. Wapner, S. Cohen & B. Kaplan (Eds), *Experiencing the environment* (pp. 55–79). New York: Plenum Press.

Dainotto, R. M. (2000). The literature of place and region. In: *Place in literature. Regions, cultures, communities* (pp. 1–33). Ithaca: Cornell University Press.

Demas, S. (2005). From the ashes of Alexandria: What's happening in the college library? In: K. Smith (Ed.), *Library as place: Rethinking roles, rethinking space* (pp. 25–40). Washington, D.C.: Council on Library and Information Resources.

Demas, S., & Scherer, J. A. (2002). Esprit de place: Maintaining and designing library buildings to provide transcendent spaces. *American Libraries*, *33*(April), 65–68.

Entrikin, J. N. (1991). *The betweenness of place: Towards a geography of modernity*. Baltimore: Johns Hopkins University Press.

Entrikin, J. N. (2001). Geographer as humanist. In: P. C. Adams, S. Hoelscher & K. E. Till (Eds), *Textures of place. Exploring humanist geographies* (pp. 426–440). Minneapolis: University of Minnesota Press.

Flay, J. C. (1989). Place and places. In: D. W. Black, D. Kunze & J. Pickles (Eds), *Commonplaces. Essays on the nature of place* (pp. 1–9). Lanham: University Press of America.

Freeman, G. T. (2005). The library as place: Changes in learning patterns, collections, technology, and use. In: K. Smith (Ed.), *Library as place: Rethinking roles, rethinking space* (pp. 1–9). Washington, DC: Council on Library and Information Resources.

Frischer, B. (2005). The ultimate internet cafe: Reflections of a practicing digital humanist about designing a future for the research library in the digital age. In: K. Smith (Ed.), *Library as place: Rethinking roles, rethinking space* (pp. 41–55). Washington, DC: Council on Library and Information Resources.

Gallagher, W. (1993). *The power of place. How our surroundings shape our thoughts, emotions, and actions*. New York: Poseidon Press.

Gorman, M. (2000). The library as place. In: *Our enduring values. Libraries in the 21st century* (pp. 43–57). Chicago: American Library Association.

Gorman, M. (2006). President's message: Get smart. *American Libraries*, *37*, 4.

Harris, M. H. (1986). State, class, and cultural reproduction: Toward a theory of library service in the United States. *Advances in Librarianship*, *14*, 211–252.

Harvey, D. (1992). From space to place and back again: Reflections on the condition of postmodernity. In: J. Bird, B. Curtis, T. Putnam, G. Robertson & L. Tickner (Eds), *Mapping the futures. Local culture, global change* (pp. 3–29). London: Routledge.

Head, H. (1920). *Studies in neurology (2 Vols.)*. London: Hodder and Stoughton.

Herrick, C. J. (1956). *The evolution of human nature.* Austin: University of Texas Press.

Jones, W. T. (1972). World views: Their nature and their function. *Current Anthropology, 13* (February), 79–109.

Klose, C. (2005). Libraries in the digital age. *NLM Newsline, 60*(Spring Special), 1–20.

Langer, S. K. (1953). *Feeling and form: A theory of art.* New York: Scribner's.

Langer, S. K. (1957). *Problems of art.* New York: Scribner's.

Levy, D. M. (2006). The place of libraries in a digital age. In: D. B. Marcum & G. George (Eds), *Digital library development* (pp. 243–252). Westport: Libraries Unlimited.

Lévy-Leboyer, C. (1982). *Psychology and environment.* Beverly Hills: Sage (Original French edition 1979).

Ley, D., & Samuels, M. S. (Eds) (1978). *Humanistic geography: Prospects and problems.* Chicago: Maaroufa Press.

Lovejoy, A. O. (1936). *The great chain of being. A study of the history of an idea.* Cambridge: Harvard University Press.

Ludwig, L., & Starr, S. (2005). Library as place: Results of a Delphi study. *Journal of the Medical Library Association, 93*, 315–326.

Lutwack, L. (1984). *The role of place literature.* Syracuse: Syracuse University Press.

Malpas, J. E. (1999). *Place and experience. A philosophical topography.* Cambridge: Cambridge University Press.

Marshall, J. D. (2004). *Place of learning, place of dreams: A history of the Seattle Public Library.* Seattle: University of Washington Press.

Metcalf, K.D. (1986). In: P. D. Leighton, & D. C. Weber (Eds), *Planning academic and research library buildings* (2nd ed.). Chicago: American Library Association.

Meyrowitz, J. (1985). *No sense of place. The impact of electronic media on social behavior.* New York: Oxford University Press.

Osburn, C. B. (2007). Corporate culture and the individual in perspective. *Advances in Library Administration and Organization, 26* in press.

Petrunkevitch, A. (1924). Environment as a stabilizing factor. In: M. R. Thorpe (Ed.), *Organic adaptation to environment* (pp. 67–110). New Haven: Yale University Press.

Pocock, D. C. D. (1981). Introduction: Imaginative literature and the geographer. In: D. C. D. Pocock (Ed.), *Humanistic geography and literature. Essays on the experience of place* (pp. 9–19). London: Croom Helm.

Price, H. H. (1953). *Thinking and experience.* London: Hutchinson House.

Proshansky, H. M., Fabian, A. K., & Kaminoff, R. (1983). Place identity: Physical world socialization of the self. *Journal of Environmental Psychology, 3*, 57–83.

Proshansky, H. M., Ittelson, W. H., & Rivlin, L. G. (1970). The influence of the physical environment on behavior: Some basic assumptions. In: H. M. Proshansky, W. H. Ittelson & L. G. Rivlin (Eds), *Environmental psychology: Man and his physical setting* (pp. 27–37). New York: Holt, Rinehart and Winston.

Relf, E. (1996). Place. In: I. Douglas, R. Huggett & M. Robinson (Eds), *Companion encyclopedia of geography. The environment and humankind* (pp. 906–922). London: Routledge.

Relph, E. (1976). *Place and placelessness.* London: Pion.

Roszak, T. (1972). *Where the wasteland ends. Politics and transcendence in post industrial society.* Garden City: Doubleday.

Rybczynski, W. (1986). *Home. A short history of an idea.* New York: Viking.

Sack, R. D. (1992). *Place, modernity, and the consumer's world.* Baltimore: Johns Hopkins University Press.

Sack, R. D. (1997). *Homo geographicus. A framework for action, awareness, and moral concern.* Baltimore: Johns Hopkins University Press.

Seamon, D. (1980). Afterword: Community, place, and environment. In: A. Buttimer & D. Seamon (Eds), *The human experience of space and place* (pp. 188–196). New York: St. Martin's Press.

Shields, R. (1991). Social spatializations and the 'sense of place'. In: *Places on the margin* (pp. 58–70). London: Routledge.

Simons, K., Young, J., & Gibson, C. (2000). The learning library in context: Community, integration, and influence. *Research Strategies, 17,* 123–132.

Smith, E. E., & Medin, D. L. (1981). *Categories and concepts.* Cambridge: Harvard University Press.

Steele, F. (1981). *The sense of place.* Boston: CBI Publishing.

Taylor, C. (1988). The moral topography of the self. In: S. B. Messer, L. A. Sass & R. L. Woolfolk (Eds), *Hermeneutics and psychological theory: Interpretive perspectives on personality, psychotherapy, and psychopathology* (pp. 298–320). New Brunswick: Rutgers University Press.

Taylor, C. (1989). *Sources of the self. The making of modern identity.* Cambridge: Harvard University Press.

Thagard, P. (1992). *Conceptual revolutions.* Princeton: Princeton University Press.

Tuan, Y.-f. (1975). Place: An experiential perspective. *Geographical Review, 65,* 151–165.

Tuan, Y.-f. (1976). Humanistic geography. *Annals of the Association of American Geographers, 66,* 266–276.

Tuan, Y.-f. (1977). *Space and place. The perspective of experience.* Minneapolis: University of Minnesota Press.

Tuan, Y.-f. (1979). *Landscapes of fear.* New York: Pantheon.

Tuan, Y.-f. (1989). *Morality and imagination. Paradoxes of progress.* Madison: University of Wisconsin Press.

Tuan, Y.-f. (1993). *Passing strange and wonderful. Aesthetics, nature, and culture.* Washington, DC: Island Press.

Vidal de la Blache, P. (1922). *Principes de géographie humaine.* Paris: Armand Colin.

Walter, E. V. (1988). *Placeways. A theory of the human environment.* Chapel Hill: University of North Carolina Press.

Wilson, B. M. (1980). Social space and symbolic interaction. In: A. Buttimer & D. Seamon (Eds), *The human experience of space and place* (pp. 135–147). New York: St. Martin's Press.

Wohlwill, J. F. (1970). The emerging discipline of environmental psychology. *American Psychologist, 25*(April), 303–312.

Wright, A. (2006). Libraries as places to linger and mingle. *Christian Science Monitor, 98* (January), 9.

Wright, J. K. (1947). Terrae incognitae: The place of the imagination in geography. *Annals of the Association of American Geographers, 37*(March), 1–15.

Zelinsky, W. (2001). The world and its identity crisis. In: P. C. Adams, S. Hoelscher & K. E. Till (Eds), *Textures of place. Exploring humanist geographies* (pp. 129–149). Minneapolis: University of Minnesota Press.

INTERACTIVE SERVICE AND PROFESSIONAL CULTURE: ACADEMIC REFERENCE LIBRARIANS IN AN EMERGING CONTEXT

Paula R. Dempsey

ABSTRACT

This study uses a microanalysis of interaction approach to study how interactive service workers collaborate with one another in conversations to construct their professional identity in the face of the rapid contextual change. The data consist of (1) a complex written exchange downloaded from an Internet listserv and (2) a mechanically recorded conversation and detailed transcript showing the exact sequence of turns in the conversation, overlapping utterances, laughter, and speech errors. Everyday descriptions in these conversations reveal how knowledge workers produce and reproduce professional identity and a shared culture in the ways they: (1) categorize themselves and other workers, (2) amend or collaborate on each other's characterizations of clients, and (3) negotiate local policies and rules as they intersect with professional values and emotional boundaries. The results demonstrate a need for opportunities to integrate the increasing complexity of interactive service into professional identity as a response to technological and social change.

Advances in Library Administration and Organization, Volume 24, 91–116
ISSN: 0732-0671/doi:10.1016/S0732-0671(06)24003-3

The service sector has emerged to dominate the US economy, with 80% of workers in service occupations (McCammon & Griffin, 2000). Service work varies from routine, highly supervised encounters to highly skilled professional service relationships. Librarians are relatively privileged, benefiting from high levels of education and association with prestigious institutions. However, service interactions in libraries are being shaped, like those in other workplaces, by accelerating technological complexity and rising consumer expectations about convenience. This study uses microanalysis of interaction to examine how academic reference librarians make sense of everyday interactions in a context of rapid change as they produce and reproduce social structure within the profession and the local institution. The data consist of unstructured conversations among librarians in temporary, voluntary groups. The value of such everyday descriptions is in how they reveal the ways in which service providers produce and repro- duce professional identity and a shared culture. These ways include how participants:

- Categorize themselves and other workers
- Amend or collaborate on one another's characterizations of clients
- Negotiate local policies and rules as they intersect with professional values and emotional boundaries

RELATED LITERATURE

Until recently, the sociology of work emphasized the manufacturing setting in which, under monopoly capitalism, management attempts to control the labor process by using scientific management to routinize tasks, allowing them to replace skilled workers with machines or unskilled, low-wage workers (Braverman, 1974; Garson, 1977). In the service economy, rout- inization and control shifts to interpersonal behavior and feelings (Hochs- child, 1983). Robin Leidner (1993) found that service interactions among low-wage, closely supervised workers (e.g., at McDonald's) are routinized by building politeness and friendliness into scripts, beginning with the fa- miliar "Welcome to McDonald's. May I take your order?" The insurance salespeople she studied, however, like librarians, worked in complex, un- predictable interactions at a distance from management. Scripts were not completely effective in routinizing service interactions in these circum- stances. Therefore, the company attempted to train workers to internalize a routinized emotional response to customers to produce higher sales. Leidner does not address the empirical question of how such emotional norms are produced and reproduced.

Leidner's (1993) service labor process theory suggests that, to reduce labor costs, the client is increasingly engaged in the production system. For example, McDonald's uses intensive advertising to teach customers what food is available. Workers are not expected to explain the menu or sell particular items, except in the most cursory fashion (e.g., "Would you like fries with that?"). In the library service process, clients must cooperate in the system to produce themselves as independent seekers and users of information. That is, the library client must be engaged in developing independent skills that at one time were the librarian's sole province. Library clients must be induced to figure out how to use systems efficiently, not tying up either computers or staff time. Therefore, librarians face simultaneous demands from administrators to encourage patron self-sufficiency and from patrons to meet expectations of efficiency and friendliness developed in the consumer service economy.

This study fills a gap in the growing literature on interactive service occupations. A few recent studies examined professional/knowledge workers in terms of emotional labor, both within the organization (Kunda & Van Maanen, 1999) and in interactions with clients (Bellas, 1999). However, no published studies examine librarians from this perspective. Moreover, limited research exists on this group of workers from any theoretical perspective. A notable exception is a stream of gender research. Of these studies, the most influential is by Christine Williams (1995), who examined male gender privilege in female-dominated professions, including librarianship. In addition, James V. Carmichael (1995) surveyed gay librarians about professional gender issues, and Sarla Murgai (1991) examined attitudes toward women managers in libraries.

Another important contribution to the knowledge of the library profession is by Annette Davies and Ian Kirkpatrick (1995), who studied the impact of government funding pressures and privatization of libraries in the United Kingdom. Davies and Kirkpatrick found that these changes caused a shift in the library profession from a traditional model to a service model. That is, the definition of quality service shifted from the professional, technical jurisdiction to the preference of the individual service-recipient, which leads to deskilling and rationalizing service routines and reducing professional power.

The goal of this study is to contribute to an understanding of how professionals interactively respond to these new pressures. This understanding will be increasingly important, because other kinds of services (e.g., financial, medical, educational) are facing or will face similar pressures. Capturing a sense of how identity is being produced during this shift will be an important point of comparison for generalization to other groups over time.

DATA AND METHODS

Most studies of interactive service work use participant observation (Leidner, 1993; McElhinny, 1995; Pierce, 1995), interviews (Wharton, 1996; Williams, 1995), or case studies (Davies & Kirkpatrick, 1995). However, rather than examining the content of interactions with clients, this study focuses on how the participants collaborate with one another in ordinary interactions to construct their professional personas. That is, their descriptions of problematic interactions with clients do not and need not convey the full picture of the relationship between worker and client. Garfinkel (1967) argued that actors' ability to intelligibly describe ordinary situations and events defines their membership in a collective or society. Thus I sought data in which participants in the library setting were engaged in making client interactions accountable to one another. The data consist of two "conversations," one online and one face to face.

The online textual interaction consists of 76 articles posted by 52 individuals in fall 1997 to an Internet discussion list for reference librarians. Excerpts from and references to the listserv discussion are numbered in brackets in this paper to represent their place in the sequence of responses. From a legal standpoint, postings to Internet discussion groups are generally considered public communication and may be analyzed freely and quoted without permission. However, to avoid the potential for chilling expression in this medium, I omit identifying institutions, and first names in all examples are pseudonyms.

The face-to-face conversation took place in fall 2000 among six librarians who provide service to clients in person at university libraries in a large metropolitan area. I elicited the conversation by recruiting participants who were willing to be recorded having a casual conversation about a topic related to their work. I did not give them the question ("What is a problem patron?") until the time of the conversation, and I left the room so they would have to negotiate its meaning on their own. The participants were aware that the researcher is also a professional librarian with a significant amount of shared knowledge, skills, and experiences. I mechanically recorded and transcribed the tape in detail to capture overlaps, pauses, breaths, laughter, repetitions, restatements, and errors. In this paper, names and other identifying features were changed for confidentiality. The appendix provides transcript conventions.

WORK CONTEXT

Academic reference librarians balance responsibility for developing the library collection, meeting with class groups to teach research skills, consulting with faculty and graduate students on research projects, fulfilling administrative duties, and working with the public on a walk-in basis at the reference desk, as well as over the phone and by e-mail. Librarians who specialize in reference work may spend a third to a half of their work hours in interactive service. For this portion of their work, they are usually alone, managing a stream of unrelated questions, demands, and difficulties from clients with varied expectations and skills.

The context of this work is shifting from the impact of two major trends. First, Internet technology is making interactions less routine and raising client expectations about convenience. As recently as 1995, academic reference librarians were responsible for mastering only the collections of their own libraries. Web-based resources mean not only that librarians have many more resources to search in response to a client request for information, but also that clients are immersed in media advertising that implies all information should be easily available (for free) online. A second trend of interest in the academic library setting is the shift in higher education to a consumer market orientation. In the late 1980s as the last Baby Boomers graduated from college, increasing competition for far fewer students led many institutions to increase their appeal to non-traditional students, such as older adults and geographically remote populations completing degrees online. Marketing appeals to these groups often emphasize convenience and personal service.

One way in which these trends affect interactive service is in speeding up emotional labor. Professional librarians (library workers who hold a Master's of Library Science (MLS) degree) adopt a philosophical commitment to presenting a "neutral" emotional stance (as defined by mainstream culture) toward diverse information needs. That is, they are committed to assist clients in finding and using even materials that offend them personally on a moral, political, religious, or aesthetic level. This ethical foundation is reinforced by the American Library Association (ALA, the accrediting body for library schools) and local administrators. The ALA Council, Office for Information Technology Policy (1996) issued a statement interpreting the

ALA "Library Bill of Rights" as it applies to access to the Internet, which reads in part:

> Libraries and librarians should not deny or limit access to information available via electronic resources because of its allegedly controversial content or because of the librarian's personal beliefs or fear of confrontation.

In addition, a document published by the Reference and Adult Services Division (RASD) of the Association of College and Research Libraries (part of the American Library Association) produced "Guidelines for Behavioral Performance of Reference and Information Services Professionals" (available online at http://www.ala.org). These guidelines are intended to allow administrators to evaluate the success of reference interactions, "measured not by the information conveyed, but by the positive or negative impact of the patron–librarian interaction" (Reference and Adult Services Division, 1996, p. 200). The 47 guidelines include displaying interest, friendliness, and reassurance (1.3, 1.4, 2.4, 3.2), concealing stress, anxiety, personal interest, distaste, or boredom (1.5, 2.5, 3.3, 3.9), and judging the patron's level of comfort, interest, or motivation (2.3, 4.14). It is important to note that unlike many other types of service workers, librarians often benefit from a "status shield" conferred by institutional authority and education in interaction with personal status markers of gender, class, race, and age (Hochschild, 1983, pp. 173–174).

The impact of emotional labor is most felt when dealing with those clients known in the library science literature as "problem patrons." This literature includes theoretical models (Hecker, 1996), case studies and practical tips (Chadbourne, 1990; Owens, 1994), humor (Manley, 1988), and library school texts (Salter & Salter, 1988). These sources describe how "problem patrons" force librarians to depart from routine practices, offend or irritate other clients, cause emotional distress, break criminal laws, and/or violate library policies. Although some of these activities are inherently disruptive, an encyclopedia entry classifies problem patrons as those who monopolize workers' time with demands for "special attention and services" (Sable, 1988, p. 171). Defining what is "special" library service requires a complex social process of negotiating what the client wants, what the worker is willing to provide, and what the institutional rules allow. Although some interactions follow a stable pattern, these standardized transactions may be a smaller proportion of service encounters, given the impact of Internet technology and customer service expectations from the consumer sector.

DEFINING THE PROFESSION

This section focuses on how the participants categorize groups of workers in the library, including reference librarians themselves. The interaction produces the boundaries of their profession and its privileges and responsibilities by delineating the boundaries of who they are (librarians, professionals) and who they are not (computer assistants, circulation staff, security guards). Although they do take on some or all of the tasks of these other groups in their everyday work, this section will show how they assert their distinction from these groups in the course of these two conversations. Harvey Sacks (1986) found that the boundaries of membership categories are shaped by "category-bound" activities, motives, rights, entitlements, obligations, knowledge, and attributes. Michael Moerman used naturally occurring conversation to show that a particular individual's membership category is not a fixed identity, but rather one that is employed by specific participants for the purposes of the occasion and its situation (Moerman, 1988, p. 7). The data suggest that what librarians think and do when working individually with clients is ratified in this kind of conversation as being within or outside the professional role.

In the online conversation, participants most often used the word "librarian" to designate library workers. A smaller number of references are to the more general term "staff," which would include both librarians and library workers who do not have the MLS degree. Following are a few examples of the many occasions on which participants make a distinction between staff in general and "real" librarians:

[2] The second time any person asks for assistance on a matter you find offense you might find another librarian or staff member who is more depraved that you are to assist the person.

[3] Censoring internet content on all machines in a library, though, should be repugnant to librarians and staff valuing the essential character of a library.

[46] A few female librarians have of late taken male librarians to task for failing to see the safety issue for female librarians and staff.

In addition to drawing a distinction between themselves and other workers, the phrases "as librarians" and "as professionals" are used to assert a shared ethical foundation:

[2] As librarians, we endeavor to make sure our personal viewpoints do not interfere with the provision of information.

[4] My personal opinion is that librarians as professionals need to be willing to look at and talk about images and issues that they do not like.

[19] As librarians we are all strong supporters of the first amendment.

The implication of these statements is that to be one of "us," the reader must subscribe to these ideals. Although the second of the three examples above frames the comment as a "personal opinion," the appeal to professionalism claims a higher ethical ground. These characterizations of librarians stand uncorrected by other participants throughout the online discussion. This is not merely a factor of overly polite discourse, given the exchanges over other characterizations, such as "public servant":

[71] It is important for us to remember that although we're "public servants" and we enter this profession to help people get the information they want, we do have rights and feelings of our own that should be taken into account as much as the patron's.

[72] We are public EMPLOYEES, not servants. Make sure you make the distinction!

The female participant who first used the term (within quotation marks) employed it not to embrace the idea but rather to assert that the nature of service work does not do away with legitimate personal boundaries. Nonetheless, the female participant who responded strongly above with words in all capitals and exclamation points challenges the term "servant" because

[74] If I wanted to be one, I never would have gone to school for most of my life. Regardless, if librarians want to be treated as professionals, a distinction must be made. The public does indeed harbor expectations and views as to what we in the service industry are doing.

In this example, the phrase "as professionals" is used once again to assert the boundary between librarians and other kinds of interactive service work. She refers to public expectations from service workers as being lower status and therefore more open to abuses. No female participant supported the use of the term "servant," but three male participants used the terms "servant" and "librarian" interactively as going "beyond the bare minimum" [73], identifying with the "ethical baggage they teach you in library school" [75], and considering service a source of power and honor.

As discussed above, participants take care to remind one another that although librarians are staff, not all staff are librarians. The groups of library staff from which the librarians distinguish themselves include computer assistants, security guards, and circulation workers. For example, a participant in the listserv discussion created distance between her role and that of computer lab assistants dispensing "technical advice."

[66] If you are going to give detailed technical advice on usage, you may well find you are turned into a computer lab tech rather than a reference librarian.

Here the participant warns against willingly adopting tasks belonging to a different membership category, one that may be lower paid or less prestigious or simply take time away from work activities she considers appropriate for her category.

One of those category-bound tasks traditionally central to librarianship is the selection of material held in the library collection. Several interactions center on the idea that the Internet calls upon librarians to assist clients in finding online material that they would not have selected for the library. One of the most active interactions in the listserv discussion focused on this issue. The participant questions why others are concerned with the issue of censorship:

[37] Librarians censor all the time; we call it book selection, collection development, whatever. I don't understand all the hand-wringing about this. And, it's interesting to me that all the people who don't understand about the safety issue (whether real or perceived) are men!

The level of response might be as much a factor of her gender analysis as her argument that the profession has always served a gate-keeping function through budget control and should also have the right to limit electronic materials to those appropriate for the library's collection.

[38] Here we're talking about trying to eliminate something that's not draining the budget and that at least some of our clientele obviously wants.

[39] The Internet is like a library full of materials that you did not select – others are doing the selecting for you and you have to manage what's there. That is not normal library practice, but that is what we're dealing with.

[41] But the main point is that you are not talking about selection – you are talking about denying patrons access to materials that are already available in the library.

In this interaction, it is possible that these three participants (all male) perceive that professional power derived from Internet technology skills is replacing bureaucratic power derived from budget control. They are encouraging others to embrace (or at least accept) the role of assisting clients with materials outside the library's walls and selection parameters. Further research is necessary to learn whether male librarians are more willing to see technological expertise as a potential power base, given traditional gender roles and perhaps increased access to training. Christine Williams' (1995) study *Still a Man's World* suggests that this is a likely gender privilege for men in a "women's profession."

In the face-to-face conversation, the two main groups set off from librarians are circulation staff and security staff. Circulation workers do not have the MLS degree required of reference librarians. They check out materials to clients, collect fines, send out notices, and give students materials held in course reserves. If only one worker is present at a library (i.e., at times of low traffic in a larger library or at any time in a smaller library), it must be someone who does circulation tasks. Two of the participants, Barbara and Frances, work at branch libraries and thus have circulation duties in addition to reference work. In addition, Evan had a job doing circulation before he earned his MLS.

Evan (E) produces a possible definition of problem patron relating exclusively to "circulation" (segment 1, lines 63–71):

63 E: I know having

64 worked in (circulation) we had an actual label you could put on

65 somebody's (.) uh (.) borrower record if#you#will (.) //basically// you- you- you got

         [   ]

66   B: hm (.) //huh {↑}//

67 that designation by not returning (.) //books//

     [ ]

68   F: //right//

69 or having an outstanding //fine// that kind of thing it basically blocked you

    [ ]

70   F: //right//

71 from borrowing (.) in the future

That is, the official "designation" related not to how clients treated staff, but how they treated library materials and obeyed rules. Circulation staff were responsible for enforcing these rules. In another segment (1, lines 26–29), Evan indicates that clients respond differently to circulation and reference workers:

26 E: I think there's a definition of what a|hə hə|problem pa(h)tron

27 is, somebody who seems to be quite irrational = in this case I've helped him

28 before and (.) to hear how he's treated (circulation) is bizarre because

29 you would not see it coming

What appears irrational in the client's behavior can be seen as a response to category-bound aspects of the two sets of tasks. Circulation work entails more routine tasks, similar to retail transactions (e.g., checking out and renewing books), whereas more complex, unpredictable service interactions are referred to professional librarians. In addition to specialized knowledge and training, the reference librarians also have the leeway to selectively enforce policies and alter procedures as necessary to provide personalized research assistance. This may result in clients finding the librarians more "helpful" than the circulation staff. It is also likely that the client's more respectful behavior was influenced by Evan's status in the organization in contrast to that of the circulation staff, who are often student workers.

This argument is supported by another turn at talk, in which Evan claims that clients in a law library "can be far more demanding and confrontational" (segment 4, lines 22–23). Although he provisionally attributes the problems to differences in the stress level among the clients of law libraries, it is also the case that he worked in circulation in that position. Similarly, Barbara (B) notes that "there's problem customers everywhere" (segment 1, lines 85–86). She makes the retail connection explicit in segment 3, lines 9–12:

9 B: Well, and having worked in a bookstore myself (.) you know there's (so

many) problem customers which I was thinking of earlier //u:m// but

        [   ]

11   ?: //m hm//

12 °°I haven't encountered the same type of people in the library

Although she could be correct in attributing the problem to the kinds of people present in the bookstore setting, the routine nature of transactions and more rigid application of policies associated with being a retail clerk, similar to the nature of circulation work, are arguably the cause of problems in the interaction.

The boundaries with respect to security staff relate to professional norms concerning the nature of the library as a "public good." In this example, Evan claims the library space as set off from private university property:

144 E: //Well security// I know has approached reference (.) at different times

145 asking if (.) we've had a problem (.) uh with certain individuals .h and I think

146 security just has a different mindset um //(.2)// they're

        [   ]

147   F: //|hə hə hə|I'm she(h)r) tha(h)t's tru(h)e//

          [   ]

148   C: //°°sher//

149 looking at the campus as a whole //(.)// and: (.) if somebody were hangin

             [   ]

150   F: //°°yeah//

151 out on the eighth floor (.) I think they would m- (.) definitely move them

152 along if they didn't have-

153 certainly#if#they#dint#have#a#(University) #ID but#of#course the

154 library is uh uh (.) public (.) //facilities we don't we

[

155   B: //right (.) right (.) right //

             [   ]

156   C: //°°yes//

157 don't card people the public-// the general public has a right to walk in so

158 I think (.) security sometimes doesn't appreciate that (.) that (.) spirit

159 //(.)// as much as perhaps we do um so we're often left (.) telling them

  [ ]

160   B://hm//

161 to-ta hold //off not// necessarily y-know roust somebody from a chair

    [   ]

162   B://m hm//

When Evan (E) claims that security staff have "a different mindset" (line 146), Frances (F) responds with laughing agreement (line 147). Evan goes on to characterize the mindset as "looking at the campus as a whole" (line 149). That is, security workers do not consider the qualitative difference between "the eighth floor" (line 151) as private property and the public nature of the library (lines 154, 157). He alludes to the category-bound nature of the problem patron concept when he suggests (line 154) that people not carrying university identification may be problem patrons for security workers but not for librarians. This difference suggests potential conflicts between the two groups of workers, with librarians claiming the authority over the space:

"we're often left telling them to hold off" (line 159). The boundary of the library's physical space, then, is also one enclosing professional norms that are in conflict with general university rules. In other spaces, people may be ejected for not carrying proper identification, but in the library, members of the general public are to be treated as clients.

CHARACTERIZING CLIENTS

The previous section illustrates how the participants negotiate categories of workers in ways that serve to define their role in the service encounter. This section focuses on how terms for clients are used in interaction to similarly define mutual roles. The participants in the online conversation most often use the term *patrons* to refer to library clients, with a smaller set of references to *student/s*, *faculty*, *person/people*, *man/men*, *public*, and *user/s*. The academic librarians in the discussion maintained a distinction not available to public librarians, that of "primary clientele" or "primary users" in statements such as the following:

> [4] the dodge that the (academic) library exists to serve its primary clientele won't solve the dilemma by itself.

> [16] basic patrons only, those being defined in writing as students, faculty, and staff of our university

> [19] who is your primary user group?

These examples show that this distinction may be important in allowing participants to set service boundaries or to restrict access to resources. Examples from the face-to-face conversation below show that rules in private institutions requiring identification cards play a role in determining primary clientele that frequently gives rise to conflict as participants negotiate service boundaries.

In comparison to the face-to-face conversation, the participants in the online discussion used a far greater range of adjectives and nouns to describe clients, and were more disparaging. Adjectives included *angry, hostile, sexually aroused, troublesome,* and *"weird"*; nouns included *"crazies," "druggies,"* and *"jerks"* [all quotes in original]. In most cases, these characterizations passed without notice in the exchange. In only one instance did a participant draw attention to a characterization of a client:

> [3] if a large bank of workstations pawed by slavering perverts creates a hazard

[4] I'm not sure what purpose it serves to characterize our patrons as "slavering perverts" because they make uses of the Internet that we would not make

It is possible that the listserv as a medium cannot support the subtle interaction by which such correction (to one's own expression or another's) can be made in a face-to-face conversation, where participants were quick to correct others or themselves to prevent appearing harsh or unprofessional toward clients. This effort introduced a stiff tone at times, rather than the natural flow of casual chat. In an example of this trouble in the talk (segment 1, lines 45–50), Barbara (B) responds to a drift in the conversation toward labeling the mentally ill and homeless as a problem.

45 B = But not everyone //who-who's// mentally unstable is a problem

      [   ]

46   C: //(   )//

47 patron //(.) sometimes// they're jus swee:t //and sort of// nice and

   [   ]   [   ]

48 C: = No#no#no#no#no //that's true// C: //that's true//

49 (.)

50 C: = That's true

In this exchange, Barbara sounds too good to be true (line 47), and Cathy (C) repeats her agreement three times (lines 48 and 50) to make sure it is heard "in the clear" in the conversation. What establishes that the conversation is not simply a false front, however, is the way participants use strategies such as laughter to hold one another accountable not just for being too harsh, as in the example above, but also for being too nice. For example, Frances (F) attempts to define problem patrons as (segment 2, lines 121–129):

121 someone from the outside, not necessarily a

122 student or professor although possibly one of those two (.) who: comes in

123 and causes °°some#kind#of disruptive behavior or confrontation (.) in the

124 library (.2) but I-I °°fortunately#have#never#encountered a professor

125 who fit (.) that description (.)nor{↑} have I encountered // a stu-

    [   ]

126 C: //(smile voice)Oh? {↑}//

       [   ]

127   E: //You havn't?|hə hə hə hə hə|//

128 F: No (.) I haven't (.) // I guess// I've just been lucky.

     [   ]

129 C: (smile voice) //Oh? {↓} //

Here, Cathy (C) and Evan (E) collaborate in good humor to prevent this attempted definition from standing. That is, professors as primary clientele may have more power in the service interaction than do students or non-affiliated clients, but it is not tenable to the group that professors are therefore never a problem.

Embedded in this careful, somewhat stiff conversation are moments of unguarded pleasure when participants recognize a description of a mutual client (segment 6, lines 36–48):

36 F: one student was someone who wanted a get into the (lab) (.) he didn't have

37 any kind of identification on him I mean not even (.) a drivers license (.)

38 identification he insisted he was (.2) an‡alum‡I‡believe (.) um (.) so I

39 was gonna have im sign in, like we normally do:? ya know and write their

40 social security number? he was adamant about not giving us his social

41 security number because he didn know what we were gonna do with that

42 //someone could take the social security number// and then use it an

   [   ]

43 C: //Oh I've helped-helped this guy before I think//

44 sell it //and// steal his identity and //so it (.) // there

   [   ]   [   ]

45 C: //m hm// C: //yeah//

46 was this whole paranoic (.) kind of qual//ity (   )//

      [   ]

47   G: //sounds like my Un(h)cle Bo:(h)b|heh heh heh//

       [   ]

48   B: //|ha ha ha ha ha|//

The transcript cannot capture the thrill in Cathy's voice at line 43, but it does show her sense of ownership in ratifying Frances's description at line 45. Even more indicative of the role of such recognitions in the conversation is Grace's contribution. Grace has had the least opportunity to serve the same clients as other participants. She introduces "Uncle Bob" as a fictive recognition that serves to bring her into the circle of laughter and mutual understanding.

Recognizing mutual clients here bolsters professional bonds and shared culture. As Moerman argues,

> A world experienced together – perceived, oriented to, felt, and meaningful in the same way–is much like what anthropologists call "a culture." In talk about the world, speakers show whether or not they share one. (Moerman, 1988, p. 112)

The pleasure of sharing a culture appears as excited vocal tone and laughter, and the further afield the tie across time and space, the more thrilling it is. In segment 9, lines 155–219, Evan and Barbara recognize a mutual client from a distant library where they had both been graduate assistants more than seven years apart.

155 E: Ya know the people that- a that research obsessively the //Kennedy (.)//

                              [   ]

156   B: //right//

157 assassination (.) for conspiracy theories and things like that (.) um-

158 B: Oh wow (.) yeah// oh man I had a guy like that at (State U) hoo: (.) yeah

159 E: = The same- y-it was //the same guy.// You knew the same //guy.//

                    [   ]   [

160   G: ///|ha ha ha ha|///   F: //Would you

161 categorize him as a problem patron?//

The ability to recognize mutual clients serves several purposes in building professional identity. First, it affirms that others working in a context of rapid, overlapping encounters with similar professional norms are irritated or offended by the same kinds of behaviors. Second, it affirms that the problem was not caused by shortcoming on their part, because another professional also struggled to meet the client's need while honoring professional norms, local policies, and personal emotional boundaries. Finally, it demonstrates the consistency of client needs and behaviors across time and location, providing a sense of continuity in a rapidly changing environment.

BEING THE BAD GUY: INSTITUTIONAL RULES AND EMOTIONAL LABOR

In the process of providing reference service, librarians loosely apply a set of rules or policies to a flow of clients to produce information users who can increasingly function independently, at least for basic tasks. The librarian is responsible for the smooth functioning of the process, for protecting resources and allocating them fairly, and for engaging clients in the process in a way that satisfies them without allocating too much time to any one client. They must ensure that only the people who are entitled to resources and services are using them, that those clients are treated fairly (not necessarily equally, because of different client categories), and that they get what they need from the institution: information resources, assistance, or a quiet place to study.

The previous two sections argued that reference librarians in these two conversations negotiated the boundaries of the service relationship by interactive characterization of library workers and clients. This section demonstrates how institutional rules function in these conversations to define working relationships with clients. The listserv discussion is primarily concerned with rules about access to the Internet: which clients should have access, under what restrictions, and how much help should they receive? Similarly, one recurring example in the face-to-face conversation is the rule that clients must have a university identification card to use the library's Internet lab. The way rules are discussed in these interactions provides evidence about the way these librarians produce themselves as "professionals" by the kinds of controls they consider appropriate as a category-bound responsibility. Discussion of rules shows the level and kinds of emotion work in the setting, where librarians must manage the client's emotional state by preventing frustration and anger as well as their own personal emotional state of approachability, patience, and friendliness.

The problem situation being discussed on the listserv is framed in a way that assumes bureaucratic control is appropriate (Edwards, 1979). That is, a librarian faced with a patron repeatedly asking for assistance in using sexually explicit Web sites appealed to her online colleagues for "documentation" in the form of legislation or established policies that would support her side against her supervisor, who claims the higher ethical ground of freedom of information. The data show that participants who responded also generally assume that bureaucratic control is possible, and they share rules they have developed and posted in their libraries:

[17] This procedure falls under our "Rules Governing the Use of the Library" of which number one states "No engaging in disorderly conduct, committing a nuisance, or unreasonably disturbing or offending library users or staff-one warning, then out."

[18] We have also posted signs that state something to the effect that the displaying of sexually explicit material may be a violation of the university's policy on sexual harassment.

[33] Our systemwide Library Code of Conduct, which is displayed for public viewing, includes under "Prohibited Activities": "Inappropriate use of library computers including ... sending, displaying, or printing obscene material" (of interest also may be to know that we include here "playing interactive games or using chat").

The sense that bureaucratic controls are appropriate and could conceivably be effective in this setting is rooted in how the workers are themselves controlled by administrators and how they perceive the appropriate role of professionals. The supervisor says he has no legal or ethical ground to create or enforce rules against the behavior the librarian experienced. That is, he has internalized the principles "as a professional," reproduces them in his interaction with her, and expects her to internalize them as well. The participants who respond in turn offer policies to be posted in the library, without any discussion of how clients might be induced to internalize them. Only the first example above [17] suggests any means of enforcement, being asked to leave the premises or be ejected by force.

Professional status in these conversations calls not only for the right to create policies, but also to enforce them selectively (segment 9, lines 83–92):

C: But I think we don enforce things jus for the sake of enforcing

them //(.)//we only enforce

      [   ]

F: //right//

them if there's a problem or the:y monopolize resources

//or infringe on other people's rights//

      [   ]

F: //Yeah an that's-that's// a good thing I think

C: I think that's good //(.)// °we tolerate a lot (as a profession)

      [   ]

E: //Well that's-that's// under the rubric of professional discretion

F://Right//

      [   ]

C: //Yeah//

That is, non-professionals would be restricted by clearly delineated rules, whereas professionals expect to be free to judge in each case whether to enforce a particular rule. The parameters given in this example are that a rule will be enforced to allocate resources fairly or to protect the rights of a larger group.

Although bureaucratic control is the first choice, the possibility of implementing technical control is of great interest to listserv participants as a way of removing themselves as enforcers of the rules. Examples proposed include password control of workstations, privacy screens on monitors, filtering software, and the humorous proposal of "ejection seats." Likewise, in the face-to-face conversation (segment 9, lines 13–22), the participants ponder the situation of a librarian in a public library being expected to enforce 30-min limits for "fair" allocation of time on Internet computers:

13 B: Gosh if they're gonna do that they should've automated it so you have to

14 log on and then it just (.) shuts you down //or something to take the//

                 [   ]

15   C: //Right {↑} so you don't have to//

16 make the person come and ya know //(.)// be the bad guy (.) right (.) I

           [   ]

17   G: //Be the bad guy//

18 thought °°oh boy that must be really hard °°(   )|hə hə|

19 F: So you're probably creating problem patrons (.) because //(.)// how nice is

              [   ]

20   C: //maybe//

           [   ]

21   G: //Yeah {↑}|hə hə hə|//

22 that patron gunna be the next time they have to use the library

This proposed technical solution implies that the computer should be the "bad guy," instead of setting up a library worker as the object of anger for the next time the person comes in. In addition to managing the client's emotional response, participants also question whether client behavior that angers them can be defined as a problem:

221 E: But w-we probably can differentiate between a problem patron and somebody

122 who's just (.) irritating I guess- //(.)// well it sounds funny to say that

          [   ]

123   B: //yeah//

          [   ]

124   G: ///\heh heh heh heh heh\///

125 (.) but I would say a problem patron is somebody whose interaction with

126 us (.) poses problems to a larger audience (.) perhaps it's (.) disruptive to

127 other patrons it's disruptive to: the work flow (.)

Here, Evan (E) implies that it might be part of the librarians' job to put up with irritation (lines 121–122), but that other clients are to be protected from it (lines 126–127). Similarly, when Barbara (B) is asked whether a persistent client was a "problem patron" (segment 9, lines 174–184), she replied not in terms of her own patience level but in terms of annoyance to other clients and control of resources:

174 B: Only {↑} because (.) not if he had been doing things independently

175 and wasn't really bothering anyone but he was-he was clearly bothering

176 others around him (.) because he'd be very agitated and irritated and start

177 talking to the computer and start talking to other people //.hh (.) and (.)//

              [   ]

178   F: //oh (.) yeah//

              [   ]

179   C: //no (.) yeah//

180 because he was (.) using (.) a- a great amount of our resources in terms

181 //of//

   [   ]

182 E: //sher//

183 asking for assistance (.) //repeatedly (.) repeatedly//

[   ]

184   F: //right (.) right (.) yeah//

Framing the problem as one of wasting resources shifts the concern from emotional labor to the traditional bureaucratic power base of institutional control. In addition to enhancing their mutual status, it also provides an acceptable reason to avoid responding to a client whose behavior is irritating or alarming. Frances (F), Cathy (C), and Evan (E) all actively ratify Barbara's framing of this interaction at lines 178, 179, 182, and 184.

In contrast, the issue of resources is absent when faculty are the clients concerned (segment 9, lines 94–102):

94   B: = I find it particularly hard (.) dealing with faculty-there's one faculty

95   member at the (branch library) who (.) comes to the library a lot- uses the

96   library a lot-which is wonderful but on the other hand (.) um (.) (haltingly)

97   isn't particularly interested in learning or applying (.)

98   what#it#is#that#I'm#trying#to#demonstrate#to#him so he just keeps coming

99   back to me and having me do it for him which (.) isn't what I'd prefer but

100   (haltingly) if that' s gonna keep him coming that's okay but-

101   I#don't#really#know#if#he's#a#problem °°so much but-I but it sorta

102   tied in with that same (.) //issue//

Here the overriding concern is to encourage the faculty member to use the library (line 96) as a client whose support is important to the institution. Because the faculty member carries more power in the interaction relative to a student, the issue of managing resources cannot be employed, even though providing the service is less preferred than demonstrating the procedure and having the client learn and apply it independently (lines 97–99). In the case of high-prestige clients like faculty, emotional labor entails managing one's own frustration or irritation. In the case of low-prestige clients, it entails managing the client's frustration or anger at not receiving the preferred level of service.

CONCLUSION: INTEGRATING CLIENTS INTO THE PROFESSIONAL IDENTITY

This study focuses on librarians as one example of a growing group of professions that provide interactive service in a context of rapid technological and social change. Developments in information technology and the accompanying increase in expectations of convenience are key sources of pressure for knowledge workers. It is important to understand how this pressure is incorporated in the construction of professional identities, which can tend either to empower the workers or to lead them into self-defeating interactions with clients and with managers.

The ways in which librarians in this study discussed encounters with difficult clients illuminate how accounting for everyday reactions and decisions contributes to the construction and reproduction of professional identities. In two conversations, one face-to-face and one online in an Internet listserv, librarians mutually reinforce a shared culture in the ways they categorize themselves and other workers, amend or collaborate on each other's characterizations of clients, and negotiate local policies and rules as they intersect with professional values and emotional boundaries.

In categorizing themselves and other workers, participants consistently set librarians off from other groups of workers in the service environment. First, they distinguished themselves as providing customized service, as opposed to workers whose interactions were routine and bound by standard policies. Second, they distinguished themselves as governing the library space by their own professional ethics, as opposed to workers to apply the general rules of the institution. The fact that customized service and professional ethics sometimes contradicted institutional rules and policies was one source of a distinct, privileged professional identity. Moreover, the terms *servant* and *librarian* were used interactively by some male librarians to define the service boundaries as going "beyond the bare minimum" and considering service a source of power and honor.

In discussing clients, the participants in the face-to-face conversation differed from those in the online listserv interaction in the way they amended or collaborated on one another's characterizations. The participants conversing face-to-face used laughter, interruptions, and silence to support or negate not only characterizations that appeared too harsh, but also those that appeared too accepting of client responses. Such amendments and collaborations were rare in the online discussion, although terms used for clients were much harsher, possibly because subtle conversational strategies are not available in written exchanges. This means that correcting another person's characterization could lead to an escalating angry exchange (known as a "flame" in listserv discussions).

Participants in the face-to-face conversation responded enthusiastically to the relatively rare opportunity to discuss shared clients in a context where most interactions with clients are brief and anonymous. Recognizing mutual clients affirmed participants' perspective of the problem and that it was not caused by shortcomings on their part. It also demonstrated the consistency of client needs and behaviors across time and location, providing a sense of continuity in a rapidly changing environment.

In negotiating local policies and rules, participants in both conversations assumed that bureaucratic approaches were appropriate to their status as professionals. However, they proposed rules and policies without accounting for the fact that bureaucratic approaches require people to internalize the rules through interactions. Clients do not share an identity with one another as "library users," and so they have limited motivation to internalize rules. This means that interactions with service workers can create conflicts in which the worker expects the client to understand and adhere to rules that oppose the client's own wants and needs. For the service worker, "being the bad guy" by enforcing rules is in conflict with the professional identity librarians work to construct in these data. Therefore, participants look to technological means of enforcing rules. This strategy is also likely to disappoint them in application, because clients see workers as being responsible for the technology present in the service context, even if the reality is that they are not trained or authorized to correct problems.

Two features of service interactions emerged in the data but cannot be fully analyzed without further research: the impact of computer mediation on service interactions, and the interwoven factor of gender. As the computer/network becomes a fourth party in the shifting service dynamics along with clients, workers, and managers, its "needs" must be attended to in order to serve the customer or to gather information for management. Being seen as a technology expert may be perceived as a way to raise prestige and/ or income. This strategy may require supporting the value of the technology even in adverse circumstances, which might increase the client's frustration. This situation requires additional emotional labor, either in facing down clients' anger or in providing reassurance and calming them down.

Hints about the role of gender in how professionals perceive and negotiate technological issues can be inferred from the relative participation of men and women in the listserv discussion. Of the 52 participants, 25 were men, 25 were women, and 2 could not be confirmed from the data. This represents far more male participation than is proportional with the profession overall. Men comprised only 16% of American librarians in 1997 (*Statistical Abstract of the United States*, 1999, p. 417), although they make up a higher percentage of academic librarians. Counting articles rather than contributors provides further evidence that men dominated the listserv discussion. Of the 76 articles, 33 were posted by women (43%) and 40 by men (53%)— the men on average took more turns in the conversation, with an average of 1.3 articles per woman and 1.6 articles per man.

I hypothesized that this dominance reflected not gender per se but organizational position. That is, I thought it is possible that administrators (those who manage other professional librarians) posted more often regardless of gender. However, the data did not bear this out. Of the 52 contributors, 14 are supervisors (27%) who posted 19 articles (25%), and 27 are non-supervisors (52%) who posted 42 articles (55%). (The organizational position of the remaining 11 contributors could not be confirmed.) The fact that non-supervisors participated at roughly twice the rate of supervisors may stem less from gender than from the uneasiness the front-line workers experienced concerning technology. With less say over how technology is implemented, they may feel more desire to interact with others in the profession to attempt to restructure their professional identity around it.

Although further research exploring the role of interactive service in professional identity is needed, these preliminary findings suggest the importance of fostering awareness of the difficulties of service in the context of rapid change. This awareness should not be aimed at developing practical techniques for dealing with idiosyncratic individuals or more effective rules and regulations, but rather a mutual foundation of shared goals and underlying professional commitments. It is vital to include in these discussions the workers least able to make exceptions to policies or to provide customized service.

Discussions of "problem patrons" as case studies can point to the growing complexity of what clients think libraries can and should provide and what workers in the library expect clients to know and be able to do. Technology is used in other knowledge contexts (e.g., real estate, travel, banking) to externalize basic interactions. Libraries have also externalized basic interactions to online settings (e.g., finding full-text articles, renewing books), leaving the more complicated and potentially more frustrating tasks to be completed in the library with the assistance of staff who must apply not only more technological skill but also more emotional labor. Posting rules and implementing technological controls will not eliminate this source of conflict in the library context. If relating to people is neglected as an aspect of professional identity as the prestige of technology grows, the stress of emotional labor will grow for those responsible for mediating the needs and expectations of clients who do not fit the institutional mold.

REFERENCES

ALA Council, Office for Information Technology Policy. (1996). Access to electronic information, services, and networks: An interpretation of the Library Bill of Rights. [Online]. Available: http://www.ala.org/ala/oif/statementspols/statementsif/interpretations/accesstoelectronic.pdf (March 14, 2006).

Bellas, M. L. (1999). Emotional labor in academia: The case of professors. *The Annals of the American Association of Political and Social Science, 561*, 96–110.

Braverman, H. (1974). *Labor and monopoly capital: The degradation of work in the twentieth century*. New York: Monthly Review Press.

Carmichael, J. V. (1995). The gay librarian: A comparative analysis of attitudes towards professional gender issues. *Journal of Homosexuality, 30*, 11–57.

Chadbourne, R. D. (1990). The problem patron: How much problem, how much patron? *Wilson Library Bulletin, 64*, 59–60.

Davies, A., & Kirkpatrick, I. (1995). Face to face with the 'Sovereign Consumer': Service quality and the changing role of professional academic librarians. *Sociological Review, 43*, 782–807.

Edwards, R. (1979). *Contested terrain: The transformation of the workplace in the twentieth century*. New York: Basic Books.

Garfinkel, H. (1967). *Studies in ethnomethodology*. Englewood Cliffs, NJ: Prentice Hall.

Garson, B. (1977). *All the livelong day: The meaning and demeaning of routine work*. New York: Penguin Books.

Hecker, T. E. (1996). Patrons with disabilities or problem patrons: Which model should librarians apply to people with mental illness? *Reference Librarian, 53*, 5–12.

Hochschild, A. R. (1983). *The Managed heart: Commercialization of human feeling*. Berkeley: University of California Press.

Kunda, G., & Van Maanen, J. (1999). Changing scripts at work: Managers and professionals. *Annals of the American Association of Political and Social Science, 561*, 64–95.

Leidner, R. (1993). *Fast food, fast talk: Service work and the routinization of everyday life*. Berkeley: University of California Press.

Manley, W. (1988). Facing the public. *Wilson Library Bulletin, 62*, 96–97.

McCammon, H. J., & Griffin, L. J. (2000). Workers and their customers and clients: An editorial introduction. *Work and Occupations, 27*, 278–293.

McElhinny, B. S. (1995). Challenging hegemonic masculinities: Female and male police officers handling domestic violence. In: K. Hall & M. Bucholtz (Eds), *Gender articulated: Language and the socially constructed self* (pp. 217–243). New York: Routledge.

Moerman, M. (1988). *Talking culture: Ethnography and conversation analysis*. University of Philadelphia: Pennsylvania Press.

Murgai, S. R. (1991). Attitudes toward women as managers in library and information science. *Sex Roles, 24*, 681–700.

Owens, S. (1994). Proactive problem patron preparedness. (Signs, brochures and staff guidelines). *Library & Archival Security, 12*, 11–23.

Pierce, J. L. (1995). *Gender trials: Emotional lives in contemporary law firms.* Berkeley: University of California Press.

Reference and Adult Services Division. Ad Hoc Committee on Behavioral Guidelines for Reference and Information Services. (1996). Guidelines for Behavioral Performance of Reference and Information Services Professionals. *RQ, 36,* 200–203.

Sable, M. H. (1988). Problem patrons in public and university libraries. *Encyclopedia of Library and Information Science.* (Vol. 43, Suppl. 8). New York: Dekker.

Sacks, H. (1986). On the analyzability of stories by children. In: J. Gumperz & D. Hymes (Eds), *Directions in sociolinguistics* (pp. 325–345). New York: Blackwell.

Salter, C. A., & Salter, J. L. (1988). *On the frontlines: Coping with the library's problem patrons.* Englewood, CO: Libraries Unlimited.

Statistical Abstract of the United States. (1999). Washington, DC: Government Printing Office.

Wharton, C. S. (1996). Making people feel good: Workers' constructions of meaning in interactive service jobs. *Qualitative Sociology, 19,* 217–233.

Williams, C. L. (1995). *Still a man's world: Men who do women's work.* Berkeley: University of California Press.

APPENDIX: TRANSCRIPT CONVENTIONS

(Words in single parentheses)	Uncertain hearings and substitutions to protect anonymity
rapid#speech	Faster than the surrounding talk
(.)	Noticeable pause
(.3)	Pause in tenths of a second
//overlapping speech//	Overlapping speech connected between lines with square brackets
(h)	Laughter within words that does not obscure speech
|hə hə|	Laughter with closed vowel; ("chuckling")
|heh heh heh|	Laughter with long "e"; ("tittering")
|ha ha|	Laughter with open vowel; ("guffawing")
word-	Abrupt ending to final sound of a word
Underscore	Emphasized word
CAPITALS	Louder than surrounding speech
= Word	Less than the usual pause between utterances
°word	Quieter than surrounding speech
°°word	Much quieter than surrounding speech
.hh	Audible in-breath
{↑}	Higher pitch than surrounding words
{↓}	Lower pitch than surrounding words

ACADEMIC LIBRARIANS' VIEWS OF THE CHAIR'S PROFESSIONAL DEVELOPMENT ROLE

Dana W. R. Boden

ABSTRACT

The purpose of this study was to determine not-yet-tenured university library faculty members' views of 27 methods their department chair may use to support and enhance the faculty member's professional development. The methods were derived from earlier qualitative research on department chairs in higher education. While academic teaching department chair roles have been the subject of the research literature for many years, little research has addressed library faculty perceptions of the department chair's role. The survey instrument used consisted of two parts: (1) a demographics section, consisting of five questions; and (2) a researcher-developed survey of faculty perceptions of the department chairs' role in faculty development. Survey participants were asked to rate the importance of methods chairs may use in enhancing the professional activities of faculty. According to the not-yet-tenured library faculty members responding to this study, a chair engaging in the most important practices to enhance their faculty's professional development would be one who utilizes good communication, while acting as an administrative advocate.

Advances in Library Administration and Organization, Volume 24, 117–149
Copyright © 2007 by Elsevier Ltd.
ISSN: 0732-0671/doi:10.1016/S0732-0671(06)24004-5

INTRODUCTION

Academic librarians are well aware of the disparity within our ranks regarding our status. Our rank, status, title, and standing within the institutions we serve vary. There is an ongoing debate among ourselves regarding whether it is best to be in tenure-leading positions (Murray-Rust, 2005), or not be burdened with those requirements (Carver, 2005). Individual views on the track academic librarians' careers should follow sometimes even change over time (Hill, 2005). Holding faculty status does not always mean the same thing from one institution to another (Cary, 2001). New hires are now given choices regarding their type of appointment at some institutions (Ruess, 2004). Even the Association of Research Libraries (ARL), in their annual survey, notes: "Since the criteria for determining professional status vary among libraries, there is no attempt to define the term "professional." Each library should report ... those staff members it considers professional(s) ..." (Kyrillidou & Young, 2005a, 2005b).

"Professional academic librarians" were welcomed into membership in the American Association of University Professors (AAUP) in 1956. It was not until 1971 that the Association of College and Research Libraries (ACRL) membership officially approved its Standards for Faculty Status for College and University Librarians (McAnally, 1975), with two revisions since (Krompart, 1994). The Standards address areas recognizable to any faculty member: professional responsibilities; governance (library, college, and university); compensation; tenure and promotion; sabbatical and other research leaves; research and development funds; and academic freedom (Association of College and Research Libraries Committee on the Status of Academic Librarians, 2001).

Today, faculty status is still not a given for librarians in higher education. In fact, among Carnegie research institutions, just over half have faculty status for their librarians. The professional librarians at a large majority of the remaining institutions have what is termed academic status (Leysen & Black, 1998; Lowry, 1993). The ACRL approved Guidelines for Academic Status for College and University Libraries in 1990. Included in the nine guidelines are recommendations for involvement in governance, research and professional activities, and protection of academic freedom (Kroll, 1994). But, whether recognized with faculty or academic status, university librarians are expected to be involved in continuing professional development.

Still we are aware of our uniqueness among our university colleagues. Women account for almost twice the percentage of library faculty members at U.S. Association of Research Libraries University Libraries (63.85%) (Kyrillidou & Young, 2005a), as compared to the percentage of all faculty at doctoral-level institutions (33%) (Curtis, 2004). A large majority of university library faculty positions require the Master of Library Science degree from an institution accredited by the American Library Association, thus most university library faculty share this disciplinary background (Lowry, 1993). Also, most of us came, and continue to come, through the program for the degree as non-traditional students and enter the profession at over 30 years of age (ALISE, 1991–2003). The disciplines represented by our other degree(s), however, are widely varied. Unlike teaching faculty in other departments across campus, we are usually employed on a 12-month basis. Yet, as with any tenure track position, participation in professional development activities is a requirement to meet the criteria for a successful bid for continuous appointment (tenure) and/or promotion (Leysen & Black, 1998; Lowry, 1993). With our varied backgrounds and life experiences, many come to librarianship having already been in the workforce and feel independent and confident in our own abilities.

The profession of librarianship is not focused simply on the academic realm, and this contributes to the contradictory views of just what is and should be our role in the academy. Our colleagues in other types of libraries, while not focused on the requirements of obtaining tenure, and the myriad of activities that demands, share our commitment to service. The organization of many libraries, no matter the type, often means supervision and management of personnel, from students to volunteers to staff to fellow professionals, is required of many the librarian. Our focus on assisting our patrons in searching the literature has meant we are most comfortable reviewing the information available to us and synthesizing it for application to our situations. Yet much of the literature we look to for guidance and application is broad-based and widely focused on the public, business world, rather than where our operations and career choice have actually placed us—on campus, in an academic setting, in professional library faculty positions.

ROLE OF THE DEPARTMENT CHAIR IN FACULTY DEVELOPMENT

The department chair position has long been recognized as an important one in post-secondary institutions (Heimler, 1967). For decades, research has been focused on department chairs, their role and functions. A role in faculty development has been a constant for chairs; however, the types of activities and the depth of involvement have evolved.

A review of the literature attests to faculty development continuing to be a concern of the academic community. Times of retrenchment and increasing numbers of mid-career faculty have brought about times of reflection and increased research on effective faculty development. In the early literature, faculty development was viewed almost exclusively in terms of how it could improve teaching (Group for Human Development in Higher Education, 1974; Bergquist & Phillips, 1975). Also, while the chair might assist and support faculty efforts, faculty development was commonly considered the responsibility of each individual faculty member (Gaff, 1975). In the mid-1980s, Eble and McKeachie's (1985) report on the Bush Foundation Faculty Development Project showed that a balance between faculty and administrative support was the key to successful faculty development and encouraged further research.

The research that followed has focused not only on the department chair's perceptions of their role, but from several levels: those of the chairs themselves (Creswell, Wheeler, Seagren, Egly, & Beyer, 1990; Gmelch & Miskin, 1993, 1995; Jennerich, 1981; Kremer-Hayon & Avi-itzhak, 1986; Lee, 1985; McLaughlin, Montgomery, & Malpass, 1975; Miles, 1983; Mitchell, 1986; Roach, 1976; Seagren, Wheeler, Creswell, Miller, & VanHorn-Grassmeyer, 1994; Smart, 1976; Wilhite, 1987); the faculty members' views (Daly & Townsend, 1992, 1994; Gordon, Stockard, & Williford, 1991; Hirokawa, Barge, Becker, & Sutherland, 1989; Knight & Holen, 1985; Moses, 1985; Neumann & Neumann, 1983; Watson, 1979, 1986); those of the chairperson's administrative supervisor – usually a dean (Jeffrey, 1985; Moxley & Olson, 1990); and across all three levels (Cohen, Bleha, & Olswang, 1981; Falk, 1979; Jones & Holdaway, 1995; Kenny, 1982; Leaming, 1998; Siever, Loomis, & Neidt, 1972; Smith, 1972; Weinberg, 1984; Whitt, 1991).

Many works cover the chairperson's entire responsibilities, but a recurrent theme presented in the literature has been the department chair's role in enhancing faculty development opportunities (Eble, 1990; Gmelch & Miskin, 1995; Leaming, 1998; McKeachie, 1990; Seagren, Creswell, & Wheeler, 1993; Tucker, 1992) or acting in a leadership role, which includes faculty professional development (Knight & Trowler, 2001; Lucas & Associates, 2000; McLaughlin et al., 1975). These works are chapters on the department chair's faculty development role, or monographs that address the overall role of the department chair, while including faculty development. There has also been research (Creswell & Brown, 1992; Seagren, Wheeler, Mitchell, &

Creswell, 1986; Wilhite, 1990), literature reviews (Scott, 1990), and administrator opinion articles (Sorcinelli, 1990; Thompson, 1990; Wheeler, 1992) specifically addressing the chair's role in faculty development.

The faculty development role has sometimes been viewed as one activity, and sometimes as multiple activities, in which a department chair may engage. The terms used for the role vary through the literature. Jennerich (1981) referred to the role as "leadership ability." "Leadership role" is the term used by McLaughlin et al. (1975). Smart (1976) and Hirokawa et al. (1989) use "faculty development." Moses (1985) refers to "encouragement" and Eble (1986) describes a role for chairs as "ingenious providers of motivation, support, and encouragement [for faculty]." Bland and Schmitz (1988, 1990a, 1990b) refer to a responsibility for taking on "faculty vitality," while Hecht, Higgerson, Gmelch, and Tucker (1999) identified the role of a "purposeful, facilitative leader." Others perceived leadership as the overarching function of the chair, which takes into account all the skills, competencies, functions, roles, or activities undertaken to guide the department's way (Coats, Lovell, & Franks, 1996; Gordon et al., 1991; Mitchell, 1986).

Specific actions chairs may use in their role in faculty leadership or development have also been identified over the years. Some of these include: "place faculty on committees" (Weinberg, 1984); "encourages faculty to participate in conventions, conferences, professional associations, etc."; "reports departmental accomplishments to [the] dean or immediate supervisor" (Smith, 1972); "commending achievement" (Moses, 1985); "delegates authority" (Kremer-Hayon & Avi-Itzhak, 1986); and "develop the potential of ... junior faculty" (McLaughlin et al., 1975).

Creswell et al. (1990) identified three levels of faculty who may need assistance: newer faculty members need assistance toward successful tenure and promotion hearings; mid-career faculty members sometimes require assistance to maintain professional involvement; and senior faculty may need assistance to give new life to their careers. Some authors have addressed specific career stages of faculty professional development needs. Boice (1992, 2000) and Bensimon, Ward, and Sanders (2000) focused on new faculty. Baldwin (1990) and Lucas and Associates (2000) note differing requirements of faculty at various points throughout their professional life. An example is the need for "nurturing faculty vitality" of post-tenure faculty (Licata, 2000).

Over the years, the emphases have expanded and shifted with the times and interests on campuses, but the department chair continues to be viewed as a mid-level administrator in a position to act as a leader, encouraging or assisting faculty members, in professional development and growth. The literature has supported the premise that the chair's role in faculty development, and as a leader, can be influential in the life of a faculty member. The chair is situated strategically to assist faculty in their development, growth, and progress professionally. As the administrative middle manager, the chair is naturally seen as in a leader position to influence subordinates. As the faculty member interacts with the chair of their department, roles are communicated and practices are observed. The faculty member's perceptions of the department chair's professional development role and leadership practices determine their professional relationship, which in turn can impact the career or, at least institutional, success of the faculty member.

Department Chairs in Academic Libraries

While research and literature exist on faculty perceptions of the chair's role in academic departments in various institution types across the United States and Canada, little research has addressed faculty perceptions of the department chair's role in non-teaching departments at the university level. The general literature on department chairs or faculty development almost never gives any indication that library personnel were considered, or included, in the research. Boice (1992) was a unique exception and also collaborated with librarians on research regarding library faculty and teaching faculty demands on scholarship (Boice, Scepanski, & Wilson, 1987). In his book on new faculty professional development, he recognized the crucial role of department chairs in the success of faculty. He addressed the work to a broad audience, but chairs were listed as "first and foremost" (p. xii). He noticed libraries within the university setting include members who have faculty status but do not teach courses on a regular basis, and observed faculty in other departments on campus may not even be aware if librarians have faculty status. His experience with researching new library faculty led him to remark that they, "more than any group ... suffered from unclear expectations" (Boice, 1992, p. 276).

Differences in the organizational setup of libraries may have delayed the focus of research from turning toward department chairs. Chief librarians at universities in the first half of the twentieth century tended to be quite autocratic, blocking the library from arranging itself along the lines of a more democratic organization similar to its teaching counterparts (McAnally, 1975). As a result, much of the research on leadership in academic libraries has been focused on the library deans or directors, not department chairs. At the same time, as has been observed, the need for support personnel to perform a myriad of duties in academic libraries has meant that librarians in their very first professional position may be called upon to be a supervisor of support staff or student workers (Bailey, 1976). The result has been literature focused on supervision of personnel and often based on a business management background. Specific department chair concerns, especially as related to leading faculty, have been addressed only to a limited extent. Excellent examples of this are the editions of *Practical Help for New Supervisors* prepared by the Supervisory Skills Committee, Personnel Administration Section, Library Administration and Management Association of the American Library Association (Giesecke, 1992, 1997). Those, as well as several others (Evans & Ward, 2003; Giesecke, 2001; Giesecke & McNeil, 2005; Gordon, 2005; Pugh, 2005) take a broad approach, across types of libraries. While they provide helpful advice, and put some focus on professionals and their development, three of the five are based on a synthesis of previous literature (Giesecke; Giesecke & McNeil; Pugh), another on the authors' "management experiences ... rooted in research" (Evans & Ward, p. vii) and the last on unscientific web surveys of "self-described library managers" and library staff (Gordon).

Among those broad-based works that do focus on the academic library setting, the authors in Mech and McCabe (1998) tend to view development as a part of leadership, with little actual text committed to how that occurs, or what is, or should be, involved. As the title states, Simmons-Welburn and McNeil's (2004) work addresses human resource management, so again, the specific needs of professionals are not a major emphasis. Even the title given to academic librarians at the department chair level in the literature varies, with some being called department chair, department head, division head, division chair, team leader, unit leader, middle manager, or supervisor.

Utilization of research instruments to determine library leadership or faculty development practices is limited, and research conducted specifically on department chairs in the academic library setting is an even smaller subset. Research on these library middle managers did not begin until the late 1960s (Bailey, 1987). Similar to the broader department chair literature, the main focus of the research and literature has been the chairs themselves or the views of higher administrators. The perceptions of faculty in university library departments regarding the department chair have not been well documented. Most publications on the topic have either been based on data gathering that used a researcher-developed instrument, surveys of the existing literature, or were basically opinion pieces.

Plate (1970) noted the predominance of library literature that focused on descriptions and applications but that included little actual research. He utilized a short questionnaire and interviews of middle managers at ARL member libraries and found that they felt professional development of those they supervised was not their responsibility, but rather the responsibility of the individuals themselves. Parallel to that finding, Stone (1969) surveyed "professional librarians" of which approximately one-half were in academic libraries, finding that, while "the ultimate responsibility for continuing education was placed by the librarians on the individual" (p. 192), the results urging administrative support for professional development included the observation "supervisors should be rewarded or promoted on the basis of how well they promote professional growth of those under them" (p. 175).

Research on perceptions of middle managers and their superiors have included Bailey's (1978, 1981) interviews of middle managers and administrators in libraries of five ARL member institutions and Mitchell's (1989) survey of academic library department heads and their immediate supervisors in 137 academic libraries, using Fiedler's Contingency Model of Leadership Effectiveness.

Several studies regarding library leadership have used the Leadership Behavior Description Questionnaire – Form XII (LBDQ-XII), developed at Ohio State University, or a modified version thereof. It examined the style of leadership as perceived by the supervisor and subordinate groups. The supervisors completed the instrument regarding themselves, while a selected number of subordinates completed it regarding the supervisor. Research on libraries in institutions of higher education included Sparks (1976), Comes (1978), and Olive (1991). Sparks utilized the instrument for a very limited study of one academic library supervisor and 15 subordinates. Comes targeted the directors at 24 institutions and eight subordinates who held supervisory responsibilities. Olive surveyed public services and technical services department heads and their subordinates, both professional and non-professional, in private Liberal Arts I institution libraries.

Focusing research on the middle managers, Person (1980) used both questionnaires and interviews and included nine large academic libraries in the Great Lakes states in her research of managerial role concepts in academic and public libraries. Interestingly, the public library managers perceived themselves having higher levels of involvement in internally oriented roles such as "leader" than did their academic library counterparts, who gave higher ratings to their involvement in externally directed areas.

Bailey and Murphy (1989) researched the "management competencies" of middle managers in 11 large ARL libraries in the Midwest, asking three managers with average performance records and three superior performers, at each institution, "to narrate three positive and three negative experiences in which they had utilized management principles." They then compared their findings to the academic portion of an earlier study. While the categories assigned differed between the two studies, they were similar, and the results of both indicated an emphasis on staffing and personnel management, which included sub-categories for motivation and staff development.

Heads of cataloging and heads of reference departments in over one hundred ARL libraries were surveyed by Wittenbach, Bordeianu, and Wycisk (1992) regarding management education and training. Their results showed that few institutions required management training when hiring department chairs, or ongoing training for the chairs.

While looking at differences among the genders, Voelck (2003) interviewed "academic library middle managers" in Michigan regarding their self-described "management style" and their use of 36 management traits. She found females saw themselves as more approachable, accessible, and cooperative than their male counterparts.

Kazlauskas (1993) specifically researched library faculty perceptions regarding department chairs' leadership practices. Surveying both non-supervisory and supervisory academic librarians regarding their supervisors, she excluded only the library directors. The research was limited to institutions in one state university system.

Bailey (1987) highlighted the need for more research regarding the leadership in library/information services, which chairs as middle managers, may provide. Sullivan (1992) observed the transition of the focus of participants in the ARL's Office of Management Services Library Management Skills Institute from the 1980s to the 1990s. Participants' focus shifted from management for the sake of advancement and higher salaries, to the desire to be effective as leaders in their new role. With the myriad of changes taking place in academic libraries, the role of the department head has been going through a time of transition (Bloss & Lanier, 1997). As we prepare for the transition of thousands of librarians to retirement (Curran, 2003), it is appropriate to look at the role our middle managers may play in the professional development, and vicariously the retention, within our ranks.

RESEARCH QUESTION

How the chair's role in enhancing the professional activities of faculty is perceived can have a profound effect upon the professional development of faculty. This is especially true of junior, not-yet-tenured faculty. Bensimon et al. (2000) noted that graduate programs (even doctoral programs) often do not do a good job of preparing or "socializing" students for the step into faculty positions and the accompanying requirements. Women and minorities are notably more vulnerable to this phenomenon. Beyond being a profession with a high percentage of women, Black and Leysen (2002) pointed to the brevity of the program of study for the MLS and the lack of requirements for a research thesis as factors making academic librarians even less prepared for their faculty roles. If these new library faculty members perceive the chair's role as one of a leader in assisting them, but the assistance is not forthcoming, the lack of leadership may lead to unfavorable tenure and promotion decisions for junior faculty.

As noted earlier, academic library middle managers and the librarians themselves have in the past considered professional development as an individual responsibility. Mitchell (1986) reported that the teaching department chairs in her initial sample indicated they believed the broader role of faculty development was "the professional obligation of the faculty themselves." More recently, McNeil (2004) broke development into three forms: staff development, "an organizational responsibility"; professional development, "a personal responsibility"; and career development, "the responsibility of both the individual and the library organization."

To determine perceptions regarding the department chair's role in enhancing the professional activities of faculty as held by not-yet-tenured library faculty, the question formulated for this research was: From the perspective of not-yet-tenured library faculty members, what are the methods department chairs should use in enhancing the professional activities of faculty?

METHODS

A survey instrument was developed which listed 27 methods department chairs may use in enhancing the professional activities of faculty. For the purpose of this study, "enhancing the professional activities of faculty" referred to activities, programs, and procedures which assist faculty in gaining knowledge, training, skills, attitudes, and insights that improve their ability to be more effective in their professional lives (Tucker, 1992, pp. 267–268; Wilhite, 1987, p. 6). The 27 methods were derived from studying the works of Boden (1994), Creswell and Brown (1992), Mitchell (1986), and Wilhite (1987). All of these works used qualitative research methods. All except Boden were studies of department chairpersons' perceptions. Boden's grounded theory study was of library faculty.

The survey instrument was distributed to all not-yet-tenured library faculty members at a land grant university in the mid-western United States. This audience was chosen because it met the criteria set out in the "Research Question" section and because of its accessibility to the researcher. The survey instrument included demographic information such as the respondents' gender, libraries department, years in the profession, years at the present institution, and educational level completed. Respondents were requested to rate each of the 27 methods a department chair might use in enhancing the professional activities of faculty based on a five-point scale. On the scale, "1" indicated the respondent felt the method was "unimportant," while a "5" indicated the method was "very important" (see Appendix A). Each of the 27 method statements was coded according to categories identified by Creswell (1991) as "practices chairs engage in in assisting faculty in their growth and development" (see Appendix B). This was done to assist any future comparisons of these methods for enhancing professional activities of non-teaching faculty to broader methods for enhancing the growth and development of teaching faculty.

The survey was distributed to 19 not-yet-tenured faculty members along with a cover letter requesting the faculty member's assistance in the research. Respondents were given one week to complete and return the survey instrument. Just prior to the deadline, an electronic mail message was sent to all possible respondents, thanking them for their response and reminding those who had not yet returned the survey instrument that they still could. This action did not result in any additional surveys being returned. Sixteen of the 19 distributed survey instruments were returned for an 84% return rate. The return rate by department varied from 67% to 100% (see Appendix C). Other tables in Appendix C show the other demographic information collected.

RESULTS

The data were first analyzed to determine the perceived importance the junior library faculty placed on each of the 27 methods chairs may use in enhancing the professional activities of faculty. Appendix D presents the rankings and mean scores of the items from the highest to the lowest ranked, or the items perceived as most important to least important. The category code is also listed for each statement. Five statements had means above four.

The methods perceived as most important were, "Provide resources to support professional activities of faculty," "Foster a professional atmosphere,
open to ideas and innovation, without fear of failure or punishment,"
"Provide ongoing feedback to faculty regarding their professional performance," "Acknowledge, compliment, and provide positive reinforcement for
good performance and accomplishments," and "Act as an advocate for
resources with the dean's office and higher administration." One method
emerged prominently as perceived as least important in the role of the department chair in enhancing the professional activities of faculty. That
method was "Spend time with faculty informally in social settings." The
rating was only 1.6875, with all other methods rated at least one full point
higher. Two other methods were rated below three. They were, "Encourage
faculty to collaborate with or assist the department head, or a senior faculty
member, on a project," and "Provide regular meetings for groups of faculty
to discuss ways to enhance faculty growth and development." The other 19
statements received ratings between 3.0 and 3.94. The overall mean for all
responses was 3.539.

Next, an analysis of the range of scores assigned to each method was
done. Four of the five top-ranked statements had no scores of "1" assigned
to them. In fact, for those four statements, a total of only two "2s" were
assigned. The lowest ranked statement received no scores above "3," and
almost half the respondents, seven of 16, gave it the lowest rating of "1," or
"unimportant." All but five of the other 22 statements received scores
ranging from either "1" to "4," or "1" to "5." Four of those five other
statements were in the top nine rated statements; however, they were subject
to one outlier which gave a "1" rating, while the rest rated the method from
"3" to "5."

Category Codes

In reviewing the category codes for each method statement as it relates to
the ranking of the statement, some interesting findings came to light. Four
of five statements with category codes of "001," identifying method statements where chairs would be "helping faculty develop and refine skills,"
were rated near the bottom on importance. The four statements were in the
bottom third of the rankings. The respondents in this research obviously see
these methods as less important than many of the other methods chairs may
use to enhance the professional activities of faculty. The means for the items,
however, were between 3.0 and 3.3 indicating faculty in this research did feel

the items were moderately important. One statement in this category code was ranked in the top ten. That method statement was "Lead by example – provide a role model" and had a mean score of 3.75. So, the non-teaching faculty, involved in this research, split the category on the basis of the individual method identified.

Splitting the statements, related to particular category codes, into different levels of importance, was the general rule with the results of this survey. Category code "002," "helping faculty relate to the organizational environment," with nine statements, finds three in the top third of the rankings, two in the middle third, and the remaining four statements in the bottom third of the rankings. Taking a look at the statements themselves, it seems the respondents perceive the chair's role more as one of an advocate promoting a professional atmosphere and encouraging and publicizing faculty activities. Less important are activities as an intermediary, or methods to promote interaction between colleagues.

Category code "004" for "relating to faculty personally" also shows a split in the rankings of the six method statements. Two are in the top third, three in the middle third, and the remaining statement is the lowest ranked item in the survey. Considering the statements in the top two-thirds with a mean of 3.3 or higher, we find the respondents desire a chair who is a good communicator. According to the statements, the chair should give positive reinforcement, keep faculty informed, be available, be a good listener, and show an interest in each faculty member. An activity the faculty in this research did not consider part of the role of the chair was informal social interaction with faculty.

The "003" category code for "helping faculty in an administrative capacity" received more consistent rankings. All seven statements are in the top two-thirds of the rankings, with means of 3.4 or above. The respondents obviously see providing resources, time, and input regarding professional performance, goals, organizational expectations; progress toward tenure and promotion; and sharing responsibilities, as important methods chairs should use in enhancing the professional activities of faculty.

Relationship to Existing Literature

The findings of this study were generally consistent with what was expected. Library faculty members, like their teaching counterparts, are most interested in growing professionally and obtaining tenure and promotion. Their perceptions of the role of the department chair are hopeful statements of a desire for support from the chairperson in obtaining those goals. Resources, academic freedom, feedback, positive reinforcement, supportive communication, and assistance are all high priorities as faculty look at actions they hope their department chair will undertake to help them enhance their professional activities.

Several activities chairs may undertake to enhance faculty members' professional activities are identified in the literature and have been outlined in the foregoing. The respondents to this survey supported the importance of these functions of the chair as well. Most notable activities, noted in the literature for years and ranked in the top third by respondents in this research, were "encourages faculty to participate in conventions, conferences, professional associations, etc." (Smith, 1972), "commending achievement" (Moses, 1985), and "maintaining a spirit of inquiry and academic freedom" (McLaughlin et al., 1975). The statements on the survey corresponding to these were numbers seven, eight, and twenty-three.

The most interesting aspects of the results of this research project were the three lowest rated method statements. The existing literature suggests the chair should have a role in assisting faculty to collaborate with senior faculty or with the chair on research projects, proposal development, publications, and the like (Creswell & Brown, 1992; Mitchell, 1986, p. 136; Seagren et al., 1986; Wilhite, 1987, p. 93). Yet, this group of respondents gave that method of enhancing the professional activities of faculty a rating placing it at 25th of the 27 methods, and a mean noting the method as less than moderately important. Perhaps this is due simply to the perception that other methods are of higher importance or, as some of the literature has suggested; perhaps these library faculty members consider this sort of activity their own individual responsibility.

The 26th rated of the 27 method statements involved providing regular meetings for faculty to discuss ways to enhance faculty growth and development. This relates to the concept of the department as a "community of scholars" (Seagren et al., 1986). Considering the context of the university libraries at the institution at the time of the survey, giving such a low rating to the possibility of more meetings may be understandable. The public services division was undergoing a multi-part analysis, while technical services were analyzing workflow issues, all in preparation for the Academic Program Review. Many meetings were being held and had been held for several months. More meetings, no matter how desirable their purpose, may have been perceived as undesirable.

The lowest ranked method a chair might use to enhance the professional activities of faculty, "Spend time with faculty informally in social settings," received a mean score indicating the method was not even "slightly important." Some research on chairs' perceptions of their role have noted that chairs perceive part of their role as handling social events for the department (Mitchell, 1986, p. 138) or informally spending time with faculty as part of an encouraging role (Creswell & Brown, 1992). Bensimon et al. (2000, pp. 49–50) noted how welcoming social gatherings and just being individually introduced to colleagues, can be for new faculty. It seems, the library faculty respondents to this survey perceived little need or desire for chairs to fulfill such a role.

SUMMARY

Much research exists regarding perceptions of the overall role of the department chair. Research has been done on academic, teaching department chairs from the perspectives of the chairs themselves, higher administrators, and faculty. More recently, research has been done on chairs' perceptions of their role in faculty growth and professional development. This research project sought to strike out in a new area in two ways: (1) the research addressed faculty perceptions of the chair's role in faculty development; and (2) the faculty members studied were in non-teaching departments in a university library setting. Also, the survey subjects were junior, not-yet-tenured library faculty members. Because faculty development often includes a teaching component, the title for the role studied was changed to "enhancing the professional activities of faculty" and a definition developed for that role.

A survey instrument designed for the study included five questions of a demographic nature and 27 statements of methods department chairs may use in enhancing the professional activities of faculty. Respondents rated each statement on a five-point scale. The respondents to the survey indicated they considered most methods outlined in the qualitative research on chairs' perceptions of the chairperson's role in faculty development moderately to very important in enhancing their professional activities.

Thoughts and Recommendations

As academic libraries look toward the future and the transition to new generations of library professionals, recruitment, socialization, acculturation, retention, development, support, and continuing revitalization will remain important. Academic library department chairs will play an important role in just how smooth that transition will be. This research has shown junior, not-yet-tenured library faculty members believe their chairs have a role in enhancing their professional development activities.

Further research regarding library faculty/academic librarians,' academic library department chairs,' and top academic library administrators' (deans or directors) perceptions of the department chair's role in professional development is needed. Perceptions of faculty beyond the junior, not-yet-tenured should be researched. Perceptions across other levels of post-secondary institutions, and across different types and sizes of institutions and libraries, should be researched as well. Research regarding possible effects of differences in the professional librarian's status on the perceptions of the professional development role of the department chair should be undertaken. For academic library department chairs to function well in support of their faculty's development activities, they must have the support of the library administration. Determination of academic library administrators' views, as well as those of the chairs themselves, regarding appropriate activities of middle level managers' in support of their faculty will advance understanding between the groups.

Over the years, library literature has contained several articles regarding mentoring. Articles regarding mentoring have focused on mentoring to develop leaders in the ranks (Cargill, 1989), chairs or higher administrators mentoring their supervisees (Fulton, 1990) or information from leaders on the mentors who impacted them (McNeer, 1988; Sheldon, 1991). More recently, there has been a shift toward general articles, or sections of articles, on mentoring with a broader focus on supporting junior faculty, guiding career development, encouraging less experienced colleagues, advising down the tenure track, retaining competent librarians, and leaders will emerge (Keyse, Kraemer, & Voelck, 2003; Martorana, Schroeder, Snowhill, & Duda, 2004; Mavrinac, 2005; Mosley, 2005; Tysick & Babb, 2006).

While many have asserted that the mentor should not be the mentee's supervisor, there are cases, including this author's, of success in opposition to that rule. In several cases, recommendations for support of mentoring includes provision of funding, travel, and release time (Keyse et al., 2003). Often it is the chairperson who informs, encourages, or plans with the faculty member regarding the activity and approves, or recommends, such activities to the higher administration. This research survey included such actions, as well as others developed from the broad department chair literature, in the 27 statements of methods department chairs may use in enhancing the professional activities of faculty.

Chairs of teaching departments have been accepted as being in a position to assist their faculty's development. Perceptions of the chair's role from the faculty's, the chair's, and higher administrators' viewpoints, and across a variety of institutional settings, have been the subject of research for decades. This research expanded the small amount of similar research that has begun regarding department chairs in academic libraries. The academic library department chairs must act as more than managers and supervisors of personnel. Library faculty, like their teaching department counterparts, should be able to view their chair as interested in the development of their faculty. The department chairs must step up and not leave their faculty to fend for themselves in these important matters. Rather, they should communicate expectations, actively mentor, and take a leadership role to support not only new faculty, but all faculty members in their department, and provide the best opportunity for their institutional success and continued professional growth throughout their careers. Professionals striving to meet the ever-changing information needs of their colleagues across the academic community deserve nothing less.

REFERENCES

ALISE Library and Information Science Education Statistical Report. (1991, 1996, 2000, 2003). Table II-8-a. Retrieved February 17, 2006 from the World Wide Web: http://ils.unc.edu/ALISE/2003/Students/Table%20II-8-a.htm.

Association of College and Research Libraries Committee on the Status of Academic Librarians. (2001). Faculty status and collective bargaining statements: Final versions. *College and Research Libraries News, 62*(3), 304–306.

Bailey, M. J. (1976, January). Some effects of faculty status on supervision in academic libraries. *College and Research Libraries, 37*, 48–52.

Bailey, M. J. (1978, September). Requirements for middle managerial positions. *Special Libraries, 69*, 323–331.

Bailey, M. J. (1981). *Supervisory and middle managers in libraries*. Metuchen, NJ: Scarecrow Press.

Bailey, M. J. (1987, September). Middle managers in libraries/information services. *Library Administration and Management, 1*, 139–142.

Bailey, M. J., & Murphy, M. (1989). Management competencies of middle managers in large academic research libraries. Paper presented at the 5th National Conference of the Association of College and Research Libraries, Cincinnati, OH. (ERIC Document Reproduction Service No. ED 314 061.)

Baldwin, R. G. (1990). Faculty career stages and implications for professional development. In: J. H. Schuster, D. W. Wheeler, & Associates (Eds), *Enhancing faculty careers: Strategies for development and renewal* (pp. 20–40). San Francisco: Jossey-Bass.

Bensimon, E. M., Ward, K. A., & Sanders, K. (2000). *The department chair's role in developing new faculty into teachers and scholars*. Bolton, MA: Anker Publishing.

Bergquist, W. H., & Phillips, S. R. (1975). *A handbook for faculty development*, Vol. 1. Washington, DC: Council for the Advancement of Small Colleges.

Black, W. K., & Leysen, J. M. (2002). Fostering success: The socialization of entry-level librarians in ARL libraries. *Journal of Library Administration, 36*(4), 3–26.

Bland, C., & Schmitz, C. C. (1988). Faculty vitality on review: Retrospect and prospect. *Journal of Higher Education, 59*(2), 190–224.

Bland, C. J., & Schmitz, C. C. (1990a). An overview of research on faculty and institutional vitality. In: J. H. Schuster, D. W. Wheeler, & Associates (Eds), *Enhancing faculty careers: Strategies for development and renewal* (pp. 41–61). San Francisco: Jossey-Bass.

Bland, C. J., & Schmitz, C. C. (1990b). A guide to the literature on faculty development. In: J. H. Schuster, D. W. Wheeler, & Associates (Eds), *Enhancing faculty careers: Strategies for development and renewal* (pp. 298–328). San Francisco: Jossey-Bass.

Bloss, A., & Lanier, D. (1997). The library department head in the context of matrix management and reengineering. *College and Research Libraries, 58*(6), 499–508.

Boden, D. W. R. (1994). A university libraries faculty perspective on the role of the department head in faculty performance: A grounded theory approach. Revised. (ERIC Document Reproduction Service No. ED 377 758.)

Boice, R. (1992). *The new faculty member: Supporting and fostering professional development*. San Francisco: Jossey-Bass.

Boice, R. (2000). *Advice for new faculty members: Nihil nimus*. Boston: Allyn and Bacon.

Boice, R., Scepanski, J. M., & Wilson, W. (1987). Librarians and faculty members: Coping with pressures to publish. *College and Research Libraries, 48*(6), 494–503.

Cargill, J. (1989). Developing library leaders: The role of mentorship. *Library Administration and Management, 3*(Winter), 12–15.

Carver, D. A. (2005). Should librarians get tenure? No, it can hamper their roles. *The Chronicle of Higher Education, 52*(6), B10. Retrieved February 17, 2006 from the World Wide Web: http://chronicle.com/free/v52/i06/06b01002.htm.

Cary, S. (2001). Faculty rank, status, and tenure for librarians: Current trends. *College and Research Libraries News, 62*(5), 510–511, 520.

Coats, L. T., Lovell, N. B., & Franks, M. E. (1996). FIRO B: Analyzing community college department chairs' effectiveness. Paper presented at the Southeastern Association for Community College Research Conference, Panama City, FL. (ERIC Document Reproduction Service No. ED 406 999.)

Cohen, W. D., Bleha, B., & Olswang, S. G. (1981). Administrative roles and perceptions of governance in the community college. *Community/Junior College Research Quarterly, 5*, 303–321.

Comes, J. F. (1978/1979). Relationships between leadership behavior and goal attainment in selected academic libraries (Doctoral dissertation, Ball State University, 1978). *Dissertation Abstracts International, 39*(10), 5782A (UMI No. 7905229).

Creswell, J. W. (1991). [Codes, categories, and illustrations: Practices chairs engage in assisting faculty in their growth and development]. Unpublished raw data.

Creswell, J. W., & Brown, M. L. (1992). How chairpersons enhance faculty research: A grounded theory study. *The Review of Higher Education, 16*(1), 41–62.

Creswell, J. W., Wheeler, D. W., Seagren, A. T., Egly, N. J., & Beyer, K. D. (1990). *The academic chairperson's handbook*. Lincoln, NE: University of Nebraska Press.

Curran, W. M. (2003). Succession: The next ones at bat. *College & Research Libraries, 64*(2), 134–140.

Curtis, J. W. (2004). American Association of University Professors. Faculty Salary and Faculty Distribution Fact Sheet 2003–04. Retrieved February 17, 2006 from the World Wide Web: http://www.aaup.org/Issues/WomeninHE/sal&distribution.htm.

Daly, F., & Townsend, B. K. (1992). Faculty perceptions of the department chair's role in facilitating tenure acquisition. Paper presented at the annual meeting of the Association for the Study of Higher Education, Minneapolis, MN. (ERIC Document Reproduction Service No. ED 352 912.)

Daly, F., & Townsend, B. K. (1994). The chair's role in tenure acquisition. *The NEA Higher Education Journal: Thought and Action, 9*(2), 125–145.

Eble, K. E. (1986). Chairpersons and faculty development. *The Department Adviser, 1*(4), 1–5.

Eble, K. E. (1990). Chairpersons and faculty development. In: J. B. Bennett & D. J. Figuli (Eds), *Enhancing departmental leadership: The roles of the chairperson* (pp. 99–106). New York: American Council on Education.

Eble, K. E., & McKeachie, W. J. (1985). *Improving undergraduate education through faculty development: An analysis of effective programs and practices.* San Francisco: Jossey-Bass.

Evans, G. E., & Ward, P. L. (2003). *Beyond the basics: The management guide for library and information professionals.* New York: Neal-Schuman.

Falk, G. (1979). The academic department chairmanship and role conflict. *Improving College and University Teaching, 27*(2), 79–86.

Fulton, T. L. (1990). Mentor meets Telemachus: The role of the department head in orienting and inducting the beginning reference librarian. In: B. Katz (Ed.), *Continuing education of reference librarians. The reference librarian* (Vol. 30, pp. 257–273). New York: The Haworth Press.

Gaff, J. G. (1975). *Toward faculty renewal: Advances in faculty, instructional, and organizational development.* San Francisco: Jossey-Bass.

Giesecke, J. (Ed.) (1992). *Practical help for new supervisors,* (2nd ed). Chicago: American Library Association.

Giesecke, J. (Ed.) (1997). *Practical help for new supervisors,* (3rd ed). Chicago: American Library Association.

Giesecke, J. (2001). *Practical strategies for library managers.* Chicago: American Library Association.

Giesecke, J., & McNeil, B. (2005). *Fundamentals of library supervision* (ALA Fundamentals Series). Chicago: American Library Association.

Gmelch, W. H., & Miskin, V. D. (1993). *Leadership skills for department chairs.* Bolton, MA: Anker Publishing.

Gmelch, W. H., & Miskin, V. D. (1995). *Survival skills for scholars: Vol. 15. Chairing an academic department.* Thousand Oaks, CA: Sage Publications.

Gordon, B. G., Stockard, J. W., Jr., & Williford, H. N. (1991). The perceived and expected roles and responsibilities of departmental chairpersons in schools of education as determined by teaching faculty. *Education, 112*(2), 176–182.

Gordon, R. S. (2005). *The accidental library manager.* Medford, NJ: Information Today.

Group for Human Development in Higher Education. (1974). *Faculty development in a time of retrenchment.* New Rochelle, NY: Change.

Hecht, I. W. D., Higgerson, M. L., Gmelch, W. H., & Tucker, A. (1999). *The department chair as academic leader* (Oryx Press series on higher education). Phoenix, AZ: American Council on Education.

Heimler, C. H. (1967). The college departmental chairman. *Educational Record, 48,* 158–163.

Hill, J. S. (2005). Constant vigilance, babelfish, and foot surgery: Perspectives on faculty status and tenure for academic librarians. *portal: Libraries and the Academy, 5*(1), 7–22.

Hirokawa, R. Y., Barge, J. K., Becker, S. L., & Sutherland, J. L. (1989). The department chair as responsible academic leader: A competency-based perspective. *ACA Bulletin, 67,* 8–19.

Jeffrey, R. C. (1985, April). A dean interprets the roles and powers of an ideal chair. *Association for Communication Administration Bulletin, 52,* 15–16.

Jennerich, E. J. (1981). Competencies for department chairpersons: Myths and realities. *Liberal Education, 67*(1), 46–70.

Jones, D. R., & Holdaway, E. A. (1995). Expectations held for department heads in postsecondary institutions. *The Alberta Journal of Educational Research, 41*(2), 188–212.

Kazlauskas, D. W. (1993). Leadership practices and employee job satisfaction in the academic libraries of the state university system of Florida (Doctoral dissertation, University of Florida, 1993). *Dissertation Abstracts International, 55*(10), 3053A (UMI No. 9505669).

Kenny, S. S. (1982). Three views of the chair: Perspectives of the department members, the dean, and the chairperson. *ADE Bulletin, 73*(Winter), 33–37.

Keyse, D., Kraemer, E. W., & Voelck, J. (2003). Mentoring untenured librarians: All it takes is a little Un-TLC. *College & Research Libraries News, 64*(6), 378–380.

Knight, P. T., & Trowler, P. R. (2001). *Departmental leadership in higher education.* Buckingham, UK: Society for Research into Higher Education and Open University Press.

Knight, W. H., & Holen, M. C. (1985). Leadership and the perceived effectiveness of department chairpersons. *Journal of Higher Education, 56*(6), 677–690.

Kremer-Hayon, L., & Avi-Itzhak, T. E. (1986). Roles of academic department chairpersons at the university level: Perceptions and satisfaction. *Higher Education, 15,* 105–112.

Kroll, S. (1994). *Academic status: Statements and resources* (2nd ed). Chicago: Association of College and Research Libraries, American Library Association.

Krompart, J. (1994). A bibliographic essay on faculty status for academic librarians. In: S. Kroll (Ed.), *Academic status: Statements and resources,* (2nd ed.) (pp. 29–38). Chicago: Association of College and Research Libraries, American Library Association.

Kyrillidou, M., & Young, M. (2005a). *ARL Annual Salary Survey 2004–05.* Washington, DC: Association of Research Libraries. Retrieved February 17, 2006 from the World Wide Web: http://www.arl.org/stats/pubpdf/ss04.pdf.

Kyrillidou, M., & Young, M. (2005b). *ARL statistics 2003–04: A compilation of statistics from the one hundred and twenty-three members of the Association of Research Libraries.* Washington, DC: Association of Research Libraries. Retrieved February 17, 2006 from the World Wide Web: http://www.arl.org/stats/pubpdf/arlstat04.pdf.

Leaming, D. R. (1998). *Academic leadership: A practical guide to chairing the department.* Bolton, MA: Anker Publishing.

Lee, D. E. (1985). Department chairpersons' perceptions of the role in three institutions. *Perceptual and Motor Skills, 61,* 23–49.

Leysen, J. M., & Black, W. K. (1998). Peer review in Carnegie Research libraries. *College & Research Libraries, 59*(6), 512–522.

Licata, C. M. (2000). Post-tenure review. In: A. F. Lucas & Associates (Eds), *Leading academic change: Essential roles for department chairs* (pp. 107–137). (The Jossey-Bass higher education series). San Francisco: Jossey-Bass.

Lowry, C. B. (1993). Research notes: The status of faculty status for academic librarians: A twenty-year perspective. *College & Research Libraries, 54*(2), 163–172.

Lucas, A. F. & Associates (2000). *Leading academic change: Essential roles for department chairs* (The Jossey-Bass higher education series). San Francisco: Jossey-Bass.

Martorana, J., Schroeder, E., Snowhill, L., & Duda, A. L. (2004). A focus on mentorship in career development. *Library Administration & Management, 18*(4), 198–202.

Mavrinac, M. A. (2005). Transformational leadership: Peer mentoring as a values-based learning process. *portal: Libraries and the Academy, 5*(3), 391–404.

McAnally, A. M. (1975). Status of the university librarian in the academic community. In: Association of College and Research Libraries Committee on the Status of Academic Librarians, *Faculty status for academic librarians: A history and policy statements* (pp. 1–30). Chicago: American Library Association.

McKeachie, W. J. (1990). Tactics and strategies for faculty development. In: J. B. Bennett & D. J. Figuli (Eds), *Enhancing departmental leadership: The roles of the chairperson* (pp. 107–114). New York: American Council on Education.

McLaughlin, G. W., Montgomery, J. R., & Malpass, L. F. (1975). Selected characteristics, roles, goals, and satisfactions of department chairmen in state and land-grant institutions. *Research in Higher Education, 3*, 243–259.

McNeer, E. J. (1988). The mentoring influence in the careers of women ARL directors. *Journal of Library Administration, 9*(2), 23–33.

McNeil, B. (2004). Managing work performance and career development. In: J. Simmons-Welburn, B. McNeil (Eds), *Human resource management in today's academic library: Meeting challenges and creating opportunities* (Libraries Unlimited library management collection). Westport, CT: Libraries Unlimited.

Mech, T., & McCabe, G. B. (Eds). (1998). *Leadership and academic librarians* (Greenwood library management collection). Westport, CT: Greenwood.

Miles, B. W. (1983). Trials and tribulations of the academic chair. *Journal of the College and University Personnel Association, 34*(4), 11–15.

Mitchell, E. S. (1989). The library leadership project: A test of leadership effectiveness in academic libraries. In: G. B. McCabe, & B. Kreissman (Eds), *Advances in library administration and organization* (Vol. 8, pp. 25–38). Greenwich, CT: JAI Press.

Mitchell, M. B. (1986). Department chairperson management strategies: Enhancing faculty performance and work satisfaction (Doctoral dissertation, University of Nebraska, 1986). *Dissertation Abstracts International, 47*(11), 3995A (UMI No. 8706240).

Moses, I. (1985). The role of head of department in the pursuit of excellence. *Higher Education, 14*, 337–354.

Mosley, P. A. (2005). Mentoring gen x managers: Tomorrow's library leadership is already here. *Library Administration & Management, 19*(4), 185–192.

Moxley, J. M., & Olson, G. A. (1990). The English chair: Scholar or bureaucrat? *The NEA Higher Education Journal: Thought and Action, 6*(1), 51–58.

Murray-Rust, C. (2005). Should librarians get tenure? Yes, it's crucial to their jobs. *The Chronicle of Higher Education, 52*(6), B10. Retrieved February 17, 2006 from the World Wide Web: http://chronicle.com/free/v52/i06/06b01001.htm.

Neumann, L., & Neumann, Y. (1983). Faculty perceptions of deans' and department chairpersons' management functions. *Higher Education, 12*, 205–214.

Olive, J. F., III (1991). Leadership styles of selected academic library department heads as perceived by self and subordinates (Doctoral dissertation, University of Alabama, 1991). *Dissertation Abstracts International, 52*(7), 2430A (UMI No. 9201175).

Person, R. J. (1980). Middle managers in academic and public libraries: Managerial role concepts (Doctoral dissertation, University of Michigan, 1980). *Dissertation Abstracts International, 41*(5), 1820A (UMI No. 8025745).

Plate, K. H. (1970). *Management personnel in libraries: A theoretical model for analysis.* Rockaway, NJ: American Faculty Press.

Pugh, L. (2005). *Managing 21st century libraries.* Lanham, MD: Scarecrow.

Roach, J. H. L. (1976). The academic department chairperson: Functions and responsibilities. *Educational Record, 57*(1), 13–23.

Ruess, D. E. (2004). Faculty and professional appointments of academic librarians: Expanding the options for choice. *portal: Libraries and the Academy, 4*(1), 75–84.

Scott, J. H. (1990). Role of community college department chairs in faculty development. *Community College Review, 18*(3), 12–16.

Seagren, A. T., Creswell, J. W., & Wheeler, D. W. (1993). *The department chair: New roles, responsibilities and challenges.* (ASHE-ERIC Higher Education Report: No. 1.) Washington, DC: The George Washington University, School of Education and Human Development.

Seagren, A. T., Wheeler, D. W., Creswell, J. W., Miller, M. T., & VanHorn-Grassmeyer, K. (1994). *Academic leadership in community colleges.* Lincoln, NE: University of Nebraska Press.

Seagren, A. T., Wheeler, D. W., Mitchell, M. B., & Creswell, J. W. (1986). Perception of chairpersons and faculty concerning roles descriptors and activities important for faculty development and departmental vitality. (ERIC Document Reproduction Service No. ED 276 387.)

Sheldon, B. E. (1991). *Leaders in libraries: Styles and strategies for success.* Chicago: American Library Association.

Siever, R. G., Loomis, R. J., & Neidt, C. O. (1972). Role perceptions of department chairmen in two land grant universities. *The Journal of Educational Research, 65*(9), 405–410.

Simmons-Welburn, J., & McNeil, B. (Eds). (2004). *Human resource management in today's academic library: Meeting challenges and creating opportunities* (Libraries Unlimited library management collection). Westport, CT: Libraries Unlimited.

Smart, J. C. (1976). Duties performed by department chairmen in Holland's model environments. *Journal of Educational Psychology, 68*(2), 194–204.

Smith, A. B. (1972). Department chairmen: Neither fish nor fowl. *Junior College Journal, 42*(6), 40–43.

Sorcinelli, M. D. (1990). Development of new faculty. *The Department Chair, 1*(2), 9.

Sparks, R. (1976). Library management: Consideration and structure. *Journal of Academic Librarianship, 2*(2), 66–71.

Stone, E. W. (1969). *Factors related to the professional development of librarians.* Metuchen, NJ: Scarecrow.

Sullivan, M. (1992). The changing role of the middle manager in research libraries. *Library Trends, 41*(2), 269–281.

Thompson, H. L. (1990). The department chairperson: An academic leader. *The Department Chair, 1*(2), 16–17, 19.

Tucker, A. (1992). *Chairing the academic department: Leadership among peers* (3rd ed). New York: American Council on Education.

Tysick, C., & Babb, N. (2006). Perspectives on ... Writing support for junior faculty librarians: A case study. *The Journal of Academic Librarianship, 32*(1), 94–100.

Voelck, J. (2003). Directive and connective: Gender-based differences in the management styles of academic library managers. *portal: Libraries and the Academy, 3*(3), 393–418.

Watson, R. E. L. (1979). The role of the department head or chairman: Discipline, sex and nationality as factors influencing faculty opinion. *The Canadian Journal of Higher Education, 9*(3), 19–28.

Watson, R. E. L. (1986). The role of the department chair: A replication and extension. *The Canadian Journal of Higher Education, 16*(1), 13–23.

Weinberg, S. S. (1984). The perceived responsibilities of the departmental chairperson: A note of a preliminary study. *Higher Education, 13*, 301–303.

Wheeler, D. W. (1992). The role of the chairperson in support of junior faculty. In: Sorcinelli, M. D., & Austin, A. E. (Eds), *Developing new and junior faculty. New Directions for Teaching and Learning* (Vol. 50, pp. 87–96). San Francisco: Jossey-Bass.

Whitt, E. J. (1991). "Hit the ground running": Experiences of new faculty in a school of education. *The Review of Higher Education, 14*(2), 177–197.

Wilhite, M. S. (1987). Department chairperson behaviors: Enhancing the growth and development of faculty (Doctoral dissertation, University of Nebraska, Lincoln, 1987). *Dissertation Abstracts International, 48*(7), 1620A (UMI No. 8722425).

Wilhite, M. S. (1990). Practices used by effective department chairs to enhance growth and development of faculty. *NACTA Journal, 34*(2), 17–20.

Wittenbach, S. A., Bordeianu, S. M., & Wycisk, K. (1992). Management preparation and training of department heads in ARL libraries. *College & Research Libraries, 53*(4), 319–330.

APPENDIX A. SURVEY OF FACULTY PERCEPTIONS OF THE ROLE OF THE DEPARTMENT HEAD IN ENHANCING THE PROFESSIONAL ACTIVITIES OF FACULTY

Demographic Information:
Please mark the correct answer with an "X."

a. Your Gender: (1) Female _____   (2) Male _____
b. Your Department:
(1) Reference Services _____
(2) Branch Services _____
(3) General Services _____
(4) Cataloging _____
(5) Serials Cataloging _____
c. Years in the Library Profession:
(1) 1–3 _____   (2) 4–5 _____
(3) 6–10 _____   (4) 11–15 _____
(5) 16+ _____
d. Time at Institution:
(1) Up to 1 year   (2) 1–2 years _____

_____
(3) 2–3 years _____   (4) 3–4 years _____
(5) 4–5 years _____   (6) More than 5 years _____
e. Education Completed:
(1) MLS _____
(2) MLS and additional coursework _____
(3) MLS and 2nd Masters degree _____
(4) MLS, 2nd Masters and additional coursework _____

Survey Statements:
    For the purpose of this study, "enhancing the professional activities of faculty" refers to activities, programs, and procedures which assist faculty in gaining knowledge, training, skills, attitudes, and insights that improve their ability to be more effective in their professional lives.
    Listed below are some methods a department chair may use in enhancing the professional activities of faculty. Please read each method and circle the

number reflecting how important you believe that method is in enhancing the professional activities of faculty.

Please rate the items based on the following five-point scale:

(1: Unimportant, 2: Slightly Important, 3: Moderately Important, 4: Important, 5: Very Important)

1.	Keep faculty informed of opportunities to participate in professional activities. (004)	1	2	3	4	5
2.	Maintain an "open door policy" so faculty can speak with her/him at any time. (004)	1	2	3	4	5
3.	Monitor faculty progress toward tenure and promotion. (0031)	1	2	3	4	5
4.	Provide ongoing feedback to faculty regarding their professional performance. (0031)	1	2	3	4	5
5.	Act as an intermediary for the faculty with the dean's office and higher administration. (002)	1	2	3	4	5
6.	Provide resources to support professional activities of faculty (funding, travel, release time, staff support, etc.). (0034)	1	2	3	4	5
7.	Encourage participation in professional peer groups at the local, state, regional, national level (committees, conferences,	1	2	3	4	5

	publishing, research, etc.). (002)					
8.	Acknowledge, compliment, and provide positive reinforcement for good performance and accomplishments. (004)	1	2	3	4	5
9.	Publicize faculty accomplishments to administrators, fellow faculty, and peer groups. (002)	1	2	3	4	5
10.	Lead by example—provide a role model. (001)	1	2	3	4	5
11.	Delegate responsibility for projects to faculty to provide growth through more and more responsible activities. (003)	1	2	3	4	5
12.	Act as an advocate by assisting faculty in getting involved in professional organizations and activities (name dropping, nominating, recommending, etc.). (002)	1	2	3	4	5
13.	Share advice, wisdom, experience, and expertise regarding carrying out professional activities. (001)	1	2	3	4	5
14.	Communicate the professional expectations of the	1	2	3	4	5

organization
(department, unit,
institution) to the
faculty. (003)

		1	2	3	4	5
15.	Help relieve pressures and stress by reducing workload to provide time for faculty to initiate research and serve on visible committees. (0033)	1	2	3	4	5
16.	Encourage faculty to collaborate with, or assist, the department head, or a senior faculty member, on a project. (002)	1	2	3	4	5
17.	Assist faculty, in setting realistic, professional goals and priorities. (0031)	1	2	3	4	5
18.	Refer faculty to workshops, centers, or training courses for improving, or providing support for, their capabilities for growth and development. (001)	1	2	3	4	5
19.	Show a personal, individual interest in faculty member's growth and development activities. (004)	1	2	3	4	5
20.	Provide regular meetings for groups of faculty to discuss ways to enhance faculty growth and development. (002)	1	2	3	4	5

21.	Encourage faculty participation in campus-wide activities and committees. (002)	1	2	3	4	5
22.	Be a good listener. (004)	1	2	3	4	5
23.	Foster a professional atmosphere, open to ideas and innovation without fear of failure or punishment. (002)	1	2	3	4	5
24.	Act as an advocate for resources with the dean's office and higher administration. (002)	1	2	3	4	5
25.	Help faculty to identify an area of expertise. (001)	1	2	3	4	5
26.	Spend time with faculty informally in social settings. (004)	1	2	3	4	5
27.	Support in-house staff development activities (instruction, training, workshops, presentations, etc.). (001)	1	2	3	4	5

Thank you for completing this survey. Please fold it with the address out, staple it, and place it in the Libraries delivery.

Remember to return the completed survey by the date requested.THANK YOU.

APPENDIX B. CODES, CATEGORIES, AND ILLUSTRATIONS – PRACTICES CHAIRS ENGAGE IN ASSISTING FACULTY IN THEIR GROWTH AND DEVELOPMENT

Content Analysis Project
Categories Findings

001   Helping faculty develop and refine skills:
-in teaching (modeling, mentoring, critiquing teaching);
-in research (modeling, help choose areas, create teams, specialities);
-through staff development activities (in-house training, speakers, meetings, attend workshops).

002   Helping faculty relate to the organizational environment.
Advocate and promote the needs of faculty: externally, enhance faculty leadership (national visibility, professional associations, off campus networks) and internally, with individuals on campus, mediate for faculty with deans the interpersonal environment (faculty to faculty, faculty to staff), the departmental environment (atmosphere, openness, friendliness).

003   Helping faculty in an administrative capacity.

0031   Evaluating faculty performance (related to the department and institution – set goals, prioritize goals; related to the individual – goal planning, student evaluations, annual appraisals, feedback; related to faculty careers – promotion and tenure)

0032   Planning the long-range needs of the department: departmental/institutional planning—goal setting, evaluation, prioritization; individual planning (goal setting, evaluation).

0033   Schedule adjustments in assignments (released time workloads and assignments).

0034   Providing material and financial resources (funds—travel, secretarial assistance, in-house, outside); equipment (laboratory, computers, materials); information (grants opportunity flyers, journals).

APPENDIX C

Table C1. Return Rate by Department.

	Department				
	A	B	C	D	E
Total distributed	8	3	2	4	2
Number of respondents	7	2	2	3	2
Percentage	87.5	66.7	100	75	100

Table C2. Gender of Respondents.

	Gender	
	Males	Females
Number of respondents	6	10

Table C3. Years in the Profession.

	Years in Profession				
	1–3	4–5	6–10	11–15	16+
Number of respondents	5	2	2	4	3

Table C4. Years at Present Institution.

	Years at Institution					
	0–1	1–2	2–3	3–4	4–5	5+
Number of respondents	2	3	4	4	1	2

Table C5. Educational Level of Respondents.

	Education			
	MLS	MLS+	2nd Masters	2nd Masters+
Number of respondents	2	9	3	2

APPENDIX D

Rank	Statement	Mean Score	Category Code
1	Provide resources to support professional activities of faculty.	4.625	0034
2	Foster a professional atmosphere, open to ideas and innovation without fear of failure or punishment.	4.25	002
3	Provide ongoing feedback to faculty regarding their professional performance.	4.125	0031
4a	Acknowledge, compliment, and provide positive reinforcement for good performance and accomplishments.	4.0625	004
4b	Act as an advocate for resources with the dean's office and higher administration.	4.0625	002
6a	Encourage participation in professional peer groups at the local, state, regional, national level.	3.9375	002
6b	Help relieve pressures and stress by reducing workload to provide time for faculty to initiate research and serve on visible committees.	3.9375	0033

8	Monitor faculty progress toward tenure and promotion.	3.875	0031
9	Keep faculty informed of opportunities to participate in professional activities.	3.8125	004
10a	Lead by example—provide a role model.	3.75	001
10b	Communicate the professional expectations of the organization to the faculty.	3.75	003
12a	Delegate responsibility for projects to faculty to provide growth through more and more responsible activities.	3.6875	003
12b	Act as an advocate by assisting faculty in getting involved in professional organizations and activities.	3.6875	002
14a	Maintain an "open door policy" so faculty can speak with her/ him at any time.	3.625	004
14b	Be a good listener.	3.625	004
16	Publicize faculty accomplishments to administrators, fellow faculty, and peer groups.	3.5625	002
17	Assist faculty in setting realistic, professional goals and priorities.	3.4375	0031
18	Show a personal, individual interest in faculty member's growth and development activities.	3.375	004
19a	Act as an intermediary for the faculty with the dean's office and higher administration.	3.25	002
19b	Share advice, wisdom, experience, and expertise regarding carrying out professional activities.	3.25	001

19c	Encourage faculty participation in campus-wide activities and committees.	3.25	002
22	Support in-house staff development activities.	3.125	001
23a	Refer faculty to workshops, centers, or training courses for improving, or providing support for, their capability for growth and development.	3.0625	001
23b	Help faculty to identify an area of expertise.	3.0625	001
25	Encourage faculty to collaborate with, or assist, the department head, or a senior faculty member, on a project.	2.9375	002
26	Provide regular meetings for groups of faculty to discuss ways to enhance faculty growth and development.	2.75	002
27	Spend time with faculty informally in social settings.	1.6875	004

MENTORING REVISITED

Deonie Botha

ABSTRACT

Mentoring is a concept that originated between 800 and 700 BC and which is still in existence in organisations irrespective of size, nature of ownership, type of industry or geographic location. In its most primal form it is regarded as a method according to which a less experienced employee (protégé or mentee) is guided and advised by a more experienced and skilled employee (mentor) in terms of life as well as professional skills. However, this definition has developed over time as organisations applied mentoring in a more structured manner and institutionalised it within formal organisational processes. Mentoring was, therefore, regarded as a method to "systematically develop the skills and leadership abilities of less experienced members of the organization" (SPA Consultants, 1995, p. 14). Mentoring has been in use within the library and information science profession from the mid-1980s and various publications have discussed the use of mentoring from an American, Australian and British perspective. However, relatively few publications are available regarding the use of mentoring within the South African contexts, and therefore an extensive discussion on the implementation of a structured mentoring scheme at the National Library of South Africa (NLSA) is included in the article. This study draws particularly on recent literature on the knowledge economy and more specifically knowledge management to suggest ways in which the concept of mentoring should be revised. Mentoring should henceforth be seen as a knowledge management technique to support the creation and sharing of tacit knowledge rather

Advances in Library Administration and Organization, Volume 24, 151–189
Copyright © 2007 by Elsevier Ltd.
ISSN: 0732-0671/doi:10.1016/S0732-0671(06)24005-7

than merely a technique to develop less experienced individuals. This revised view of mentoring is of particular importance to ensure the sustainability of library and information service organisations in the knowledge economy.

INTRODUCTION

There are only a small number of concepts from the managerial sciences that have stood the test of time beyond any doubt. Concepts like business process engineering, the learning organisation, six sigma, business and competitive intelligence and, more recently, knowledge management are in abundance in management literature but are often viewed as fads rather than fact and whether they will continue to appear in the literature on management remains to be seen. Although it is beyond the scope of this article to deliberate on the merit of these concepts, they all seem to have had a fleeting moment of glory before they got "shelved" on the bookcase of many an executive, with more pressing managerial issues such as an ever shrinking budget or an unmotivated workforce to attend to. However, it seems as if there is one concept, which has had the ability to reinvent and transform itself and has survived three major revolutions, namely the industrial (1750–1880), production (1880–1945) and management revolutions (1945–) (Andriessen, 2004). The concept of mentoring not only has survived three revolutions but is also used by organisations, public or private, large or small, global or local, irrespective of the services they deliver or the products they manufacture.

Although various definitions are found in the literature, mentoring is regarded as a method of human resource development whereby a more experienced and usually senior staff member (mentor) takes responsibility for and becomes actively involved in the personal and/or professional development and empowerment of a less experienced and usually younger staff member (protégé or mentee). The development and empowerment of the protégé takes place within the context of a comprehensive and mutual relationship that evolves between the mentor and protégé. Such a relationship can evolve spontaneously and informally between two people and is then known as unstructured mentoring, but it can also evolve as part of a structured process implemented by an organisation to foster the development and empowerment of its human resources. The applicability and relevance of mentoring, irrespective of time period, geographic area, organisation or industry, are therefore ascribed to the fact that it is a highly adaptable technique for developing and empowering the human resources of an organisation.

Organisations can apply mentoring for different reasons. To some, mentoring is a means of identifying and developing human resources with the potential to move into management positions. To others it is a means of facilitating the induction of new human resources; it can also be applied to develop and empower human resources from previously disadvantaged groups and eventually bring them into the management structure. Irrespective of the reason(s) why mentoring was implemented, the value of this method of human resource development lies therein that it enables human resources to work more effectively and efficiently. It is therefore beneficial to the mentor, the protégé, the organisation and the profession in which the organisation is actively involved.

In this article, which is a position paper on the nature and scope of mentoring, the author examines and defines the concept of mentoring, both in general terms and in the context of the library and information science profession. The aim of the article is to discuss the use of mentoring in broad terms but specific emphasis is placed on the use of mentoring as a knowledge management technique in libraries and information services. This however necessitates an understanding of the dual function of libraries and information services in terms of information and knowledge. Information and knowledge not only are a product of libraries and information services, but also should be managed as a process within the context of libraries. Once libraries and information services have developed an understanding of this duality in terms of information and knowledge they will be able to make use of mentoring in its most recent manifestation, namely as a method to create new knowledge or to innovate and to share knowledge. This also explains the transformation of mentoring as a human resource development concept into a concept that is associated with information and knowledge management.

Although a variety of aspects regarding mentoring are discussed, emphasis is placed on mentoring as a knowledge management technique and the importance that libraries and information service have an understanding of the knowledge-based view of their human resources. The article includes a case study on the use of mentoring in the National Library of South Africa (NLSA). This discussion outlines the needs that prompted the implementation of such a process at the NLSA, the manner in which the process was implemented, and describes the results. The case study is included in the article due to the fact that in 1999 the author was responsible for launching a structured mentoring process at the NLSA in order to address the professional development and empowerment of the human resources of this national institution.

The origin of the mentoring process at the NLSA is ascribed to two factors, namely:

- The mentorship process was linked to the NLSA's employment equity programme, which revealed a need to accelerate the development of high-potential employees from previously disadvantaged groups.
- The author conducted empirical research for a Masters Degree in Information Science on the topic of mentoring as a method of human resource development in the context of the library and information science profession.

The NLSA's project was a groundbreaking exercise because the use of structured mentoring is a relatively uncommon method of staff development in the library and information science profession in South Africa.

DEFINING MENTORING

There is no single, generally accepted operational definition of mentoring. The definition of the term mentoring is therefore considered as vague and diverse and it has even been described as a definitional dilemma. However, for the purposes of this article, some definitions from the disciplines of management and organisational behaviour are quoted to explain what is implied by the concept of mentoring:

> Mentoring is defined as the growth of protégés with the primary purpose of systematically developing the skills and leadership abilities of less experienced members of the organization. (SPA Consultants, 1995, p. 14)

> Mentoring is the process by which the knowledge, skills and life experience of a selected, successful manager are transmitted to another employee in the organisational system, for the purpose of growing that employee for greater efficiency and effectiveness. (Nasser, 1987, p. 12)

> Mentoring is a special relationship within an organization. It extends only to a hand-picked few the counseling, role modeling, and interest that might benefit every motivated young employee. (Harris, 1993, p. 37)

> Mentoring deals with individuals who are mentors in terms of their overall life adjustment behavior in order to advise, counsel and/or guide mentees [protégés] with regard to problems that may be resolved by legal, scientific, clinical, spiritual and/or other professional principles. (Jesudason, 1997, p. 23)

Although mentoring is regarded as definitional vague, consensus exists on the manifestations thereof, namely structured or formal and unstructured or informal. This implies that a difference exists in the formality according to which the mentoring process is managed as well as the manner in which the mentoring relationship is maintained.

In the literature on the library and information science profession the term mentoring is rarely defined; even where it does exist, it often relates more to the management and organisational behavioural disciplines than specifically to library and information science, as the following definition of mentoring from the library and information science literature indicate:

> Mentoring is a special relationship within an organisation. It extends only to a hand-picked few the counseling, role modeling, and interest that might benefit every motivated young employee. (Harris, 1993, p. 37)

This explains why Golian and Galbraith (1996, p. 99) state that "no operational definition for mentoring currently exists within library science".

HISTORICAL OVERVIEW

The concept of mentoring is not new but, as previously indicated, it is still as relevant and applicable as it was many centuries ago. Mentoring originated in Greek mythology and the word "mentor" was first used by the Greek poet Homer in his epic poem the *Odyssey* between 800 and 700 BC. The saga of Mentor was continued in *Les Adventures de Telemaque* by Fénélon (Dreyer, 1995, p. 142). In both these tales Mentor was appointed to accompany Telemachos on his adventures in search of his father, King Odysseus. However, Mentor was more than merely escorting Telemachos, since he advised and prepared him for his role as future king of Ithaca. The relationship between Mentor and his protégé was of such a nature that it included the development of Telemachos in terms of both his personal as well as his professional competencies. This explains the origin of the word "mentor", which is synonymous with words such as trusted, wise and experienced adviser or even friend. Clawson (1985, p. 36) and Dreyer (1995, p. 42) are of the opinion that the type of relationship that existed between Mentor and Telemachos reappeared during the Middle Ages (500–1500) in the context of apprenticeships. Clutterbuck (1991, p. 1) explains:

> In the days when the guilds ruled the commercial world, the road to the top in business began in an early apprenticeship to the master craftsmen, a trader, or a ship's captain. This older, more experienced, individual passed down his knowledge of how the task was

done and how to operate in the commercial world. Intimate personal relationships
frequently developed between the master (or mentor) and the apprentice.

Although Carrell et al. (1997, p. 320) states that: "Informal mentoring relationships seem to have always existed" the origin of both unstructured and
structured mentoring can be traced back to the relationship between Mentor
and Telemachos as described in the *Odyssey* by Homer and *Les Adventures
de Telemaque* by Fénélon. The relationship between Mentor and Telemachos is regarded as the first manifestation of unstructured mentoring based
on the following characteristics:

1. The mentoring relationship did not originate and was not maintained
   within a clearly defined contextual environment.
2. There were no predetermined aims and objectives that had to be achieved
   in order for the mentoring relationship to be regarded as effective.
3. The mentoring relationship did not develop according to a particular
   structure, and the extent and nature thereof was spontaneous and informal.
4. The participants in the mentoring relationship were limited to the mentor
   and the protégé.

The unstructured or informal approach towards mentoring has continued
to exist through time and characteristics thereof are often recognised in
relationships between prominent figures such as Socrates and Plato, Haydn
and Beethoven, and Freud and Jung, as well as that of Annie Sullivan and
Helen Keller (Shea, 1992, p. 3). Zey (cited in Dreyer, 1995, p. 42) explains
that the population explosion after World War II gave rise to an increase in
labourers who had to be trained as swiftly and as effectively as possible.
Organisations identified and implemented mentoring in a purposeful manner in order to address the training needs of labourers. However, due to the
number of labourers that had to be trained, organisations were forced to
follow a structured approach towards mentoring. This approach only made
provision for the development of human resources in terms of their professional needs, and mentoring as it manifested in the days of the guilds
ceased to exist.

The structured approach towards mentoring was further encouraged by a
publication edited by Levinson (1978). This publication was entitled *The
seasons of a man's life* and focused on the contribution of mentoring to
develop the maturity of human resources. The popularity of the publication
by Levinson led to a conference paper delivered by Zey (1985) on the impact
of structured mentoring on the professional environment. These

publications established structured mentoring as a technique to develop human resources in a professional capacity.

MENTORING IN THE LIBRARY AND INFORMATION SCIENCE LITERATURE

Mentoring has been a well-known concept in the managerial sciences and management literature since the 1960s, but Jesudason (1997, p. 24) remarks that library and information science literature did not include any extensive coverage of mentoring as a human resource development strategy until the mid-1980s or later, and even then it was only discussed in terms of American, Australian and British library and information science professionals. This is confirmed by Nankivell and Shoolbred (1997, p. 97) which states that: "After that time [the early 1980s] mentoring literature specific to the LIS community grew slowly in the United States, although little was published in the UK".

Mentoring has been used for human resource development in the British library and information science profession for many years, but it became more commonplace after 1981 when the Library Association encouraged pre-registration candidates to use their supervisors as mentors throughout the pre-registration process. The use of mentoring was also strongly encouraged by the Library Association (1992) through its *Continuing Professional Development Framework*. The first book on mentoring specifically for the library and information science profession was published in Britain in 1994, but there seems to have been few formal mentoring schemes as Fisher writes: "Despite many leads, it was not possible to trace one library organization which used a formal mentoring scheme" (Nankivell & Shoolbred, 1997, p. 98). A 14-month (May 1995–July 1996) investigation into the extent and nature of mentoring as well as the experiences of those who had been involved in it was funded by the British Library Research and Innovation Centre. The investigation report concluded: "Mentoring can be an extremely valuable tool for change and development of both individuals within the library and information profession and of the profession as a whole".

Another early example of a contribution to the library and information science literature on the use of structured mentoring was written by Cargill and was entitled: *Developing library leaders: the role of mentorship* (1989). In this groundbreaking article Cargill (1989, pp. 12–15) expresses the need for a

method of human resource development, which would allow the identification and development of promising individuals within the profession.
However, of equal importance was the fact that Cargill also explored and
voiced the contribution that professional associations should make in terms
of the development and especially the empowerment of human resources
involved in the library and information science profession. It was this article
by Cargill and others (e.g., *The role of mentorship in shaping public library
leaders* Chatman (1992)) which characterises the literature on the applicability of mentoring as a method of developing and empowering library and
information science professionals in terms of their professional and/or personal skills.

In terms of the use of mentoring in the Australian library and information
science profession, the Victoria Branch of the Australian Library and Information Association applied an unstructured mentoring process to address the needs of student members in 1993. This mentoring process is an
important example of mainstream mentoring and the application thereof
specifically to the library and information science profession, because of its
treatment of the matching of mentors and protégés. However, in 1996 Golian and Galbraith (1996, p. 116) report on the practical use of a mentoring
process in *Effective mentoring programs for professional library development.*
In this publication, the authors comment on the implementation of a structured mentoring programme by the American Council on Library Resources
in association with the Association of College and Research Libraries of the
American Library Association. Golian and Galbraith (1996, p. 116) explain:

> First time library directors are paired with experienced directors who serve as coaches,
> guides, and peers for a designated one-year period. New directors begin the program
> with an intense three-day seminar, which is then followed-up with campus visits, tel-
> ephone support, and electronic mail communications. This successful project has gen-
> erated interest in, and acts as a model for, other groups who are considering
> incorporating mentoring into their programs.

This contribution was of particular importance due to the fact that Nankivell and Shoolbred (1997, p. 97) are of the opinion that the literature is
lacking in terms of discussions on actual mentoring programmes within the
library and information science profession. The lack of practical programmes in the American library and information science profession is further emphasized in an article by Linda Marie Golian and Michael W.
Galbraith, which is regarded as "the most detailed contribution to the
mentoring issue in US library literature" (Nankivell & Shoolbred, 1997, p.
97). However, the existing shortage of literature in which practical mentoring programmes are discussed is partly alleviated through an article by

Wojewodzki, Stein and Richardson entitled *Formalizing an informal process*, published in 1998. In this publication the authors discuss the implementation of a structured mentoring programme in the library of the University of Delaware, Newark, Delaware.

The prevailing situation in terms of the British, American and Australian literature on mentoring, specifically within the library and information science profession, also seems to be applicable to South Africa. The literature on mentoring as a method of human resource development for library and information professionals seems to be limited to a report by Botha and Van Zyl (2001, pp. 10–16) in 2000. In this publication, entitled *Mentoring: a new approach to staff development at the National Library of South Africa*, the authors describe the implementation of a structured mentoring process at a national library. Although the Foundation of Tertiary Institutions of the Northern Metropolis (FOTIM), in conjunction with the Gauteng and Environs Library and Information Consortium (GAELIC), presented the *Mentoring: an instrument for transformation* conference in October 2005, it remains to be seen if any formal publication would appear as a result of this conference and act as a catalyst for the use of structured mentoring within the library and information science profession in South Africa.

The above-mentioned selection of publications provides a brief overview of contributions that exist on mentoring specifically within the library and information science profession. However, it is evident that the literature on this topic has grown significantly since the 1980s as Gibson's bibliography (2003) on mentoring and libraries contain more than a hundred titles.

MANIFESTATIONS OF MENTORING

Mentoring, as previously indicated, is primarily characterised in terms of the manner in which it manifests within organisations, namely in a structured or unstructured form by two approaches. Structured, formal or institutionalised mentoring (Nasser, 1987, p. 12) entails that the needs of the protégé are addressed in a purposeful manner according to a detailed and specific development plan which forms part of a formal mentorship process, while unstructured or natural mentoring involves an informal relationship or in some instances even a friendship which develops between two individuals. Although these manifestations of mentoring chiefly vary in terms of the level of formality according to which the mentoring process are managed and maintained, they also vary in terms of the duration thereof and are either short term or long term in nature. Hunt (1991b, p. 31) and Shea (1992, p. 8) describe the various occurrences of structured and unstructured mentoring in the following manner:

1. Highly structured, short-term mentoring is formally established for an introductory or short period, often to meet clearly defined and specific organisational objectives. This type of mentoring is also referred to as planned project mentoring.
2. Highly structured, long-term mentoring is often used for succession planning, and the relationship frequently involves grooming an individual to take over a specific position or to master a craft. This type of mentoring is also referred to as planned career mentoring.
3. Unstructured, short-term mentoring ranges from ad hoc or spontaneous to occasional or as-needed counselling. There may be no ongoing relationship between the mentor and protégé. This type of mentoring is also referred to as informal career mentoring.
4. Unstructured, long-term mentoring or "friendship" mentoring consists of being available as needed. This type of mentoring is also referred to as informal life mentoring.

Structured Mentoring

The extremely formal nature of structured mentoring or institutionalised mentoring is a result of the following typical characteristics of a structured mentoring process:

1. A clearly defined and formally agreed upon objective that has to be achieved by the mentor and protégé through their participation in the mentorship process.
2. A particular timeframe within which the objectives should be achieved and on conclusion of which the formal relationship between the mentor and protégé officially ends.
3. The involvement of a variety of stakeholders (mentor, protégé, coordinator of the mentorship process, manager of the protégé, management) in the mentorship process.
4. A structured mentoring programme which consists of successive phases.

Although a variety of terms are found in the literature to refer to the various phases which constitute a typical mentoring programme, it seem as though most programmes consist of four phases, as indicated in Table 1.

Table 1. Phases of a Structured Mentoring Programme (adapted from Hunt & Michael, 1983; Kram, 1985; Nasser, 1987; Healy, 1977; Fourie, 1991; Hunt, 1991).

Phase 1	Phase 2	Phase 3	Phase 4	Publication date of model
Initiation	Protégé	Breakup	Friendship	1983
Initiation	Cultivation	Breakup	Redefining	1985
Need Seeking	Sparkling Establishing/optimising	Maturity	Decline	1987
Initiation	Developing Disillusionment	Breakup	Changing	1977
Initiation	Cultivation	Breakup	Redefining	1991
Selection and initiation	Protégé	Breakup	Friendship	1991
Duration: 6–12 months	Duration: 2–5 years		Duration: 6 months–2 years	

Phase 1: Awareness Phase

The first phase of the mentoring programme is chiefly characterised by the protégé developing an awareness of a particular need in terms of his professional skills. However, in some cases the organisation can become aware of the need for the development of a particular individual or groups of individuals for a particular organisational purpose. Interaction is established between the mentor and protégé and their roles and responsibilities in terms of the mentoring programme are determined. However, during this phase the mentor is acknowledged as the more skilled and knowledgeable party involved in the mentoring relationship.

Phase 2: Developmental Phase

The second phase of the mentoring programme is primarily characterised by an intense involvement that develops between the mentor and protégé. This phase is regarded as the most important phase of the mentoring programme since both the mentor and protégé should experience it as rewarding in terms of their roles and responsibilities as identified during the awareness phase (Dreyer, 1995, p. 56). The mentor and protégé should have frequent interaction and their involvement should be characterised by mutual trust. During this phase the protégé develops from merely an "apprentice" or learner, who demonstrates a particular potential to acquire an identified skill or set of skills, to a fully fledged protégé, who should accept and take responsibility for the development of his/her professional skills. Hunt and Michael (1983, p. 483) refer to the second or the developmental phase of the mentoring programme as the protégé phase due to the significant increase in the skills of the protégé during this stage. The second phase is concluded when the protégé can perform independently and without the guidance of the mentor.

Phase 3: Parting Phase

The third phase of the mentoring relationship is mainly characterised by a significant decrease in the intensity and frequency of the interaction between the mentor and protégé. During the third or parting phase of the mentoring programme the role and responsibilities of the mentor is more of a participatory than a leading nature. The protégé becomes aware of his ability to act independently and values the active involvement of the mentor in terms of the development of his/her skills to a lesser degree. Although the protégé prefers to act independently from the mentor, he/she acknowledges the contribution of the mentor in terms of the development of his/her skills and might in some instances even experience a feeling of loss due to the decrease in the involvement of the mentor. This emotion can also be experienced by the mentor, as Kram (1985, p. 57) indicates:

> The senior manager (mentor) loses direct influence over the young manager's (protégé's) career and personal development as well as the technical and psychological support of someone valued for high performance and potential. The young manager loses the security of having someone looking out for his career by providing developmental functions that enhance one's self-image and ability to navigate in the organization.

Hunt and Michael (1983, p. 483) explain that the parting between the mentor and protégé is important since it prevents the relationship that exists between the mentor and protégé to become stagnated and superfluous. The official relationship that has developed between the mentor and protégé is now terminated, since the objectives were achieved and the protégé has developed the ability to act independently from the mentor.

Phase 4: Redefining Phase
The final phase of the mentoring programme is chiefly characterised by redefining the official nature of the relationship that developed between the mentor and protégé. A mutual awareness and understanding exist between the mentor and protégé, which give rise to them acknowledging each other as peers (Fourie, 1991, p. 38; Hunt, 1991a, p. 16; Dreyer, 1995, p. 58).

The mentoring programme is developed within the larger contextual framework of a structured mentoring process or rather the mentoring process serve as the blueprint for the development of the mentoring programme. This type of mentoring process typically consists of ten generic steps. However, these steps should be customized according to the requirements of the specific organisation in which the process will be implemented. These ten generic steps are:

1. Ensuring senior management commitment as well as their visible support for the process.
2. Defining the aims and objectives of the mentoring process.
3. Appointing a mentoring coordinator or champion for the process.
4. Creating organisational readiness by means of information sessions.
5. Identifying the criteria for the inclusion of mentors and protégés.
6. Selection of mentors and protégés.
7. Training of mentors and protégés, the mentoring coordinator as well as the managers of the protégés.
8. Matching of mentors and protégés based on a set of predetermined criteria, including skills, experience, gender or location.

9. Initiating introductory meetings between the mentors and protégés and setting up of mentoring agreements.
10. Monitoring and evaluation of the programme.

Unstructured Mentoring

In contrast to the formal nature of structured mentoring, the informal manifestation of mentoring is characterised by:

1. The absence of an organisationally defined objective that has to be achieved by the mentor and protégé through their participation in the mentorship programme.
2. The nature of the relationship between the mentor and protégé is not dictated by the organisation and is therefore unstructured.
3. The involvement of stakeholders is limited to the mentor and the protégé.

The informal and spontaneous nature of unstructured mentoring is best described by the following statement by Golian and Galbraith (1996, p. 103): "However, it is very difficult to explain how the mentoring relationship began, developed, and sustained itself".

VARIATIONS OF MENTORING

Although mentoring can manifest in a structured or unstructured manner, both these manifestations can demonstrate variations in terms of the nature and extent of the mentoring relationship that is formed between the mentor and the protégé. These variations are as follows.

Homogeneous Mentoring Relationships

A homogeneous mentoring relationship is characterised by the mentor and protégé being of the same gender. Logsdon (1992, p. 95) is of the opinion that homogeneous mentoring relationships are more effective, since both members of the mentoring relationship experience the same demands in terms of gender roles and responsibilities.

Heterogeneous Mentoring Relationships

A heterogeneous mentoring relationship is characterised by the mentor and protégé differing in terms of their gender. Ragins (1989, p. 12) explain the challenges of this particular variation of mentoring:

> In sum, the empirical studies in this area indicate that female protégées may be less likely than their male counterparts to be selected by either male or female mentors. Male mentors may not perceive females as potential protégées, and may be reluctant to mentor them because of fear of sexual involvement and innuendos. Female mentors are scarce, and may not be able to afford the time or the risks associated with mentoring a male protégé. Although a comparative empirical analysis of the benefits of male and female mentors needs to be conducted, extrapolation from existing data indicates that male mentors may provide more power for female protégées, while female mentors may provide more support and role-modeling functions.

Cross-Cultural Mentoring Relationships

A cross-cultural mentoring relationship is characterised by the mentor and protégé differing in terms of the cultural group to which they belong. The literature on cross-cultural mentoring relationships is characterised by opposing perspectives on the effective use of cross-cultural relationships. Nankivell and Shoolbred (1997, p. 103) explain that cross-cultural mentoring relationships are exposed to the same challenges as heterogeneous mentoring relationships. However, Shea (1992, p. 85), Teke (1996, p. 16) and Tsukudu (1996, p. 16) are of the opinion that cross-cultural mentoring relationships are of exceptional value to organisations. Shea explains (1992, p. 85):

> As we move from a society focused on things to one focused on human values, mentoring offers a powerful tool for benefiting from cultural diversity. By carefully listening, by respecting our differences and by practicing the art of inclusion, we can build a stronger, more rewarding organization and society.

Group Mentoring

The typical one-to-one mentoring relationship between the mentor and the protégé can be extended to include a "one mentor to many protégés" type of mentoring relationship. The Business Management Institute (1997, p. 91) explains that the group should ideally consist of four to six protégés. This particular variation in the nature of the mentoring relationship is beneficial due to the level of interaction, which is established between the protégés within the context of the so-called learning group. A few additional benefits of the group in this type of mentoring is:

"... less chance of falling into dependencies";
"... diffuse issues of personal-chemistry mismatch";
"... group bond emphasizes interrelationships among all group members"; and
"spreads responsibility for learning and leading" (Business Management Institute, 1997, p. 91).

However, Norry (1997, p. 544) is of the opinion that group mentoring is characterised by a lesser degree of closeness in the relationship between the individual protégés and the mentor.

Telephonic and Electronic Mentoring Relationships

Although mentoring relationships are primarily characterised by face-to-face interaction between the mentor and protégé, they can be conducted effectively by means of telephonic or electronic (e-mail and list servers) interaction according to Pantry (1995, p. 12), Nankivell and Shoolbred (1997, p. 104) as well as Woodd (1999, p. 140).

Apart from the above-mentioned variations mentoring relationships also differ in terms of the nature and extent of the role of the mentor as well as his/her position in the organisation.

External or Co-Mentors

Mentoring relationships can be characterised by a mentor and protégé differing in terms of the organisation by which they are employed or the profession which they represent. The terms and conditions of this type of mentoring relationship are to a lesser extent dictated and influenced by organisational requirements. However, Lewis (1996, p. 62) is of the opinion that the mentor might lack the necessary insight into the culture and nature of the organisation and, more importantly, might not have the ability to promote the career of the protégé. The appointment of co-mentors entails that the protégé is paired with two mentors with a similar level of seniority or, as Nankivell and Shoolbred (1997, p. 103) explain "using peers, unrelated work colleagues and external mentors to create alliances –

developmental alliances". Nankivell and Shoolbred (1997, p. 103) are also of the opinion that co-mentors alleviate the shortage of effective mentors and:

> ...because anyone can be a mentor, developmental alliances do not have some of the difficulties associated with traditional mentoring (i.e., pressures on managers and gender issues) and suit multi-cultural societies.

Peer Mentors

Although a mentoring relationship is traditionally characterised by a senior or more experienced mentor being responsible for the development of the professional and personal skills of a more junior or less experienced protégé, some mentoring relationships entail the mentor and protégé being of equal seniority or level of experience. This type of mentoring relationship is referred to as buddy mentoring or peer mentoring, according to Moerdyk and Louw (1989, p. 24).

Position of the Mentor

Mentoring relationships often vary in terms of the position of the mentor in relation to the protégé in terms of the organisational structure. Effective mentoring relationships do not necessarily require that the protégé be directly in line to the mentor in terms of the organisational structure.

In conclusion to the above-mentioned discussion on the manifestations and variations of mentoring it is important to explain that a structured mentoring process is not always conducted in a formal style and an unstructured mentoring process is not necessarily characterised by an informal mentoring style. This implies that the level of formality maintained during the mentoring relationship is determined by the mentor. However, mentors should take cognizance of the impact of the mentoring style on the effectiveness of the relationship. Nankivell and Shoolbred (1997, p. 101) explain:

> In the US, over-formalising has sometimes stifled the mentoring relationship while in the UK it is the reverse and some schemes have suffered from lack of structure.

CLASSICAL FUNCTIONS OF MENTORING

Although organisations frequently make use of the structured manifestation of mentoring to support the professional and personal development of the skills of its human resources, it is not necessarily of more significance or more beneficial than the unstructured manifestation of mentoring. Some of the more traditional or rather classical functions of the various manifestations of mentoring are summarised as follows:

1. The structured mentoring process develops and empowers the human resources of the organisation both as a person and as a worker, since it focuses on the development of personal and professional skills.
2. Mentoring supports the recruitment and retention of skilled human resources, since their potential is identified and developed.
3. Mentoring supports the accelerated development of human resources, which enables them to acquire a particular position(s) in the organisation.
4. Mentoring supports and enhances the effective utilisation of the skills of the senior as well as the junior human resources of the organisation.
5. Mentoring is used as reward mechanism, since senior members are offered the opportunity to participate in a mentoring programme as an alternative to promotion.
6. Mentoring supports the development of both the professional and personal skills of the human resources within an unthreatening and tranquil environment.
7. Mentoring also supports the initiation of new human resources into the ethos and the manner in which business is conducted in the organisation, as stated by Burrington (1993, p. 226):

> Wise or helpful seniors are particularly influential to people in their first post, or to newcomers to a library system: they inspire enthusiasm for the work and the library and encourage those they mentor to develop the skills they need for making their full contribution to developments in libraries and librarianship. This is a significant benefit to employers, since staff who are enthusiastic about the library service will give it their best effort; they will also be less likely to move elsewhere just for the sake of a change.

However, the benefits of mentoring are not limited to the organisation concerned. Golian and Galbraith (1996, p. 113) show that the benefits of mentoring extend beyond library and information service organisations to the library and information science profession as a whole. The benefits of mentoring for library and information service organisations as well as the library and information science profession include:

1. Competent and dependable human resources who continue to grow and meet new challenges and obligations.
2. Increased productivity.
3. Increased commitment, especially from beginner professionals.
4. Lower rates of staff turnover.
5. Team-based/facilitative management.
6. Establishment of an organisational esprit de corps.
7. Increased effective communication and cooperation among staff and administrative units.
8. Lower incidence of burnout for senior-level professionals.
9. Improved community relations, awareness and support.

The benefits for the library and information science profession include:

1. Developing a unified professional reputation.
2. Supporting a professional code of ethics.
3. Sharing a vision of professional services.
4. Fostering an understanding of changing trends and technologies within the profession.
5. Building essential communication and negotiation skills.
6. Supporting social responsibility and the need to incorporate global views.
7. Developing professionals for their next career move.
8. Cultivating a sense of inquiry necessary for the growing knowledge base of the profession.
9. Cultivating workplace diversity by empowering minorities and women.

Although it is apparent from the above discussion on the significance of mentoring that this method of human resource development is beneficial to the mentor, protégé as well as the organisation and the library and information science profession, Harris (1993, p. 37) warns about the use of mentoring to solve managerial inadequacies:

> ... libraries should not depend on the goodwill of seasoned professionals who are willing to take an active interest in the career development of younger or less experienced employees. In fact, by encouraging the mentoring system, library managers may run the risk of supporting a process through which the establishment of special relationships is a means of overcoming difficulties within the organization as a whole.

CONTEMPORARY VIEW ON THE FUNCTIONS OF MENTORING

Recently it became clear that a shift has taken place in the way that mento-ring is viewed and applied within organisations. This shift entails that mentoring is no longer simply regarded as a technique for enabling the development of the human resources of the organisation but rather as a knowledge management technique that support the creation of knowledge or innovation in organisations. This shift is a result of the increasing view of organisations – and including library and information service organisations – from a resource-based view to a knowledge-based view of the organisa-tion. The resource-based view entail that the organisation consists of bun-dles of resources which can only be developed internally and which have the potential to positively differentiate the organisation from others. However, the knowledge-based view of the firm suggests that it is not merely the resources of the organisation which differentiate it from others but rather the ability to create internally the knowledge required to adapt to the in-ternal and external strategic environment of the organisation. Grant (1998, p. 110) explains the resource-based view of the organisation as follows:

> ... establishing competitive advantage through the development and deployment of resources and capabilities, rather than seeking shelter from the storm of competition, has become the primary goal for strategy formulation.

In contrast to the resource-based view of the firm, Grant (1998, p. 433) defines the knowledge-based view of the organisation in the following man-ner:

> A number of recent books have suggested that the most important resource of the firm is the knowledge embedded within the firm's people and its systems. The resulting surge of interest in knowledge as the critical resource of the firm and the fundamental manage-ment challenge, has resulted in an emerging conceptualisation of the firm and the nature of management identified as the knowledge-based view of the firm.

Organisations, and especially library and information service organisations, should increasingly take cognizance of the knowledge-based view of the organisation since Tissen (cited by Andriessen, 2004, p. 5) is of the opinion that, in the knowledge economy, services and thus service-based organisa-tions are equally important as products and thus production-based organ-isations. The author states: "Not only do products get more knowledge intensive, knowledge itself has become an important product, as shown by the rise of the services industry". This dual quality or rather paradoxical nature of knowledge as part of a process to enhance the value of products as well as a product in its own right is also deliberated by Snowden (2002, p. 2). Snowden (2002, p. 2) are of the opinion that knowledge is either a thing or product as well as a flow or process. Library and information service organisations should develop the ability to make use of knowledge as a flow or process to increase the value of the service they deliver to clients as well as to view knowledge as a thing or product that they deliver to clients.

The knowledge-based view of organisations and the paradoxical nature of knowledge require service industries such as library and information services organisations to view mentoring, not only as a method to merely develop and empower human resources but also as a technique to support knowledge creation, thus enabling human resources to be innovative. Line, Mackenzie, and Feather (1998, p. 22) explain the importance for libraries, and more specifically national libraries, to take cognizance of their changing environment and thus also the demands that are placed on them. These authors state:

> ... the changing circumstances facing national libraries are forcing a re-evaluation of their role. The fact of increasing competition on quality of service and on cost, sometimes from other national libraries, is an inevitable result of globalization.

Mentoring as a knowledge management technique, and more specifically as a technique that supports knowledge creation, must therefore be considered within the broader context of knowledge management.

A multitude of definitions is available in the literature to describe the concept "knowledge management". A few of these definitions are:

> The management function that creates or locates knowledge, manages the flow of knowledge within the organization and ensures that knowledge is used effectively and efficiently for the long-term benefit of the organization. (Darroch & McNaughton, 2002, p. 228)

> Knowledge management enables the creation, distribution and exploitation of knowledge to create and retain greater value from core business competencies. (Tiwana, 2002, p. 4)

> Treating the knowledge component of business activities as an explicit concern of business reflected in strategy, policy, and practice at all levels of the organization; and; making a direct connection between an organization's intellectual assets – both explicit (recorded) and tacit (personal know-how)-and positive business results. (Barclay & Murray, 1997)

It can therefore be concluded that knowledge management entails the creation of an environment in which the knowledge strategy of the organisation is enabled by means of related knowledge processes in order to ensure a competitive advantage for the organisation.

These five knowledge processes are as follows:

1. The creation or generation of knowledge or innovation.
2. The capturing or coding of knowledge.
3. The organisation of knowledge.
4. The sharing, distribution, dissemination or transfer of knowledge.
5. The use or application of knowledge.

The above-mentioned knowledge processes are largely enabled and supported by means of the knowledge spiral, SECI spiral, SECI model or the SECI process (Nonaka & Takeuchi, 1995, p. 14; Darroch & McNaughton, 2002, p. 231; Takeuchi & Nonaka, 2004, p. 8; Dalkir, 2005, p. 56). The spiral depicts how tacit and explicit knowledge or information is amplified in terms of quality and quantity, as well as from the individual to the group and then to the organisational level. The four modes included in the spiral are known as socialisation, externalisation, internalisation and combination.

Socialisation

This activity entails the transfer of tacit knowledge between the trainer and learner(s) and/or between individual learners or the sharing and creation of tacit knowledge through direct experience (Takeuchi & Nonaka, 2004, p. 8). During this process tacit knowledge is not transformed into explicit knowledge. Thus, knowledge is not articulated or encoded. The transfer of knowledge takes place mainly through techniques such as imitation, observation and practice (Nonaka, 1991, p. 28). Nonaka and Konno (1998, p. 40) explain:

> We use the term socialization to emphasize that tacit knowledge is exchanged through joint activities such as being together, spending time, living in the same environment – rather than through written or verbal instructions.

The learner's personal knowledge base increases due to the "new" knowledge he has acquired. This knowledge is, however, only available to the learner and does not form part of the knowledge base of the organisation (Nonaka, 1991, p. 28).

Externalisation

This activity entails the conversion of the tacit knowledge of the trainer and/ or individual learner(s) into explicit knowledge or the articulation of tacit knowledge through dialogue and reflection (Takeuchi & Nonaka, 2004, p. 8). During this process, tacit knowledge is articulated and can thus be shared with other learners and/or individuals. Nonaka and Konno (1998, p. 43) explain:

> During the externalization stage of the knowledge-creation process, an individual commits to the group and thus becomes one with the group. The sum of the individuals' intentions and ideas fuse and become integrated with the group's mental world.

Knowledge is shared through a variety of structured (for example communities of practice, expert forums, training, meetings, think tanks, knowledge cafes) or unstructured techniques (for example discussions, water coolers) and the use of a variety of media. Knowledge thus does not only form part of the personal knowledge base of the trainer or learner, but is now shared with other learners and is therefore part of the knowledge base of the organisation (Nonaka, 1991, p. 29).

Combination

This activity occurs when discrete parts of explicit knowledge are combined and integrated in order to form a more complex whole or systemising and applying explicit knowledge and information (Nonaka & Takeuchi, 2004, p. 9). Combination also indicates that knowledge that was created during the externalisation activity is disseminated or diffused throughout the organisation (Nonaka & Konno, 1998, p. 44). Although "new" explicit knowledge can be created through this activity, it contributes to the expansion of the knowledge base of the learner but not that of the organisation (Nonaka, 1991, p. 29).

Internalisation

This activity entails the conversion of the explicit knowledge of the trainer and/or individual learner(s) into tacit knowledge or learning and acquiring new tacit knowledge in practice (Takeuchi & Nonaka, 2004, p. 9). During this process explicit knowledge is internalised and the personal knowledge base of the learner is expanded by the "new" knowledge he or she has acquired. As Nonaka and Konno (1998, p. 45) explain: "This requires the individual to identify the knowledge relevant for one's self within the organizational knowledge". If the learner does not internalise the knowledge that has been transferred to him or her, learning does not take place.

The challenge for organisations in terms of the effective execution of knowledge processes is largely dependent on the creation of an environment which is conducive to the above-mentioned knowledge processes and the use of appropriate tools and techniques to enable employees to share their knowledge with one another in order for it to benefit the organisation in its entirety (Nonaka, 1991, p. 29).

Darroch and McNaughton (2002, pp. 231–234) provide specific examples of knowledge management tools and techniques, which are applicable to each of the four modes in the SECI model. Socialisation, or the mode where tacit knowledge interacts with tacit knowledge and individuals share experiences, is enabled by means of mentoring, coaching, apprenticeship and other forms of on-the-job training; imitating and developing shared mental models. Externalisation, or the mode where tacit knowledge converts into explicit knowledge, is enabled by creating metaphors and analogies, capturing best practices and developing an organisational memory. Combination, or the mode where explicit knowledge is converted into other sets of explicit knowledge, is enabled by combining discrete pieces of explicit knowledge or information:

> Combination is typical in information processing situations and might include reconfiguring existing knowledge bases through sorting, adding, combining, and categorizing explicit knowledge. Therefore, combination will make heavy use of databases and computerized communication networks, as these will make capturing, storing, retrieving, and transmitting of codified knowledge easier. (Darroch & McNaughton, 2002, p. 233)

Internalisation, or the mode where newly created explicit knowledge is converted into tacit knowledge, is enabled by learning by doing and having access to technical libraries.

In response to the importance of the adoption of a knowledge-based view of the organisation, the paradoxical nature of knowledge as well as the increasing importance of knowledge processes for all organisations, the role of mentoring has undergone a significant transformation. This transformation entails two aspects, namely:

1. Mentoring is regarded as a knowledge management technique and largely supports "the creation and sharing of tacit knowledge through direct experience" rather than merely an approach to develop the professional and personal skills of employees (Takeuchi & Nonaka, 2004, p. 9).

2. Mentoring in its structured manifestation is increasingly used by organisations, since the creation of knowledge cannot be left to chance as is the case when knowledge is created by means of mentoring in its unstructured manifestation.

STAFF DEVELOPMENT AT THE NATIONAL LIBRARY OF SOUTH AFRICA (PRETORIA CAMPUS)

Until 1 November 1999, for historical reasons, South Africa had two national libraries, the South African Library, founded in 1818, in Cape Town, and the State Library, founded in 1887, in Pretoria. In terms of South African legal deposit legislation, each of the national libraries was a legal deposit library, entitled to receive from the publishers a gratis copy of every book, serial, newspaper, government publication or other printed items published in South Africa. In South Africa, legal deposit, in some form or another, dates back to 1842. As a result, extensive collections of material of great scholarly value have been built up in the former national libraries. During the 1990s the Department of Arts, Culture, Science and Technology began a review of all legislation under its jurisdiction, including the *National Libraries Act, No. 56 of 1985* (South Africa, 1985). The Minister of Arts, Culture, Science and Technology in 1996 appointed a Working Group on the National Libraries of South Africa to advise him on the future of the two national libraries. The most important recommendation of the Working Group was that the two national libraries be amalgamated to form a dual-site (Cape Town and Pretoria) national library, to be known as the National Library of South Africa. The creation of the new National Library looks ahead to a revitalisation and transformation that will align the new institution with the goals of the new democracy. The new institution was constituted on 1 November 1999. On that day the South African Library and the State Library ceased to exist as separate entities and became, respectively, the Cape Town and Pretoria campuses of the NLSA (National Library of South Africa, 2000).

INVESTIGATION INTO THE USE OF MENTORING AT THE NATIONAL LIBRARY OF SOUTH AFRICA (PRETORIA CAMPUS)

The implementation of a structured mentoring process at the NLSA (Pretoria Campus) came as a result of a recommendation by the Employment Equity Committee to investigate mentoring as a possible method to develop employees from the previously disadvantaged groups and to empower them accordingly by appointing them in junior and senior management positions should these become available. An in-depth study (1998–2000) on the concept of mentoring was done, which included a discussion as well as an analysis of the manner in which it is currently applied within the library and information science profession. The study concluded with the findings of empirical research that was done in order to determine whether the employees of the NLSA (Cape Town and Pretoria Campuses) would be willing to participate in a structured mentoring process and to determine whether the NLSA could be regarded as a suitable environment for the implementation of structured mentoring. The primary objective of the study was to ascertain whether mentoring was an appropriate method of human resource development to extend the professional and personal skills of the employees of the NLSA. The secondary objectives were to determine if the NLSA could be regarded as a contextual environment which is conducive to the implementation of a structured mentoring process, as well as to determine whether employees would be willing to participate in a structured mentoring process. The "willingness" of employees to participate in the mentoring process can be translated into their willingness to act as a mentor to a junior or less-experienced staff member or to act as a protégé and to consent to the guidance of a more senior or experienced employee. The research was conducted within the theoretical framework provided by Hunt and Michael (1983) in *Mentorship: a career training and development tool*. This framework was specifically developed for research on mentor–protégé relationships for both men and women. Critical dimensions of this framework include the context within which a mentor–protégé relationship exists, the gender of these role partners, the characteristics each partner seeks in the other, the stages of the relationship, and the positive and negative outcomes accruing to the mentor, the protégé, and to their organisation (Table 2).

Table 2. Conceptual Framework for Research on Mentoring (Hunt & Michael, 1983, p. 478).

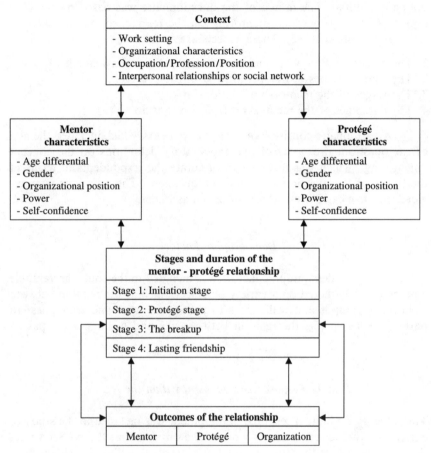

RESEARCH METHODOLOGY

Data on mentoring in general, and on the specific use of mentoring within the library and information science profession, were collected by means of a comprehensive literature study. The findings of the literature study were tested by means of empirical research that was conducted at both the Cape

Town and Pretoria campuses of the NLSA. The data for the empirical component of the study were gathered by means of the structured questionnaire method. The design of the questionnaire was based on the four aspects according to which mentoring can be researched, as identified by Hunt and Michael (1983). These aspects are as follows:

1. The context within which mentor–protégé relationships emerge.
2. The characteristics of the mentor and of the protégé.
3. The stages of the mentorship relationship.
4. The outcomes of the mentor–protégé relationship.

The questionnaire consisted of three components, which included the aim of the questionnaire, a set of five explanatory definitions on the concept "mentoring" which was included to orientate the respondents in terms of the theme of the questionnaire, and the questions. The questions were divided into five categories, which are given as under.

Demographic Factors

The category on demographic factors was included in the study, as valuable data could be gathered on a variety of aspects such as the relation between location of campus and willingness to participate, race and willingness to participate, as well as the relation between age and willingness to participate.

Human Resource Development within the NLSA

The category on human resource development was included in the study to determine whether respondents were of the opinion that the NLSA values the development of their professional and personal skills. This category of questions relates to the "context within which mentor–protégé relationships emerge" aspect, as included in the Hunt and Michael (1983) framework.

Participation of Employees in Mentoring as a Method of Human Resource Development

The category on participation of employees was included in the study to determine the willingness of employees to participate in a structured mentoring process. Questions were also included to determine whether employees experienced a need to develop their skills, as well as the nature and scope of the skills that needed to be developed. Although this category of questions formed the core of the questionnaire, it does not relate to any particular aspect included in the Hunt and Michael (1983) framework and is therefore regarded as an addition to their model.

Manifestations of Mentoring Relationships

The category on manifestations of mentoring was included in the study to determine the preferences of respondents in terms of the various manifestations and variations of mentoring. This category of questions relates to "the characteristics of the mentor and of the protégé" aspect as included in the Hunt and Michael (1983) framework.

Effect of Mentoring

The category on the effect of mentoring was included in the study to determine the expectations of respondents in terms of their participation in a structured mentoring process. This category of questions relates to "the outcome of the mentor–protégé relationship" aspect, as included in the Hunt and Michael (1983) framework.

The questionnaires were distributed to a randomly selected sample at both the Cape Town and Pretoria campuses of the NLSA. However, the sample was not limited to employees of the NLSA who have a professional qualification or who are responsible for library and information science activities within the setting of the NLSA. This is due to the fact that the primary objective of the study was to conduct research on the conduciveness of the NLSA as an environment to implement a structured mentoring process rather than to limit the research to the use of mentoring as a method of human resource development to extend the professional and personal skills of library and information science professionals employed by the NLSA. In total, 62 self-administered questionnaires were distributed to a representative sample of the NLSA staff, and all were returned to the researcher in person or by means of the internal mail system of the NLSA. This represents 39.7% of the staff employed by the NLSA. The data that were gathered by means of the questionnaires were processed by means of a

software package known as the Statistical Package for Social Sciences
(SPSS) (Botha, 2000, pp. 22, 204).

ANALYSIS AND INTERPRETATION OF THE FINDINGS

Some of the most significant findings of the study on mentoring at the
NLSA are indicated according to each of the categories of questions included in the questionnaire:

Demographic Factors

Most of the respondents (67.7%), as well as the majority of the senior
managers of the NLSA, were female (57.1%), while 32.3% of the respondents were male. Only 42.9% of the senior management of the NLSA represented the male gender group, indicating that the NLSA's staffing reflects
findings in the literature that the majority of employees within the library
and information science profession are female (Nankivell & Shoolbred,
1997, p. 102). However, it does not support the statement by Nankivell and
Shoolbred (1997, p. 102) that the majority of senior management positions
in the library and information science profession are occupied by males.
Irrespective of the findings by Nankivell and Shoolbred (1997, p. 102) regarding gender disparities in the library and information science profession
mentoring is regarded as a method to develop the skills of minority groups
such as women and members of previously disadvantaged groups. This implies that particular focus should be placed on the use of mentoring to
develop the skills of males in the context of the NLSA. It also implies that
some heterogeneous mentoring relationships had to be formed between
mentors and protégés. The respondents representing the white population
group totalled 46.7%, while 33.3% of the respondents represented the black
population group and 20.0% of the coloured (a group of non-white, non-
black South African who originates from and are primarily resident in the
Western Cape and Northern Cape provinces of South Africa) population
group. This finding reflects the unique nature of South African history, since
the economy has been dominated by the white population group and most
positions were filled by employees from the white race group before 1994.
Measures such as the *Employment Equity Act, No. 55 of 1998* (South Africa,
1998a), the *Skills Development Act, No. 97 of 1998* (South Africa, 1998b)

and related policies of affirmative action stipulated that the economy had to become more representative in terms of the demographics of the South African population. This brought forth the need for methods of human resource development, such as mentoring, to develop the professional and personal skills of members of the previously disadvantaged race groups. This finding indicated that the developmental needs of members of the previously disadvantaged groups had to be addressed by means of cross-cultural mentoring relationships (Botha, 2000, p. 207).

Most respondents (30.6%) were from the age category 35–44, while 27.7% of the respondents represented the 45–54 and 55 + age category. This finding indicated that there was more or less an equal distribution of junior or less experienced employees who were in an early career phase and sought the advice and guidance of a mentor, and senior and experienced employees who were willing to act as mentors (Botha, 2000, p. 205).

The findings of the study indicated that the biggest challenge posed to the implementation of a structured mentoring programme at the NLSA was the heterogeneous and cross-cultural nature of mentoring relationships rather than the availability of mentors and protégés who were willing to participate in the programme.

Human Resource Development within the NLSA

Three aspects were identified that impact on the manner in which human resource development manifests in the NLSA. These factors are the nature and structure as well as the culture of the organisation. A large number of respondents (66.7%) indicated that the management of the NLSA valued the development of their skills. This was also confirmed by the fact that 56.5% of the respondents indicated that they regard the NLSA as a learning organisation. However, 41.7% of the respondents were of the opinion that the NLSA does not provide employees with enough opportunities for the development of their skills, which clearly indicated the need for human resource development initiatives.

The structure of the NLSA is regarded as bureaucratic in nature by 71.7% of the employees. This type of organisational structure is not always regarded as conducive to the implementation of a mentoring programme due to the fact that it is characterised by centralised management and decision making, a variety of managerial layers, rigid and hierarchical relations that have to be adhered to, as well as tasks and activities which have to be completed within specific timeframes. These aspects pose unique challenges to mentors and protégés and necessitate the involvement of the manager of the protégé in the process.

Almost all the respondents (80.0%) indicated that the culture of the NLSA was conducive to the implementation of mentoring, since they were able to identify an experienced individual who had a particular skill in terms of which they would like to be developed. In addition to this overwhelmingly positive response, 56.5% of the respondents indicated that they were of the opinion that employees of the NLSA are supportive of one another in terms of the development of their skills. The findings indicated that, although respondents were of the opinion that there was a lack of opportunity for employees to develop their skills, they are willing to participate in existing as well as new initiatives created by management in order to expand their skills (Botha, 2000, pp. 212–215).

Participation of Employees in Mentoring as a Method of Human Resource Development

The respondents who indicated that they would be willing to participate in a mentoring process at the NLSA totalled 83.6%, while 4.9% of the respondents showed a lack of interest in participating in a structured mentoring programme, either as mentors or as protégés. A profile was compiled of the characteristics of a typical respondent who would be interested to participate in a structured mentoring process. These characteristics are as follows:

1. Gender: male (94.7%) versus female (78.6%).
2. Race: black (94.7%) versus coloured (91.7%) versus white (71%).
3. Participation as a mentor: + 15 years of service at the NLSA (88.9%).
4. Participation as a protégé: 0–5 years of service at the NLSA (84.6%).
5. Nature of work at the NLSA: employees responsible for non-professional or non-library and information science-related activities (84.2%) versus employees responsible for library and information science-related activities (82.5%).
6. Participation as a mentor: responsible for current position: 11–+15 years (100%).
7. Participation as a protégé: responsible for current position: 0–5 years (84.2%).
8. Qualification: unqualified or not a library- and information science-related qualification (85.7%) versus a library- and information science-related qualification (80.8%).

In addition to the above-listed characteristics of a typical respondent who would be interested in participating in a structured mentoring process, a total of 80.3% respondents indicated that they were interested in participating as a mentor, while 86.7% respondents indicated that they would like to participate as protégés (Botha, 2000, pp. 215–219).

Manifestations of Mentoring Relationships

As indicated in the literature and as discussed earlier [see manifestations and variations of mentoring], mentoring relationships can manifest in a variety of ways. Some of the most significant findings in terms of the manner in which a structured mentoring process should manifest at the NLSA are:

1. Heterogeneous mentoring relationships: A total of 65.6% of the respondents indicated that they did not have any specific gender preferences and indicated that they would be willing to participate in a heterogeneous mentoring relationship.
2. Position of the mentor in the organisational structure: A total of 63.9% of the respondents indicated that they did not have any preferences in terms of the position of their mentor in the structure of the organisation and that their mentor did not have to be directly in line with them in terms of the organisational structure. This finding indicated that mentors should be included in the programme based on their experience and skills rather than their seniority within the organisation.
3. Group mentoring: A total of 41.0% of respondents indicated that they did not have any objection to being mentored in a group context which correlates with the finding that the NLSA is regarded as a learning organisation and that employees are supportive of one another in terms of the development of their skills.
4. Cross-cultural mentoring relationships: The opinion of respondents was not tested in terms of their willingness to participate in a cross-cultural mentoring relationship due to the sensitivity of racial issues at the time the research was conducted (Botha, 2000, pp. 220–221).

Effect of Mentoring

The majority (42.8%) of the respondents indicated that they did not expect to be promoted as a result of their participation in a structured mentoring process, while 32.8% regarded it as a realistic outcome of their willingness to participate. Although a large number of employees (85.0%) were of the opinion that the satisfaction they would possibly experience as a result of their participation in the mentoring programme was sufficient compensation, 29.3% of the respondents expected to be compensated in financial terms for their participation in the mentoring programme (Botha, 2000, pp. 221–222).

Although the research project focused on the use of mentoring in terms of its classical function or as a method to develop the professional skills of employees rather than the more modern or contemporary view of mentoring as a knowledge management technique, the findings of the research were overwhelmingly in favour of the implementation of a structured mentoring process at the NLSA.

RECOMMENDATIONS: IMPLEMENTATION OF A STRUCTURED MENTORING PROCESS AT THE NLSA (PRETORIA CAMPUS)

The findings of the research project and the recommendations made by the researcher regarding the implementation of a mentoring process led the management of the NLSA to invite an external consultant from the National Productivity Institute (NPI) to submit proposals on the implementation of a structured mentoring process. In this way, the NLSA supported the idea of the Employment Equity Committee to apply mentoring for the accelerated development of high-potential employees from the previously disadvantaged groups.

In October 1999, a climate for mentoring was created at the NLSA (Pretoria Campus) when management and employees were informed of the "what, why and how" of the process at a mentoring workshop facilitated by the NPI. At the workshops, employees had to consider whether they would like to participate in the process either as mentors or as protégés. Employees who indicated that they were willing to serve as mentors, and therefore take the responsibility for and to become actively involved in the development of another employee, were further trained at 3-day workshops presented in December 1999. A Mentorship Steering Committee was appointed early in 2000 to coordinate and steer the mentoring process together with the NPI consultant. The Committee consisted of representatives from management, trade unions, the Employment Equity Committee and the NLSA Human

Resources Section with other interested members of staff. The functions of the Mentorship Steering Committee were to:

1. Determine the criteria for protégés.
2. Match mentors and proteges.
3. Design and implement the mentoring programme.
4. Deal with issues which could have a negative influence on the outcome of the process.
5. Monitor and evaluate the progress of the programme.

The Mentorship Steering Committee presented a progress report to all staff members as an opportunity for the Management of the NLSA (Pretoria Campus) to show their support and commitment to the development of the professional and personal skills of employees. During the presentation the proposed mentorship strategy was explained and employees were invited to become protégés and to have their skills developed by a more experienced and skilled member of staff. Interested staff members had to complete an application form so that the Mentorship Steering Committee could establish their development needs and their preferences regarding a possible mentor. Thirty-seven applications were received and, after consideration of each application in terms of the criteria set for protégés, 26 protégés were assigned to individual mentors.

The Mentorship Steering Committee was also responsible for matching protégés with their first or second choice of mentor. The appointment of a particular mentor to a protégé depended on the preference of the protégé, the suitability (according to the criteria set for mentors) of the mentor, and whether he/she had attended the 3-day NPI workshop. In the few cases where it was impossible to assign either a first or second choice of mentor, a match was made according to the nature of the development need and the personality of the protégé. Mentors and protégés were informed of the outcome of the matching process. Both groups could inform the Mentorship Steering Committee if they felt hesitant about the mentor/protégé assigned to them. In such cases the reasons for a particular match were given and, if necessary, a new mentor/protégé was assigned.

A generic mentoring programme was designed by the Mentorship Steering Committee in consultation with the NPI and was included in the NLSA Mentor Manual. The programme made provision for mentors to assume the role of either counsellor or trainer, but should the development needs of the protégé require it, the mentor could assume both these roles.

In the role of counsellor, the mentor addresses the career and longer term goals of the protégé. Specific skills such as computer literacy can be covered.

Usually the mentor will not teach these skills, but will rather help the protégé to find the right teacher at the right time and assist the protégé to learn effectively. In the role of teacher, the mentor covers specific skills, such as typing, filing or cataloguing, and the mentor provides the teaching. The NLSA Mentor Manual provided guidance to mentors on the manner in which they should go about in developing the personal and professional skills of the protégés. Progress was monitored by means of report forms in the manual which mentors and protégés had to complete and return to the Human Resources Section.

The mentoring process of the NLSA (Pretoria Campus) reached its final phase in January 2001 when a questionnaire, compiled by the Mentorship Steering Committee, was completed by mentors and protégés in order to measure the successes and failures of the process. Botha and Van Zyl (2001, p. 16) indicate that the questionnaire was completed by 84.61% of the mentors and protégés. The majority (68.19%) of these respondents indicated that the mentorship process contributed to the development of their personal and professional skills and can thus be regarded as a success.

The following statistics further illustrate the success of the process:

1. The percentage of respondents (mentors and protégés) who were of the opinion that the mentoring process should be repeated during 2001 was 63.64%.
2. The percentage of mentors who were of the opinion that the mentoring process contributed to the development of their skills was 57.14%.
3. The percentage of protégés who were of the opinion that the mentoring process contributed to the development of their skills was 60.87%.
4. The percentage of protégés who were of the opinion that they were ready to participate in the mentoring process as a mentor was 63.03%.

However, the importance of the implementation of a structured mentoring process for the employees of the Pretoria Campus is defined by the following quote from the questionnaire of a protégé:

> I found the mentoring process to be the best way of skills sharing between colleagues and also as a strategy that gives us fidelity which leads us to change and to build our human dignity.

CONCLUSION

This article offers a contribution to the process of understanding the value of mentoring for organisations. Mentoring has traditionally been regarded as a method to develop and empower the human resources of organisations in terms of their professional and personal skills in all types of organisations including libraries and information services. However, the author explains that a shift has occurred in the economy and therefore organisations, and more specifically service-based organisations like library and information services, must redefine their role and thus also the manner in which they regard their human resources. Human resources are no longer simply an asset that contributes to the competitive advantage and therefore the sustainability of the organisation, but rather emphasis is placed on the value of the knowledge of these resources. This shift from the resource-based towards the knowledge-based view of the organisation necessitates definite measures to "manage the knowledge" of human resources.

Knowledge management entails the creation of an environment in which knowledge processes are conducted by means of a variety of tools and techniques in order to contribute to the competitiveness of the organisation. The knowledge-based view of the organisation has brought about a transformation in the way organisations apply mentoring. Mentoring is currently viewed as a knowledge management technique which supports the creation of the knowledge of employees. Libraries and information service organisations should therefore regard "knowledge" as a process that needs to be enhanced and supported in the organisation as well as their primary product.

The article concludes with a report on an in-depth research project that was conducted at the NLSA in order to determine the applicability of mentoring as a technique to develop the professional and personal skills of employees within this particular setting, as well as the implementation of a structured mentoring process resulting from the findings of the research project. This provides valuable guidelines on the importance of ascertaining the suitability of the context within which mentoring will be implemented as a first step to ensure the effective use of this knowledge-management technique.

REFERENCES

Andriessen, D. (2004). *Making sense of intellectual capital: Designing a method for the valuation of intangibles*. Burlington: Elsevier, Butterworth-Heinemann.

Barclay, R., & Murray, P. (1997). *What is knowledge management?* Retrieved January 14, 2006, from http://www.media-access.com/whatis.html.

Botha, D. F. (2000). *Mentorskap as metode van menslike hulpbronontwikkeling – met spesiale verwysing na die toepassing daarvan binne die Nasionale Biblioteek van Suid-Afrika.* Unpublished masters dissertation. University of South Africa, Pretoria.

Botha, D. F., & Van Zyl, J. P. (2001). Mentoring: A new approach towards staff development at the National Library of South Africa. *Meta-info Bulletin, 10,* 10–16.

Burrington, G. (1993). Mentors: A source of skill, strength and enthusiasm. *Library Association Record, 95,* 226–227.

Business Management Institute. (1997). *Education, training and development in business.* Business Management Institute Rivonia.

Cargill, J. S. (1989). Developing library leaders: The role of mentorship. *Library Administration and Management,* (Winter), *3,* 12–15.

Carrell, M. D., Elbert, N. F., Hatfield, R. D., Grobler, P. A., Marx, M., & Van der Schyf, S. (1997). *Human resource management in South Africa.* Cape Town: Prentice Hall, SA.

Chatman, E.A. (1992). The role of mentorship in shaping public library leaders. *Library Trends,* (Winter), *40,* 492–512.

Clawson, J. G. (1985). Is mentoring necessary? *Training and Development Journal,* (April), 36–39.

Clutterbuck, D. (1991). *Everyone needs a mentor.* London: Institute of Personnel Management.

Dalkir, K. (2005). *Knowledge management in theory and practice.* Amsterdam: Elsevier, Butterworth-Heinemann.

Darroch, J., & McNaughton, R. (2002). Developing a measure of knowledge management. In: N. Bontis (Ed.), *World congress on intellectual capital readings* (pp. 226–242). Boston: Butterworth-Heinemann.

Dreyer, J. M. (1995). *Mentorskap as begeleidingshandleiding.* Unpublished masters dissertation. University of South Africa, Pretoria.

Fourie, N. (1991). Mannekragontwikkeling: Mentorskap of toesighouding? *Nexus,* (June), 36–38.

Gibson, R. (2003). *Mentoring & libraries: A bibliography.* Retrieved February 1, 2006, from http://colt.ucr.edu/bibmentoring.html.

Golian, L. M., & Galbraith, M. W. (1996). Effective mentoring programs for professional library development. *Advances in Library Administration and Organisation, 14,* 95–124.

Grant, R. M. (1998). *Contemporary strategy analysis: Concepts, techniques, applications* (3rd ed.). Malden, MA: Blackwell.

Harris, R. M. (1993). The mentoring trap. *Library Journal,* (October), 118(17), 37–39.

Hunt, D. M. (1991a). Mentoring and Machiavelli. *IPM Journal,* (July), 11–16.

Hunt, D. M. (1991b). Trust: Essential to effective mentoring. *IPM Journal,* (November), 29–39.

Hunt, D. M., & Michael, C. (1983). Mentorship: A career training and development tool. *Academy of Management Review, 8,* 475–485.

Jesudason, M. (1997). Mentoring new colleagues: A practical model from the University of Wisconsin-Madison. *Illinois Libraries, 79,* 23–120.

Kram, K. E. (1985). *Mentoring at work.* Glenview, IL: Scott, Foresman & Co.

Levinson, D. J. (1978). *The seasons of a man's life.* New York, NY: Ballantine Books.

Lewis, G. (1996). *The mentoring manager.* London: Pitman Publishing.

Library Association. (1992). *Framework for continuing professional development.* London: LA Publishing.

Line, M. B., Mackenzie, G., & Feather, J. (1998). *Librarianship and information work worldwide: An annual survey.* London: Bowker-Saur.

Logsdon, J. (1992). Need help? … ask your mentor. *Journal of Library Administration, 17,* 87–101.

Moerdyk, A., & Louw, L. L. (1989). Mentoring: A powerful tool in the career development process. *IPM Journal*, (October), 24–27.

Nankivell, C., & Shoolbred, M. (1997). Mentoring in library and information services. *New Review of Academic Librarianship, 3*, 91–114.

Nasser, M. (1987). Mentoring: The key to optimizing your corporate talent. *IPM Journal*, (November), 12–15.

National Library of South Africa. (2000). The national library of South Africa. Retrieved February 8, 2006, from http://www.nlsa.ac.za.

Nonaka, I. (1991). The knowledge-creating company. *Harvard Business Review*, (November–December), 21–47.

Nonaka, I., & Konno, N. (1998). The concept of "Ba": Building a foundation for knowledge creation. *California Management Review, 40*, 40–54.

Nonaka, I., & Takeuchi, H. (1995). *The knowledge creating company: How Japanese companies create the dynamics of innovation.* New York: Oxford University Press.

Norry, J. (1997). Working together, not in line. *Library Association Record, 99*, 544.

Pantry, S. (1995). Personnel development in information management. *Information Management Report*, (September), 11–13.

Ragins, B. R. (1989). Barriers to mentoring: The female manager's dilemma. *Human Relations, 42*, 1–22.

Shea, G. F. (1992). *Mentoring: A practical guide.* Menlo Park, CA: Crisp Publications.

Snowden, D. (2002). Complex acts of knowing: Paradox and descriptive self-awareness. *Journal of Knowledge Management, 6*, 100–111.

South Africa. (1985). *National Libraries Act, no. 56, 1985.* Pretoria: Government Printer.

South Africa. (1998a). *Employment Equity Act, no. 55, 1998.* Pretoria: Government Printer.

South Africa. (1998b). *Skills Development Act, no. 97, 1998.* Pretoria: Government Printer.

SPA Consultants. (1995). *Human resources procedures and best practices handbook.* SPA Consultants Rivonia.

Takeuchi, H., & Nonaka, I. (2004). Knowledge creation and dialectics. In: H. Takeuchi & I. Nonaka (Eds), *Hitotsubashi on knowledge management* (pp. 1–27). Singapore: Wiley.

Teke, M. (1996). Develop your internal talent and achieve targets. *People Dynamics*, 14(4), (May), 18–21.

Tiwana, A. (2002). *The knowledge management toolkit: Orchestrating IT, strategy, and knowledge platforms* (2nd ed.). Upper Saddle River, NJ: Prentice Hall.

Tsukudu, T. (1996). Mentoring for career advancement in South Africa. *People Dynamics*, 14(3), (April), 14–18.

Wojewodzki, C., Stein, E., & Richardson, T. (1998). Formalizing an informal process. *Technical Services Quarterly, 15*, 1–19.

Woodd, M. (1999). The challenges of telementoring. *Journal of European Industrial Training, 23*, 140–144.

THE WORK PROCESS OF RESEARCH LIBRARIANS, ELICITED VIA THE ABSTRACTION–DECOMPOSITION SPACE

Kevin J. Simons, Marvin J. Dainoff and Leonard S. Mark

ABSTRACT

Cognitive work analysis (CWA) is a method of understanding and documenting the constraints inherent in a work domain, irrespective of the actions undertaken within the work domain and the actors who undertake them. The keystone of CWA is the abstraction–decomposition space (ADS), which provides a constraint-based overview of the system. CWA has been successfully applied in a variety of settings to create tools that make the underlying goals and constraints of the system more apparent, and allow a worker the flexibility to perform his or her job in a manner appropriate to the current conditions, without being restricted to a particular task flow. In the current study, semistructured protocol analysis was conducted with six research librarians in order to create an ADS representing the information research work domain. The resulting ADS was reviewed with the participants, who confirmed its accuracy. Insight provided by the ADS regarding the work domain of research librarians is discussed, as are implications for tools to support information research.

Advances in Library Administration and Organization, Volume 24, 191–230
Copyright © 2007 by Elsevier Ltd.
All rights of reproduction in any form reserved
ISSN: 0732-0671/doi:10.1016/S0732-0671(06)24006-9

INTRODUCTION

Tools to support information research have traditionally been developed using a process that seeks to add new features without looking at the larger context in which those features will be used. Therefore, while these research tools provide a certain level of support for research activities, they may do so in a piecemeal manner that fails to integrate related tasks. This paper develops a methodology to identify and better understand the constraints inherent in the entire system in which a researcher performs his or her job. Such a method could facilitate the development of products that address a greater range of issues and make the system constraints more evident to the information workers, thereby providing tools necessary for the workers to more fully utilize their skills and expertise to work in a way that addresses these issues.

The inadequacy of traditional methods is particularly evident in the context of what Vicente (1999) has termed a "complex sociotechnical system." Vicente notes 11 factors that serve to increase the complexity of a system involving both automation and interpersonal relations, including a dynamic system, distributed work systems, and mediated interaction via computers. As a system becomes more complex and unpredictable, it is more important for workers to be able to adapt the process to meet unexpected demands of the work environment. In such situations, traditional methods fail to provide the information necessary to create products that fully meet users' needs.

For instance, normative approaches seek to determine how work *should* be done, which would allow one to define the best tools to support this ideal work process (e.g., traditional task analysis), but they tend to limit the worker to a single course of action, which leaves workers unprepared to deal with unexpected situations. Descriptive approaches seek to determine how work *is* done, with the goal of creating new products to make it easier for workers to do what they are already doing. However, descriptive approaches assume that workers have a complete understanding of the system, an assumption that may not be warranted in light of the complexity of today's work environments. Another problem with a descriptive approach is that it encourages the development of tools to support the current work process but does not encourage the development of new and improved work processes.

A formative approach, however, seeks to understand how work *could* be done. Cognitive work analysis (CWA; Rasmussen, Pejtersen, & Goodstein, 1994; Vicente, 1999) is a formative approach that considers the entire system in order to reveal the goals and constraints therein, rather than focusing solely on what workers are doing or how they should be doing it. In the process, CWA seeks to reveal the higher-order goals of the system and the way in which these relate to the specific actions that are undertaken to complete a job, so that an individual can better perform his or her job in spite of disturbances and the context-specific variation inherent to the system.

Formative approaches, such as CWA, which both encompass and supersede normative and descriptive approaches, can be particularly valuable in information-dense and dynamic environments such as modern research libraries. In a world of Internet-accessible electronic media with constantly changing formats, information search tools designed on the basis of previously successful methods (normative) or current practice (descriptive) are bound to run into unanticipated variants for which they are unsuited. CWA provides a solution to this problem via an analytic architecture which is simultaneously abstract enough to encompass unanticipated variations, but specific enough to design new products.

The keystone of CWA is the abstraction–decomposition space (ADS), which provides an overview of the system in terms of the constraints inherent to the system at several different levels of means–end relationships and part–whole decompositions. Means–end relationships are determined by three goal-oriented questions: "how," "what," and "why." For any given level of the ADS ("what"), the level above provides information about why this "what" is desirable; the level below provides information about how one accomplishes this "what." Specifically, the ADS represents structural means–end relationships, or means–end relationships between nouns. This is important, as the work domain consists of the objects of action, rather than the specific actions themselves. This is the foundation of the constraint-based approach of the ADS, which only specifies the constraints on action, but does not delineate the specific actions to be undertaken. It contrasts with task analysis, which seeks to capture the actions undertaken. A graphical representation of structural means–end relationships is shown in Fig. 1, an adaptation of a figure from Vicente (1999, p. 166).

Fig. 1 represents a sample domain analysis related to buying a house. Traditionally, Vicente and Rasmussen have used five levels of means–end abstraction in the ADS, but Vicente (1999) notes that this number can vary depending on the system captured and the level of detail with which it is captured. Part–whole, or decomposition, relationships are relationships between an entity and the components of which it is made. An example of part–whole relationships is shown in Fig. 2.

Thus, the ADS is a logical system, defined by (and constrained by) means–end and part–whole relationships. By starting with an understanding

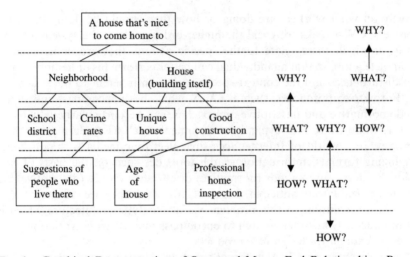

Fig. 1. Graphical Representation of Structural Means–End Relationships, Based on a Sample Domain Analysis Related to Buying a House. Adapted from Vicente (1999, p. 166).

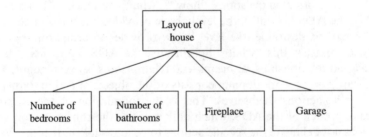

Fig. 2. Graphical Representation of Part–Whole Relationships, Based on a Sample Domain Analysis Related to Buying a House.

of these higher order constraints, one then can better determine a physical environment (tools) that will enable a worker to complete his or her job effectively. Additionally, the ideal physical environment would provide the worker with insight into the conceptual functioning of the system and thereby help the worker to deal with unexpected problems in the system.

Again, the dynamic nature of electronic media guarantees that unanticipated problems will emerge. Consider the rapid transformation of databases from paper (card catalogs) to punched card-based large computers through tape, floppy disks, CDs, and transportable plug-in hard drives. Each of these forms of media has certain constraints, which effect search tools. At the same time, the virtualization of informational databases through world-wide Internet access introduces a different set of constraints and potential problems. Issues of search engine structure and comprehensiveness, password access, capability and format for retrieval (print, plain text, PDF), and even socio-political constraints become relevant. CWA can be a useful tool in visualizing this complex world and helping to develop stable tools for information literacy.

The current study will use a semistructured method of protocol analysis that, unlike many methods, provides the foundation for a formative model of work. (As noted above, traditional task analysis – and the traditional use of protocol analysis – is normative, seeking to define behaviors needed to accomplish a task, whereas the current model seeks to be formative by focusing on the work domain constraints on behavior that provide boundaries for the range of activities that can be used to accomplish a task.) The process outlined in this study is a variation of protocol analysis in which subject matter experts' problem-solving actions on the work domain are used to extract elements of the domain. Work domain analysis then is used as the organizing framework for understanding the behavior-shaping constraints within the work domain.

Outline of the Current Study

The current study sought to understand the work process of research librarians by conducting semistructured protocol analysis with librarians as they performed information research. Data from these sessions were used to construct an ADS for the process of conducting information research. This ADS, in turn, was reviewed with the participants, as a vehicle for verifying and revising the information obtained from the initial interviews.

METHOD

Participants

The study was conducted at Miami University in Oxford, Ohio. Participants included six subject-specialist librarians (four men and two women) recommended by the Dean of University Libraries for the broad range of library functions they represented. Participant librarians supported a wide variety of academic areas, including Black World Studies, Communications, East Asian Languages, French, German, Interactive Media Studies, Interdisciplinary Studies, International Studies, Italian, Law, Library Science, Mathematics & Statistics, Philosophy, Political Science, Psychology, Religion, Speech Pathology and Audiology, and Theater. Additionally, two of these librarians regularly performed material acquisition work; two librarians had expertise in information creation (Information Commons) activities; one librarian had an extensive background in dataset acquisition, manipulation, and analysis; and another librarian coordinated digital library activities and had focused on developing a cross-institutional cataloging system for geospatial data. All participants had spent part of their time working at the library help desk, where students and faculty can obtain assistance in formulating and conducting an information search.

Procedure

Preparation

Participants initially were contacted by email to request their participation in a study of the process of information research by professional librarians. In the initial contact, each participant was contacted by phone, given a brief explanation of the study, and invited to schedule a 2 hour session in which he or she was asked to explain/demonstrate the information research activities related to his or her job.

Initial Sessions

Introduction. The primary investigator met librarian participants at their desks, and they were able to use any resource within the library. The primary investigator read a short explanation of the study to each participant.

Demonstration of Typical Research Scenarios. The primary investigator then reviewed the list of job-related information research tasks identified by the participant in the initial phone interview. The participant was asked to demonstrate a typical process that he or she would undertake to address each information research task. As the participant was demonstrating, the primary investigator asked "how" and "why" questions to elicit additional information.

Protocol Record. A protocol record was constructed during the session to provide a written record of the participant's actions and comments. The protocol record contained preliminary information about means–end and part–whole relationships, derived from questions asked by the investigator concerning "how" and "why" the participant proceeded as he or she did. Sessions were audio taped, and each session lasted approximately 120 min.

Analysis

Identifying Elements of Information. The primary investigator listened to the audio tape of each session and compared the audio record to the written protocol record for the purpose of identifying anything that was omitted or erroneously recorded in the protocol record. The next step in data analysis was the identification of elements of information. A given item was considered an element of information if it could be characterized as either a "why," "what" or "how" item with respect to the overall work domain. The primary investigator used both the protocol record and the audio tape of each session to identify elements of information. A second investigator independently reviewed the audio tape of each session to identify elements of information. Then, the investigators conferred about the elements of information captured. Both investigators had to agree about an item for it to be included as an element of information. An example extraction of elements is shown in Appendix A.

Constructing the Abstraction—Decomposition Space. Next, an ADS was constructed, based on the elements of information extracted from the protocol records. In determining the appropriate placement for elements of information and ADS items, it was helpful to develop some guiding principles for these levels: *Functional Purposes* are the highest-level purposes for which the system exists (the ultimate goals). *Priorities and Values* are the basic principles that govern the operation of the system. *Purpose-Related Functions* are the basic functions the system is intended to achieve. *Physical Functions* are components used to bring about the system's intent. And *Physical Forms* are the specific embodiments of the components described at the "Physical Functions" level. These guiding principles are based upon Naikar and Sanderson (1999). A tabular representation of this is shown in Fig. 3.

To create the ADS, the primary investigator began by reviewing all of the protocol records (and the lists of research activities in which participants reported engaging, from the initial phone contacts) to determine some subsystems of information research. Having identified some subsystems, the primary investigator began mapping elements of information onto the ADS, beginning with the protocol record for one representative participant and

Level	Description
Functional Purposes	Highest-level purposes for which the system exists
Priorities & Values	Basic principles that govern the operation of the system
Purpose-Related Functions	Basic functions the system is intended to achieve
Physical Functions	Components used to bring about the system's intent
Physical Forms	Specific embodiments of the components described at the "Physical Functions" level

Fig. 3. Guiding Principles Used in Determining Appropriate Placement of Elements of Information and ADS Items in the ADS.

then continuing the process for other participants. Elements of information that seemed to be related were grouped together into ADS items.

Next, a topological mapping was created among the ADS items in a given cell of the ADS. These mappings showed some of the more prominent relationships among items within a given cell. Then, for each subsystem a separate topological ADS representation was created, consisting solely of that subsystem and the Total System level. These topological, subsystem-specific ADS representations then were used to drive discussion in follow-up sessions with the original participants.

Follow-Up Sessions
In order to assess the validity of the ADS, a follow-up session (lasting approximately 1 hour) was held with each librarian. Each librarian first was given an overview of ADS. Then, the librarian was shown the topological, subsystem-specific ADS representation for each subsystem discussed with the librarian in the initial session, one subsystem at a time. The librarian was asked to provide his or her overall impression of the fit between the ADS representation and his or her actual experience of information research, as well as feedback on some specific questions:

- Do the relationships described between items within a level look accurate?
- Does each item in a level provide the means (the "how") to the level above it?
- Does each item in a level provide the rationale (the "why") for the level below it?
- Are there any items that appear to be in the wrong location (needing to be either relocated or removed)?
- Are there any items that are missing?

The feedback provided by the librarians was used as a measure of the accuracy of the ADS created in this study. It was assumed that, with a brief overview of ADS representations, librarians would be able to provide meaningful feedback on the topological, system-specific ADS representations. Their feedback then was used to make revisions to the ADS.

RESULTS

Abstraction–Decomposition Space

The full ADS, capturing the six subsystems that emerged from the sessions with librarians, is presented in Appendix B. Topological, subsystem-specific ADS representations (consisting of the Total System level paired with a given subsystem level) are presented in Appendixes C–H. The Collection Building subsystem captures activities related to identifying materials important for the library collection and purchasing those materials, either at the direct request of students/faculty or in anticipation of future student/faculty needs. Bibliographic Training refers to formal training opportunities, either through regular courses taught by librarians or through special lectures librarians provide in classes taught by other faculty at the university. Quick Answer involves answering a specific question brought by a client. Detailed Research, on the other hand, incorporates a process of going beyond a simple question to refine client needs via reference interviews with clients and evolution of the research problem as the client assimilates and analyzes more and more information. Information Creation is the process of helping clients take information they have gathered and publish it in a new form (e.g., video, web pages). And Classification includes the process of creating classification systems and using classification systems to assign metadata to information so that it can be retrieved at a later point.

At the Functional Purposes level, two ultimate goals emerged: supporting faculty research and teaching, and supporting student education. The Priorities and Values that expressed themselves across all subsystems included ensuring one's workload does not exceed the amount of time available, and, therefore, balancing one's time among the various activities that need to be completed. Additionally, the librarians all expressed a shift within the department from physical materials (e.g., hard copies of books on library bookshelves) to online/digital resources (e.g., online full-text journal articles). Other priorities were more specific to one or more subsystems, but were not critical to all subsystems. The Purpose-Related Functions level captures the systems necessary for each subsystem to function properly. The ADS then is rounded out by the tangible items/concepts that interact to enable each subsystem to operate (captured at the Physical Functions level), as well as specific examples of these items (detailed at the Physical Forms level). The items at the Physical Forms level are not intended to constitute an exhaustive list of all embodiments of the items at the Physical Functions level; rather the items at the Physical Forms level are exemplars that happened to be mentioned by the librarians in the sessions. Furthermore, the topological lines that appear within a cell indicate some typical relationships between items, but are not meant to be exhaustive. Footnotes at the bottom of each topological, subsystem-specific ADS representation provide further clarification for selected items.

Participant Evaluation of Topological Abstraction–Decomposition Space Representations

In follow-up interviews, the librarians verbally indicated that they understood the structure of the ADS; they seemed comfortable recommending substantive changes to it. Overall, these follow-up interviews indicated that the information obtained from the initial sessions was valid and comprehensive. Appendix I shows the feedback librarians provided. Only 12 of the 133 items in the final ADS were added by librarians in the follow-up interviews, while one item in the original ADS was removed at participants' recommendations. Another 14 recommendations involved repositioning/renaming items, adding topological relationships, or adding explanatory footnotes to items. And all of the librarians' recommendations were made at the intermediate levels that were difficult to abstract from the initial interviews (the Priorities & Values level and the Physical Functions level). However, the basic structure of the ADS was not affected by the changes suggested by the librarians.

DISCUSSION

The intent of this study was to better understand the work process of research librarians, by conducting a CWA and constructing an ADS. Through semistructured interviews with research librarians representing a variety of information research activities, the primary investigator obtained the information necessary to create an ADS covering six subsystems of information research. Follow-up interviews in which librarians reviewed topological representations of the ADS indicated that they felt the ADS was an accurate representation of their work domain.

The follow-up interviews regarding the ADS revealed that librarians in the current study were passionate about their role as educators. The information at the Functional Purposes level captured the general mission of the library and their roles as librarians. And the lower levels captured the items related to the work they do in support of this general mission. However, the librarians also recognized that the Priorities and Values level could capture the objectives of librarian-educators in ways that other representations of their work domain would be likely to omit. The ADS items librarians added at the Priorities and Values level were things like "Educational opportunity" (the basis for determining whether to turn a given interaction with a client into a "teachable moment") and "Foster critical thinking/evaluation of information." They added items like "Movement from information consumption to information creation," which indicated their view of themselves as not simply supporting information retrieval, but also supporting clients' ability to take the information they obtain, evaluate/assimilate it, and transform their resulting knowledge into a publishable form in order to contribute to an intellectual discussion. The librarians also noted, with regret, the constraints that sometimes prevent them from fulfilling their ideals (e.g., "Budget" and "Availability/access restrictions on information"), though they were quick to point out that these were just incidental constraints in their work, not driving factors. Thus, the ADS served to stimulate very meaningful dialog regarding the librarians' views of themselves and their work, and how this was reflected in their Priorities and Values. By delving further into the exact nature of the ADS items at the Priorities and Values level, one could get a much better idea of the organizing principles in participants' work (i.e., why they do what they do), and thereby allow one to provide tools/resources to better meet participants' needs. *This abstraction beyond the day-to-day workflow of the participant is what makes CWA unique.*

The ADS from this study may be specific to the work environment of the librarians interviewed. Alternatively, it may be a model that applies to the work domain of librarians at other institutions, as well. Therefore, to further understand the work domain of librarians, it would be helpful to conduct similar studies in other places of work. As Burns, Bisantz, and Roth (2004) showed, it is expected that there will be significant overlap between ADS representations for work domains of people who perform similar work in similar environments (e.g., for research librarians at various institutions). However, differences in organizational factors (organizational purpose/mission, organizational structure, resources available) as well as differences in the intent of the CWA itself (e.g., level of specificity desired) could lead to differences in the resulting CWAs. Nevertheless, as Burns et al. note, these differences would not necessarily be detrimental, but rather would show the flexibility of CWA and would lead to a richer understanding of the work domain of librarians across institutions.

Having such knowledge of the work domain of research librarians then would allow for the creation of innovative tools to better support the research process. By understanding the constraints, values, and priorities inherent in the work domain, companies can go beyond just building a new feature that people will buy, to creating a research system that makes the system constraints apparent and then allows the worker to complete the system by maneuvering within those constraints. For instance, the current study indicates that librarians often are focused on providing educational opportunities for their clients. This may mean teaching students how to determine where to begin their research, depending on their ultimate goal; how to discern the reputability of online information (cf., Nunberg, 2005); and/or what to do when an information search provides too much or too little information (in which case the librarian may need to get the student into a difficult situation in order to teach him or her how to get out of it). Long-term research solutions would need not only to provide for these options, but also to make the underlying Priorities and Values more evident. The current CWA also revealed that there are several distinct, yet intertwined, subsystems in which librarians work, and that research tools need to support the distinct needs of each subsystem while allowing for the transfer of information between subsystems. For instance, powerful search tools (including tools for manipulating search results) are necessary for the Detailed Research subsystem. However, once information is obtained in the Detailed Research subsystem, there must be a way to use this information in the purchase of new materials for the library (Collection Building) and the creation of research reports (Information Creation), whether these reports are presented on paper, in web pages, in videos, or in an alternate format.

In summary, CWA provides a methodology for revealing and making more transparent the complex and dynamic structure comprising the modern research library. As such, it can reveal the constraints of this system at different levels of abstraction. This permits a formative approach to work analysis and design which can encompass unanticipated changes and events.

The current study serves to inform the specific work domain of university librarians, as well as document a process by which the initial stages of CWA can be accomplished. Future studies may wish to replicate this work with librarians in other settings, to determine whether the ADS created in this study is exhaustive, or whether it is specific to the institution in which these librarians work. Additionally, it would be beneficial to try to take the information gleaned from this study and apply it to the development of tools to support information research activities, as noted earlier.

REFERENCES

Burns, C. M., Bisantz, A. M., & Roth, E. M. (2004). Lessons from a comparison of work domain models: Representational choices and their implications. *Human Factors*, *46*(4), 711–727.

Naikar, N., & Sanderson, P. (1999). Work domain analysis for training-system definition and acquisition. *The International Journal of Aviation Psychology*, *9*(3), 271–290.

Nunberg, G. (2005). Teaching students to swim in the online sea. *The New York Times*, February 13 (sect. 4), p. 4.

Rasmussen, J., Pejtersen, A., & Goodstein, L. (1994). *Cognitive Systems Engineering*. New York: Wiley.

Vicente, K. J. (1999). *Cognitive Work Analysis: Toward Safe, Productive, and Healthy Computer-Based Work*. Mahwah, NJ: Erlbaum.

APPENDIX A. SAMPLE EXTRACTION OF ELEMENTS FROM THE PROTOCOL RECORD

The following is a sample extraction of elements of information from a protocol record. The protocol record (left column) is a written record of the participant's actions and comments. The elements of information (right column) are the "why," "what," or "how" items identified in the protocol record by the primary investigator and validated by a second investigator.

Protocol record	Elements
• I'm an information services librarian	Librarian
○ Basically, I'm a subject specialist for several departments	Subject specialist
• I'm also on the consultation desk downstairs several times a week	Consultation desk
• As a subject specialist,	Subject specialist
○ I select books for the library	Books/Stacks of books
○ I use my interactions with students and faculty to see what kinds of things I want to collect	Student, Faculty member
○ I look through different databases to find out what is available	Databases/multiple databases
○ I have set up profiles in different subject areas, so certain things come in automatically	Profile, Subject area
	Bibliographic instruction
	Boolean search logic
	Overcoming information overload, Information, Knowledge (end goal)

- ○ I also do bibliographic instruction in the departments I work with
  - I may be giving a basic overview of strategy and Boolean logic to an introductory class
  - My main focus is how to get beyond information overload; turning information in to knowledge
- • Information – all that stuff
- • Knowledge – the integration of information in consciousness
- • I try to bring students to a stage of information literacy

Knowledge (end goal)
Information literacy

APPENDIX B. FULL ABSTRACTION–DECOMPOSITION SPACE WITHOUT TOPOLOGICAL MAPPINGS

The following is the full abstraction–decomposition space (ADS), capturing the total system level and the six subsystems that emerged from the sessions with librarians. Topological mapping is not captured in this representation, but is shown in Appendixes C–H.

	Total System (T)	Subsystem: Collection Building (C)	Subsystem: Bibliographic Training (B)	Subsystem: Detailed Research (D)	Subsystem: Quick Answer (Q)	Subsystem: Classification (Cl)	Subsystem: Information Creation (I)
Functional Purposes (FP)	Support faculty research and teaching (T-FP1) Support student education (T-FP2)						
Priorities and Values (PV)	Time ≥ workload (T-PV1)	Budget ≥ cost of resources (C-PV1)	Positive research experience (B-PV1)	Materials available ≥ client needs (D-PV1)	Materials available ≥ client needs (Q-PV1)	Positive research experience (Cl-PV1)	Budget ≥ cost of resources (I-PV1)
	Balance of time among necessary activities (T-PV2)	Materials available ≥ client needs (C-PV2)	Foster critical thinking/evaluation of information (B-PV2)	Positive research experience (D-PV2)	Positive research experience (Q-PV2)	Budget ≥ cost of resources (Cl-PV2)	Positive research experience (I-PV2)
	Movement toward online/digital resources (T-PV3)	Balance of usability/accessibility issues between traditional paper materials and online/digital resources (C-PV3)		Educational opportunity (D-PV3)	Educational opportunity (Q-PV3)	Movement from collection orientation to service orientation (Cl-PV3)	Movement from collection orientation to service orientation (I-PV3)

Purpose-Related Functions (PRF)					
Balanced information (among different points of view) (C-PV4)	System of client requests for training (B-PRF1)	Availability/access restrictions on information (D-PV4)	System of locating materials (Q-PRF1)	System of cataloging previously unclassified materials (CI-PRF1)	System of creating physical information (by clients) (I-PRF1)
Movement from collection orientation to service orientation (C-PV5)	System of providing training to clients (B-PRF2)				
System of locating materials: Searching (C-PRF1)		System of locating materials (D-PRF1)		System of creating [systems of cataloging materials] (CI-PRF2)	System of creating digital information (by clients) (I-PRF2)
System of locating materials: Foraging (C-PRF2)		System of distributing materials to clients (D-PRF3)	System of distributing materials to clients (Q-PRF3)	System of acquiring previously unclassified materials (CI-PRF3)	System of converting physical information to digital information (I-PRF3)
System for purchasing materials (C-PRF3)		System of client requests for information: Detailed Research (D-PRF4)	System of client requests for information: Quick Answer (Q-PRF4)		
System for requesting specific materials from librarian (C-PRF4)		System of client requests for materials (D-PRF5)	System of client requests for materials (Q-PRF5)		
System of automatically recommending materials (C-PRF5)		System of providing information to clients (D-PRF6)	System of providing information to clients (Q-PRF6)		

Physical Functions (PFu)						
	Web site (C-PFu1)	Web site (B-PFu1)	Web site (D-PFu1)	Web site (Q-PFu1)	Material metadata (Cl-PFu1)	Materials/information and their characteristics (I-PFu1)
	Search functionality (C-PFu2)	Search functionality (B-PFu2)	Search functionality (D-PFu2)	Search functionality (Q-PFu2)	Metadata assignment tool (Cl-PFu2)	Clients (I-PFu2)
	Search query (C-PFu3)	Search query (B-PFu3)	Search query (D-PFu3)	Search query (Q-PFu3)	Catalogs/indexes of material and their characteristics (Cl-PFu3)	Client needs (I-PFu3)
	Search results (C-PFu4)	Search results (B-PFu4)	Search results (D-PFu4)	Search results (Q-PFu4)	Materials/information and their characteristics (Cl-PFu4)	Budget (I-PFu4)
	Catalogs/indexes of material and their characteristics (C-PFu5)	Catalogs/indexes of material and their characteristics (B-PFu5)	Catalogs/indexes of material and their characteristics (D-PFu5)	Catalogs/indexes of material and their characteristics (Q-PFu5)	Clients (Cl-PFu5)	Tools for publishing information (I-PFu5)
	Materials and their characteristics (C-PFu6)	Materials/information and their characteristics (B-PFu6)	Materials/information and their characteristics (D-PFu6)	Materials/information and their characteristics (Q-PFu6)	Client needs (Cl-PFu6)	Tools for accessing/capturing information (I-PFu6)
	Vendor (C-PFu7)	Clients (B-PFu7)	Clients (D-PFu7)	Clients (Q-PFu7)	Budget (Cl-PFu7)	Multimedia help desk (I-PFu7)
	Clients (C-PFu8)	Client needs (B-PFu8)	Client needs (D-PFu8)	Client needs (Q-PFu8)	Cataloging/indexing standards (Cl-PFu8)	Project (I-PFu-8)
	Client needs (C-PFu9)	Assignments (B-PFu9)	People to aid in locating materials (D-PFu9)	People to aid in locating materials (Q-PFu9)	Search functionality (Cl-PFu9)	Facilities (Information Commons) (I-PFu9)
	Budget (C-PFu10)	Training facilities (B-PFu10)	Reference interview (D-PFu10)	Help desk (Q-PFu11)	Search query (Cl-PFu10)	Tools for manipulating information (I-PFu10)

People to aid in locating materials (C-PFu11)	Subject-specialist librarian (B-PFu11)	Help desk (D-PFu11)	Research project (Q-PFu-12)	Search results (CI-PFu11)
Information about available materials (C-PFu12)	Access to information/materials (B-PFu12)	Research project (D-PFu-12)	Facilities (Q-PFu13)	Web site (CI-PFu12)
Subject-specialist librarian (C-PFu13)	Results management functionality (B-PFu13)	Facilities (D-PFu14)	System-recommended sources (Q-PFu15)	People to help develop classification standards (CI-PFu13)
Results management functionality (C-PFu14)	Assessment of instruction (B-PFu14)	System-recommended sources (D-PFu16)	Access to information/materials (Q-PFu16)	Uncataloged materials/information and their characteristics (CI-PFu14)
		Subject-specialist librarian (D-PFu17) Access to information/materials (D-PFu18) Results management functionality (D-PFu19)	Results management functionality (Q-PFu17)	Results management functionality (CI-PFu15)

Physical Forms (PFo)

Amazon.com (C-PFo1)	Academic Search Premier (B-PFo2)	Academic Search Premier (D-PFo2)	Academic Search Premier (Q-PFo2)	Google (CI-PFo1)	Center for Information Management (CIM) (I-PFo1) BarnesAndNoble.com (C-PFo2)

Academic Universe (B-PFo3)

Academic Universe (Q-PFo3) Google (C-PFo3) Yankee Book Peddler (C-PFo4)	Alta Vista (B-PFo4) AP photo database (B-PFo5)	Alta Vista (D-PFo4) AP photo database (D-PFo5)	Alta Vista (Q-PFo4) AP photo database (Q-PFo5)

Academic Universe (D-PFo3)

Applied Science and Technology (database) (B-PFo6)	Applied Science and Technology (database) (D-PFo6)	Applied Science and Technology (database) (Q-PFo6)
Blackboard (B-Pfo7)	Center for Information Management (CIM) (D-PFo7)	Blackboard (Q-PFo7)
Center for Information Management (CIM) (B-Pfo8)	ChemAbstracts (database) (D-PFo8)	ChemAbstracts (database) (Q-PFo8)
ChemAbstracts (database) (B-Pfo9)	COMPENDEX (database) (D-PFo9)	COMPENDEX (database) (Q-PFo9)
COMPENDEX (database) (B-Pfo10)	Congressional Universe (D-PFo10)	Congressional Universe (Q-PFo10)
Congressional Universe (B-Pfo11)	Endnote (D-PFo11)	ERIC (Specific database) (Q-PFo11)
Endnote (B-PFo12)	ERIC (Specific database) (D-PFo12)	Google (Q-PFo12)
ERIC (Specific database) (B-Pfo13)	Google (D-PFo13)	MathSciNet (database) (Q-PFo13)
Google (B-Pfo14)	Electronic Data Center (D-PFo14)	MEDLINE (Q-PFo14)
MathSciNet (database) (B-Pfo15)	jake.net.yale.edu web site (D-PFo15)	Newsweek (Q-PFo15)
MEDLINE (B-Pfo16)	MathSciNet (database) (D-PFo16)	ProCite (Q-PFo16)
Newsweek (B-Pfo17)	MEDLINE (D-PFo17)	PsychInfo (Q-PFo17)
ProCite (B-Pfo18)	Newsweek (D-PFo18)	

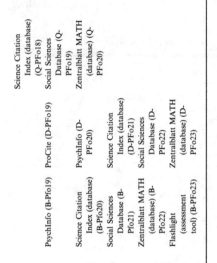

PsychInfo (B-Pfo19)

Science Citation Index (database) (B-Pfo20)
Social Sciences Database (B-Pfo21)
Zentralblatt MATH (database) (B-Pfo22)
Flashlight (assessment tool) (B-PFo23)

ProCite (D-PFo19)

PsychInfo (D-PFo20)
Science Citation Index (database) (D-PFo21)
Social Sciences Database (D-PFo22)
Zentralblatt MATH (database) (D-PFo23)

Science Citation Index (database) (Q-PFo18)
Social Sciences Database (Q-PFo19)
Zentralblatt MATH (database) (Q-PFo20)

APPENDIX C. TOPOLOGICAL ABSTRACTION–DECOMPOSITION SPACE FOR COLLECTION BUILDING SUBSYSTEM

The following is the topological representation of the Collection Building subsystem, paired with the Total System. The Collection Building subsystem captures activities related to purchasing materials, either at the direct request of students/faculty or in the anticipation of future student/faculty needs. The following includes both the original ADS items (solid lines) and ADS items added per librarian feedback in follow-up interviews (dashed lines).

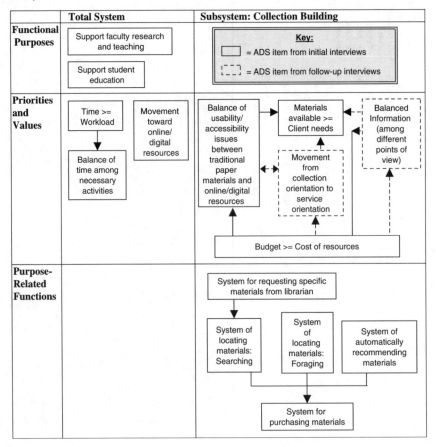

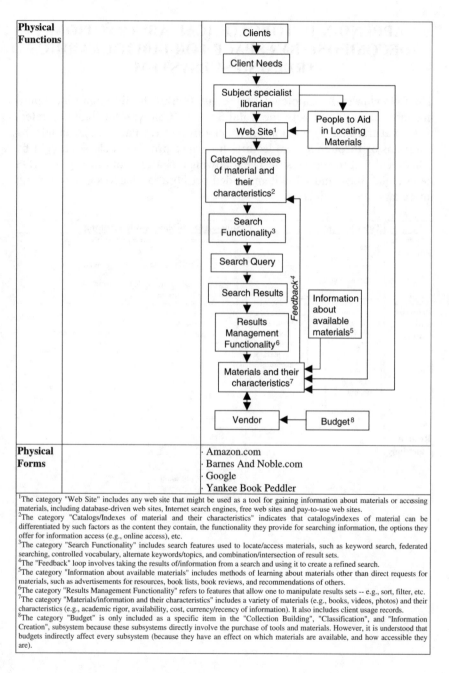

Physical Functions	

Clients

Client Needs

Subject specialist librarian

Web Site[1]

People to Aid in Locating Materials

Catalogs/Indexes of material and their characteristics[2]

Search Functionality[3]

Search Query

Search Results

Feedback[4]

Results Management Functionality[6]

Information about available materials[5]

Materials and their characteristics[7]

Vendor

Budget[8]

Physical Forms	· Amazon.com · Barnes And Noble.com · Google · Yankee Book Peddler

[1]The category "Web Site" includes any web site that might be used as a tool for gaining information about materials or accessing materials, including database-driven web sites, Internet search engines, free web sites and pay-to-use web sites.

[2]The category "Catalogs/Indexes of material and their characteristics" indicates that catalogs/indexes of material can be differentiated by such factors as the content they contain, the functionality they provide for searching information, the options they offer for information access (e.g., online access), etc.

[3]The category "Search Functionality" includes search features used to locate/access materials, such as keyword search, federated searching, controlled vocabulary, alternate keywords/topics, and combination/intersection of result sets.

[4]The "Feedback" loop involves taking the results of/information from a search and using it to create a refined search.

[5]The category "Information about available materials" includes methods of learning about materials other than direct requests for materials, such as advertisements for resources, book lists, book reviews, and recommendations of others.

[6]The category "Results Management Functionality" refers to features that allow one to manipulate results sets -- e.g., sort, filter, etc.

[7]The category "Materials/information and their characteristics" includes a variety of materials (e.g., books, videos, photos) and their characteristics (e.g., academic rigor, availability, cost, currency/recency of information). It also includes client usage records.

[8]The category "Budget" is only included as a specific item in the "Collection Building", "Classification", and "Information Creation", subsystem because these subsystems directly involve the purchase of tools and materials. However, it is understood that budgets indirectly affect every subsystem (because they have an effect on which materials are available, and how accessible they are).

APPENDIX D. TOPOLOGICAL ABSTRACTION–DECOMPOSITION SPACE FOR BIBLIOGRAPHIC TRAINING SUBSYSTEM

The following is the topological representation of the Bibliographic Training subsystem, paired with the Total System. Bibliographic Training refers to formal training opportunities, either through regular courses taught by librarians or through special lectures librarians provide in classes taught by other faculty at the university. The following includes both the original ADS items (solid lines) and ADS items added per librarian feedback in follow-up interviews (dashed lines).

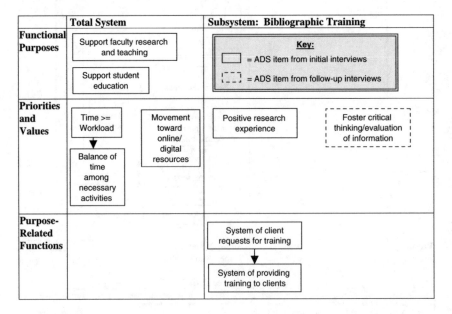

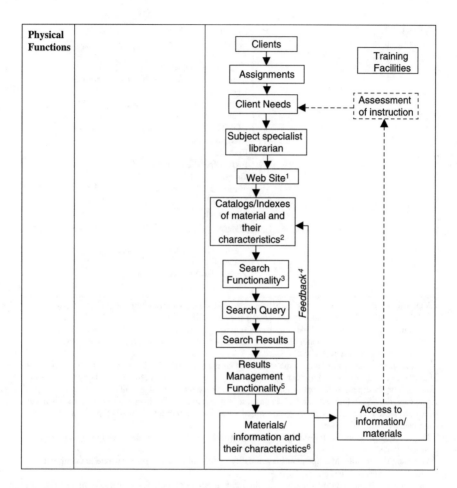

Physical Forms		· Academic Search Premier
		· Academic Universe
		· Alta Vista
		· AP photo database
		· Applied Science and Technology (database)
		· Blackboard
		· Center for Information Management (CIM)
		· Chem Abstracts (database)
		· COMPENDEX (database)
		· Congressional Universe
		· Endnote
		· ERIC (Specific database)
		· Google
		· MathSciNet (database)
		· MEDLINE
		· Newsweek
		· ProCite
		· PsychInfo
		· Science Citation Index (database)
		· Social Sciences Database
		· Zentralblatt MATH (database)
		· Flashlight (assessment tool)

Note: This subsystem includes classes that are a part of the Miami curriculum (taught by librarians), as well as training sessions provided in response to client needs/requests.

[1]The category "Web Site" includes any web site that might be used as a tool for gaining information about materials or accessing materials, including database-driven web sites, Internet search engines, free web sites and pay-to-use web sites.

[2]The category "Catalogs/Indexes of material and their characteristics" indicates that catalogs/indexes of material can be differentiated by such factors as the content they contain, the functionality they provide for searching information, the options they offer for information access (e.g., online access), etc.

[3]The category "Search Functionality" includes search features used to locate/access materials, such as keyword search, federated searching, controlled vocabulary, alternate keywords/topics, and combination/intersection of result sets.

[4]The "Feedback" loop involves taking the results of/information from a search and using it to create a refined search.

[5]The category "Results Management Functionality" refers to features that allow one to manipulate results sets-- e.g., sort, filter, etc.

[6]The category "Materials/information and their characteristics" includes a variety of materials (e.g., books, videos, photos) and their characteristics (e.g., academic rigor, availability, cost, currency/recency of information).

APPENDIX E. TOPOLOGICAL ABSTRACTION–DECOMPOSITION SPACE FOR DETAILED RESEARCH SUBSYSTEM

The following is the topological representation of the Detailed Research subsystem, paired with the Total System. Detailed Research goes beyond a simple question, refining client needs via reference interviews with clients and following the evolution of the research problem as the client assimilates and analyzes more and more information. The following includes both the original ADS items (solid lines) and ADS items added per librarian feedback in follow-up interviews (dashed lines).

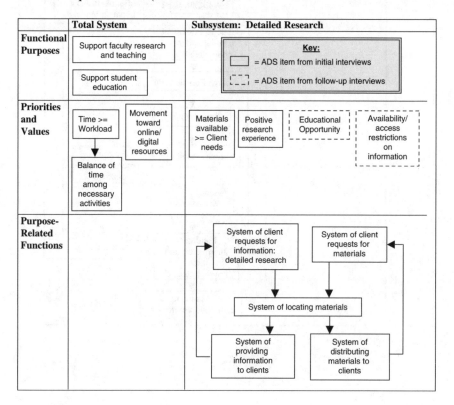

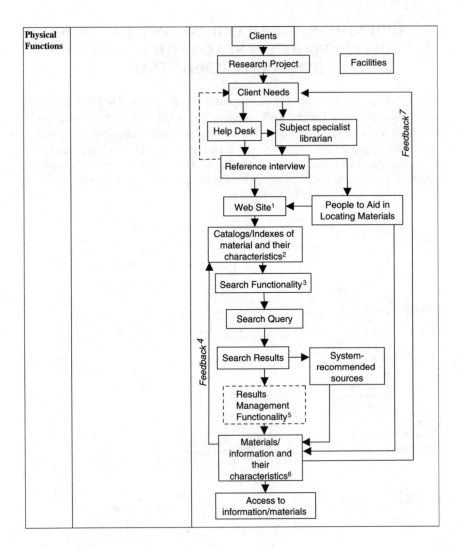

Physical Forms		· Academic Search Premier
		· Academic Universe
		· Alta Vista
		· AP photo database
		· Applied Science and Technology (database)
		· Center for Information Management (CIM)
		· ChemAbstracts (database)
		· COMPENDEX (database)
		· Congtressional Universe
		· Endnote
		· ERIC (Specific database)
		· Google
		· Electronic Data Center
		· jake.net.yale.edu web site
		· MathSciNet (database)
		· MEDLINE
		· Newsweek
		· ProCite
		· PsychInfo
		· Science Citation Index (database)
		· Social Sciences Database
		· Zentralblatt MATH (database)

[1] The category "Web Site" includes any web site that might be used as a tool for gaining information about materials or accessing materials, including database-driven web sites, Internet search engines, free web sites and pay-to-use web sites.

[2] The category "Catalogs/Indexes of material and their characteristics" indicates that catalogs/indexes of material can be differentiated by such factors as the content they contain, the functionality they provide for searching information, the options they offer for information access (e.g., online access), etc.

[3] The category "Search Functionality" includes search features used to locate/access materials, such as keyword search, federated searching, controlled vocabulary, alternate keywords/topics, and combination/intersection of result sets.

[4] The first "Feedback" loop involves taking the resultsof/information from a search and using it to create a refined search.

[5] The category "Results Management Functionality" refers to features that allow one to manipulate results sets--e.g., sort, filter, etc.

[6] The category "Materials/information and their characteristics" includes a variety of materials (e.g., books, videos, photos) and their characteristics (e.g., academic rigor, availability, cost, currency/recency of information).

[7] The second "Feedback" loop involves taking the information from a search and/or the materials obtained via a search and using it to refine the client's research problem.

APPENDIX F. TOPOLOGICAL ABSTRACTION–
DECOMPOSITION SPACE FOR QUICK ANSWER
SUBSYSTEM

The following is the topological representation of the Quick Answer subsystem, paired with the Total System. Quick Answer involves answering a specific question brought by a client. The following includes both the

220   KEVIN J. SIMONS ET AL.

original ADS items (solid lines) and ADS items added per librarian feedback in follow-up interviews (dashed lines).

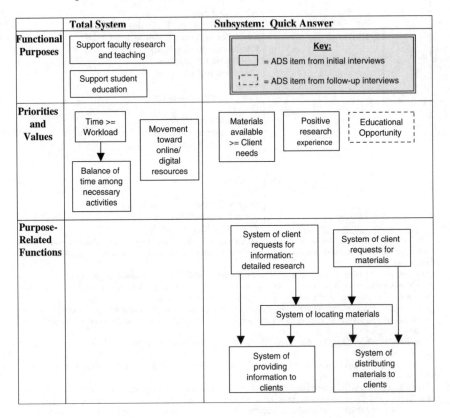

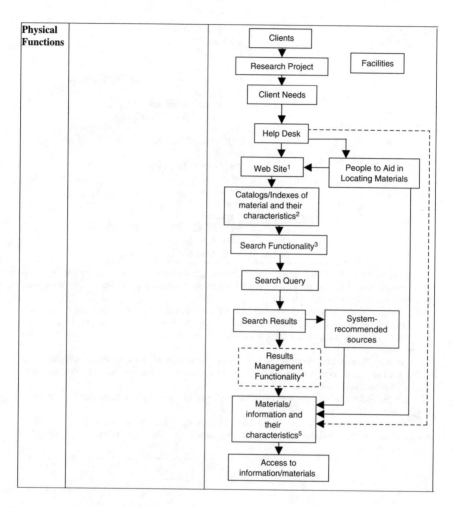

Physical Forms		· Academic Search Premier · Academic Universe · Alta Vista · AP photo database · Applied Science and Technology (database) · Blackboard · ChemAbstracts (database) · COMPENDEX (database) · Congressional Universe · ERIC (Specific database) · Google · MathSciNet (database) · MEDLINE · Newsweek · ProCite · PsychInfo · Science Citation Index (database) · Social Sciences Database · Zentralblatt MATH (database)

[1]The category "Web Site" includes any website that might be used as a tool for gaining information about materials or accessing materials, including database-driven web sites, Internet search engines, free web sites and pay-to-use web sites.

[2]The category "Catalogs/Indexes of material and their characteristics" indicates that catalogs/indexes of material can be differentiated by such factors as the content they contain, the functionality they provide for searching information, the options they offer for information access (e.g., online access), etc.

[3]The category "Search Functionality" includes search features used to locate/access materials, such as keyword search, federated searching, controlled vocabulary, alternate keywords/topics, and combination/intersection of result sets.

[4]The category "Results Management Functionality" refers to features that allow one to manipulate results sets -- e.g., sort, filter, etc.

[5]The category "Materials/information and their characteristics" includes a variety of materials (e.g., books, videos, photos) and their characteristics (e.g., academic rigor, availability, cost, currency/recency of information).

APPENDIX G. TOPOLOGICAL ABSTRACTION– DECOMPOSITION SPACE FOR CLASSIFICATION SUBSYSTEM

The following is the topological representation of the Classification subsystem, paired with the Total System. The Classification subsystem includes the process of creating classification systems and using classification systems to assign metadata to information so that it can be retrieved at a later point.

The following includes both the original ADS items (solid lines) and ADS items added per librarian feedback in follow-up interviews (dashed lines).

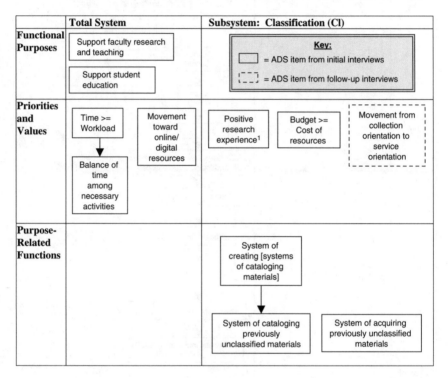

	Total System	**Subsystem: Classification (Cl)**
Functional Purposes	Support faculty research and teaching Support student education	**Key:** ▢ = ADS item from initial interviews ⌐ ¬ = ADS item from follow-up interviews
Priorities and Values	Time >= Workload → Balance of time among necessary activities Movement toward online/ digital resources	Positive research experience[1] Budget >= Cost of resources Movement from collection orientation to service orientation
Purpose-Related Functions		System of creating [systems of cataloging materials] ↓ System of cataloging previously unclassified materials System of acquiring previously unclassified materials

Physical Functions		

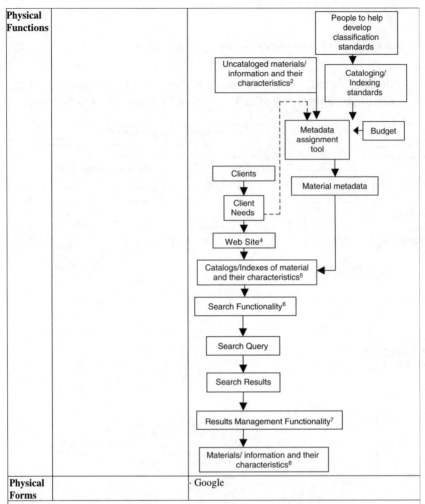

People to help develop classification standards

Uncataloged materials/ information and their characteristics[2]

Cataloging/ Indexing standards

Metadata assignment tool ← Budget

Clients

Client Needs

Material metadata

Web Site[4]

Catalogs/Indexes of material and their characteristics[5]

Search Functionality[6]

Search Query

Search Results

Results Management Functionality[7]

Materials/ information and their characteristics[8]

Physical Forms	· Google	

[1]The category "Positive Research Experience" encompasses the goal of Continuous Quality Improvement.

[2]The category "Uncataloged materials/information and their characteristics" includes materials that have not previously been classified (e.g., satellite and other geospatial data) and their characteristics

[3]The category "Budget" is only included as a specific item in the "Collection Building", "Classification", and "Information Creation", subsystem because these subsystems directly involve the purchase of tools and materials. However, it is understood that budgets indirectly affect every subsystems (because they have an effect on which materials are available, and how accessible they are).

[4]The category "Web Site" includes any web site that might be used as a tool for gaining information about materials or accessing materials, including database-driven web sites, Internet search engines, free web sites and pay-to-use web sites.

[5]The category "Catalogs/Indexes of material and their characteristics" indicates that catalogs/indexes of material can be differentiated by such factors as the content they contain, the functionality they provide for searching information, the options they offer for information access (e.g., online access), etc.

[6]The category "Search Functionality" includes search features used to locate/access materials, such as keyword search, federated searching, controlled vocabulary, alternate keywords/topics, and combination/intersection of result sets.

[7]The category "Results Management Functionality" refers to features that allow one to manipulate results sets--e.g., sort, filter, etc.

[8]The category "Materials/information and their characteristics" includes a variety of materials (e.g., books, videos, photos) and their characteristics (e.g., academic rigor, availability, cost, currency/recency of information).

APPENDIX H. TOPOLOGICAL ABSTRACTION– DECOMPOSITION SPACE FOR INFORMATION CREATION SUBSYSTEM

The following is the topological representation of the Information Creation subsystem, paired with the Total System. Information Creation is the process of helping clients take information they have gathered and publish it in a new form (e.g., video, web pages). The following includes both the original ADS items (solid lines) and ADS items added per librarian feedback in follow-up interviews (dashed lines).

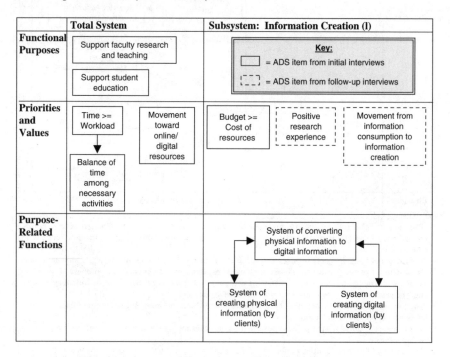

	Total System	Subsystem: Information Creation (I)	
Functional Purposes	Support faculty research and teaching Support student education	**Key:** ☐ = ADS item from initial interviews ⌐ ¬ = ADS item from follow-up interviews	
Priorities and Values	Time >= Workload → Balance of time among necessary activities	Movement toward online/ digital resources	Budget >= Cost of resources	Positive research experience	Movement from information consumption to information creation
Purpose-Related Functions		System of converting physical information to digital information → System of creating physical information (by clients) / System of creating digital information (by clients)	

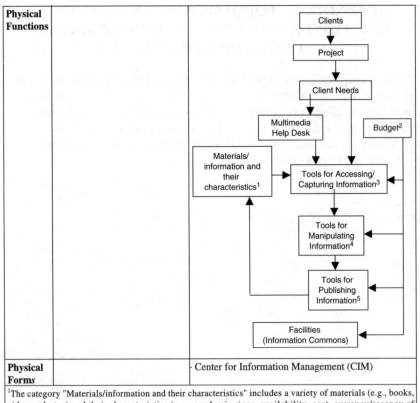

Physical Functions		

| **Physical Forms** | | · Center for Information Management (CIM) |

[1] The category "Materials/information and their characteristics" includes a variety of materials (e.g., books, videos, photos) and their characteristics (e.g., academic rigor, availability, cost, currency/recency of information).

[2] The category "Budget" is only included as a specific item in the "Collection Building", "Classification", and "Information Creation", subsystems because these subsystems directly involve the purchase of tools and materials. However, it is understood that budgets indirectly affect every subsystems (because they have an effect on which materials are available, and how accessible they are).

[3] The category "Tools for Accessing/Capturing Information" includes tools such as digital cameras, online image capturing tools, sound recording tools, etc.

[4] The category "Tools for Manipulating Information" includes tools such as image editing software, sound editing software, etc.

[5] The category "Tools for Publishing Information" includes tools such as CD burners, web creation tools, etc.

APPENDIX I. PARTICIPANT FEEDBACK ON TOPOLOGICAL ABSTRACTION–DECOMPOSITION SPACE REPRESENTATIONS

In follow-up interviews, librarians first were given a brief explanation of ADSs, then shown the topological ADS representations to which their initial interview contributed. During these follow-up interviews, the six librarian participants recommended the following revisions to the topological ADS representations. Checkboxes indicate which participants recommended each modification, while grayed-out cells indicate that a given participant's original interview did not contribute to this subsystem, so the participant did not provide feedback on this subsystem in the follow-up interview.

Key:

☑	= Participant recommended this modification
(gray)	= Participant did not report on this subsystem

		Participant					
		1	2	3	4	5	6
Quick Answer							
Priorities & Values							
	Added "Educational Opportunity"	☑	☑				☑
	Put each P&V side-by-side, to avoid unintentional perception of hierarchy	☑				☑	
Physical Functions							
	Removed "Reference Interview"		☑				
	Added loop from "Help Desk" to "Materials/information and their characteristics"		☑				
	Changed "Catalog/Index of Material" to "Catalogs/indexes of material and their characteristics"	☑			☑		
	Added "Results Management Functionality"	☑					

Detailed Research					
Priorities & Values					
Added "Educational Opportunity"					
Added "Availability/access restrictions on information"	☑				☑
Put each P&V side-by-side, to avoid unintentional perception of hierarchy					
Physical Functions					
Added feedback loop from Reference Interview to Client Needs		☑	☑		
Changed "Catalog/Index of Material" to "Catalogs/indexes of material and their characteristics"	☑			☑	
Added "Results Management Functionality"	☑				
Information Creation					
Priorities & Values					
Added "Positive Research Experience"		☑			☑
Added "Movement from information consumption to information creation"					☑
Physical Functions					
Changed "Tools for Capturing Information" to "Tools for Accessing/Capturing Information"		☑			
Changed "Research Project" to "Project"					☑
Changed "Facilities" to "Facilities (Information Commons)"					☑

Collection Building						
Priorities & Values						
Moved "Budget" below "Materials available >= Client Needs" and "Balance of usability issues"	☑					☑
Change "Balance of usability issues between traditional paper materials and online/digital resource" to "Balance of usability/accessibility issues between traditional paper materials and online/digital resource"	☑					
Added "Balanced Information (Among Different Points of View)"						☑
Added "Movement from collection orientation to service orientation"	☑					
Physical Functions						
Added indication in note on "Materials and their characteristics" that this also included Client Usage Records.						☑
Bibliographic Training						
Priorities & Values						
Added "Foster critical thinking/evaluation of information"		☑				
Physical Functions						
Added "Assessment of Instruction"				☑		

Classification								
Priorities & Values								
Added a note to "Positive Research Experience" that this encompasses the goal of Continuous Quality Improvement			☒					
Added "Movement from collection orientation to service orientation"			☒					
Physical Functions								
Added a feedback loop from Client Needs to Metadata Assignment Tool			☒					

LIBRARY MANAGEMENT EDUCATION AND REALITY: A CLEARER CONNECTION

Rich Gazan

ABSTRACT

The results of a study of a collaborative digital library development project suggested that activities positively associated with project success included various forms of connection work, such as integrating diverse people, organizations, and collections of information. The digital library study results are juxtaposed with the results of a survey of the skills and interests of 106 library school students, which revealed that though few aspire to be library managers per se, students reported strong interest in the type of collaborative and synthetic work found to be success factors in the digital library project. The comparison suggests a disconnection between theoretical management concepts, student perceptions of library management, and real-world practice in library management education. A hybrid library management course and practicum is proposed, one which de-emphasizes fictional case studies in favor of providing opportunities for students to evaluate management concepts by observing practice, and to challenge their perceptions of what management is.

Advances in Library Administration and Organization, Volume 24, 231–248
Copyright © 2007 by Elsevier Ltd.
All rights of reproduction in any form reserved
ISSN: 0732-0671/doi:10.1016/S0732-0671(06)24007-0

INTRODUCTION

A recent Library Journal article (Jacobsen, 2004) tracked 40 members of the UCLA MLS class of 1988 15 years into their professional careers. While the entire article provides a unique and effective reality check about career paths and expectations, relevant here is the graduates' consensus opinion about the relative value of their coursework:

> When asked about meaningful library school coursework, the Class of '88 said that cataloging was the acknowledged foundation ... followed by information-seeking behavior and a good solid handle on the reference interview. Management courses were the big question mark. Some respondents felt they were out of step with what graduates needed, while others lavished praise on their management professors' ability to teach from experience.

This conclusion should not surprise anyone familiar with management education in LIS. While current students might understandably view management as a required course that has little immediate relevance to the career they wish to pursue, the fact that this attitude persists a decade and a half into students' professional careers is more troubling.

Budd (2003) reviewed courses and syllabi from 50 ALA-accredited master's programs in LIS to address the question of how well the subtle and varied skills required in library management are being taught in MLS programs. While cautioning the extent to which syllabi are reliable indicators of course content, he writes:

> ... courses tend to focus considerably more on specific processes that arise in libraries, and less on the conceptual bases for addressing the processes. (p. 162)

While it is outside the scope of this chapter to rehash the larger schism between the diverse views of students, professionals, and researchers about how any subset of the LIS curriculum should be taught, understanding and articulating the difference between student perceptions of management and real-world practice is conceptual work, and should be one of the primary goals of library management education.

This chapter begins by reviewing some recent research that has called for an expanded view of library management, then juxtaposes the results of a study of the management of a digital library design project with the results of a 3-year survey of library school student attitudes about various aspects of library operations. Though students reported little interest and skill in management per se, they reported strong interest in management success factors found in the literature and identified in the digital library design project as forms of "connection work": creating connections across diverse people, organizations, and collections of information. The chapter concludes with a brief discussion of the implications of recasting library management education to reflect these results via a management practicum component.

BACKGROUND

Budd is certainly not the only researcher to have identified weaknesses in library management education as a whole. Frye (2001) reflects on emerging management challenges in academic libraries, where new university norms include for-profit models, lower budgets, supporting undergraduates with high technological needs and expectations, and undermining the "hegemony" of existing departmental boundaries by catalyzing cross-disciplinary research. Frye identifies several characteristics of an academic library leader, surprisingly few of which involve library-specific skills or knowledge: crafting a coherent vision and persuading talented people to embrace and work toward it, understanding and overcoming institutional resistance and creating relationships across diverse organizations. Similarly, Mosher (2001) sees a transformation of the role of research library directors from "keepers" of texts to "agents provocateur":

> By 'agent-provocateur' we mean nothing hostile or anti-social, but a role for the library director as teacher, philosopher of values, instigator, innovator, and provocative administrator: the librarian as a "change agent" on the university stage. (p. 313)

Kingston (2002) focused on the job tasks of five library managers at different levels of management, from a supervisor of a single individual to a supervisor of 141, and found that at all levels, relationship management was critical. Buckland (2003) seeks both "bolder" and more focused library research in his discussion of five "grand challenges" for library research, the first of which is the question of how library services might be made more meaningful to the people they serve. Buckland discusses bibliotherapy and affective factors related to information seeking as being of primary importance, providing another dimension to Kingston's relationship management: that of the relationship between people and the information they seek, a much subtler form of understanding the library customer than is generally taught in library management courses.

According to Budd, the most commonly used textbook in library management courses is Robert Stueart and Barbara Moran's *Library and Information Center Management* (Stueart & Moran, 2002). Currently in its sixth edition, the Stueart and Moran textbook is divided into seven sections:

Evolving, Planning, Organizing, Human Resources, Leading, Coordinating, and Managing in the 21st Century (which spans less than 10 pages). Though it contains an impressive distillation of management theory and tools, its main focus is on the practicalities of running a library: funding, staffing, mission statements, and so on. One would be hard pressed to imagine it as a manifesto for an aspiring agent-provocateur.

> Management isn't primarily about supervising others ... management's real genius is turning complexity and specialization into performance. (Magretta, 2002, p. 6)

You will not find Joan Magretta's name on an LIS faculty Website, but you will find it on the editorial masthead of *Harvard Business Review*. Her book *What Management Is* (Magretta, 2002) is an example of an alternative or complementary textbook that might be used as a non-library-centric introduction to management concepts and realities, with its focus on management challenges of well-known companies in a variety of industries. For example, branding is one of the most important concepts in management. It is the institutional identity, purposefully packaged and projected to its target audience via words, images, and everyday experience. All organizations— for profit or not—attempt to create and perpetuate a brand identity, and one of the primary factors for the success of any organization is the extent to which its brand is known and embraced by its target audience.

The library "brand" is connected with the core value of the institution: providing access to information. Introducing the concept of branding by starting with library values might seem the logical approach in a library management course, but introducing the general concept of branding with examples from outside the library allows students to evaluate for themselves which aspects of the concept relate to libraries, and which do not. Airlines, clothing companies, motorcycle manufacturers—all attempt to emphasize or de-emphasize particular aspects of their product or service and transform it into an identity bestowing object. Who flies British Airways as opposed to Southwest? Who rides a Harley versus a Triumph? Who uses the library? Who are our competitors? What aspects of our service should we emphasize or de-emphasize accordingly?

All organizations struggle to differentiate and communicate their brand, and all have obstacles to overcome. An overly library-centric view risks the perpetuation of the notion that due to their unique mission, libraries cannot learn from, or be compared with, other types of organizations. However, from a branding standpoint, it is precisely that uniqueness that should be actively compared.

> **habit,** *n.* A shackle for the free. Bierce (1911)

Overall, there is a sense in the literature that library management, like librarianship itself, has been limited primarily by external forces, such as university administration, or a social environment that deprivileges those in service professions. However, the individuals within the library and information professions must accept some responsibility as well. The foundation for any kind of change must arise from a more nuanced understanding of what management is – and can be – both inside and outside the library. One way to gather such data is to observe innovative library management projects.

CASE STUDY: THE MANAGEMENT OF A DIGITAL LIBRARY DEVELOPMENT PROJECT

This section will discuss the management implications of a digital library development project where a diverse array of environmental scientists, librarians, archivists, educators, managers, and system builders from a variety of different institutions came together to build a university-based environmental science digital library. The investigation was focused on the concept of connection work, defined as activity creating opportunities for the exchange of diverse types of knowledge. Data were collected via fieldwork, observations, interviews, and document analysis, resulting in a series of social network diagrams depicting information sharing relationships at four critical points in the project as identified by the participants, and a narrative of the first grant-funded year of the project. Narrative analysis revealed several management-related activities that participants believed contributed to the success of the project, which can be summarized as the ability to see connections between diverse people, organizations, and collections.

Whether weaving together disparate types of knowledge or simple pieces of cloth, connections are made at the boundaries. The concept of a boundary object is useful not just to draw conceptual borders between communities or knowledge forms – an inherently inexact activity – but to examine areas of interaction and how meaning is negotiated across them. People from different backgrounds are "often helped to communicate by a shared object: a rock, a diagram, a collection of stories and observations, a pile of computer code, and so on" (Agre, 2000). Bowker and Star (1999, pp. 15–16), provide a more formal definition of boundary objects:

> ... we speak of classifications as objects for cooperation across social worlds, or as boundary objects (Star & Griesemer, 1989). Drawing from earlier studies of

interdisciplinary scientific cooperation, we define boundary objects as those objects that
both inhabit several communities of practice *and* satisfy the informational requirements
of each of them … [they are] both ambiguous and constant; they may be abstract or
concrete.

It is important to note that the word "satisfy" is not used here in the sense of
total fulfillment as when repaying a loan, but in the weaker sense of in-
complete, though passable, success (OED, 2003). Boundary objects mediate
the different goals and perspectives of diverse actors, and serve as a means
of coordination, alignment, and translation. They are dynamic, adjusted as
needed to fit changing situations.

Klein (1990, pp. 189–190) offers a list of "integrative techniques" people
use to work toward integrative synthesis in multidisciplinary environments.
Note that most of these techniques involve boundary objects and connection
work of some sort:

- Regular meetings
- Internal and external presentations
- Joint organizing and planning
- Periodic reports and reviews
- Joint presentations, publications, and papers
- Common data
- Common vocabulary
- Common equipment
- Common facilities
- Common objectives
- Articulating differences among team members
- Performing iterations
- Involving the client/user/customer
- Using established techniques
- Analysis of common object/objective
- Focusing on a common enemy
- Informal gatherings
- Role negotiation

The environmental information system that is the object of this study
brings together environmental data sets, archival photographs, mission logs
of research expeditions, oral histories, and other diverse content into a single
merged collection. It was imagined from the beginning not just as a collection of disparate items, but also as an integrated resource that would
present a more holistic and realistic view of environmental science to both
researchers and the general public. Having researchers and professionals

come together to help design the system and combining the disparate collections was supposed to create new knowledge, in the sort of "integrative synthesis" that typifies true interdisciplinarity (Klein, 1990, p. 118). This was one of the most captivating rationales for the project: the potential for a university library to create "hybrid knowledge" (Gazan, 2004) by the juxtaposition and integration of diverse resources. This was a ripe environment in which to observe innovative library management practice.

Though it is always debatable to identify one moment when a project begins, the first seeds of the environmental information system were sown 2 years before the grant proposal was written. The University[1] had hired a new University Librarian who had a strong background in digital libraries. One of his goals was to provide better access to the disparate and unique collections of the University, many of which had been underutilized.

> [The University Librarian] provided the initial focus. From day one, he wanted to innovate in digital libraries ...
>
> Associate University Librarian

Shortly after arriving at the University, the University Librarian formed the Digital Library Innovation Team (DLIT). As a starting point, the DLIT developed a mission statement to describe the University's digital library effort:

> The [University] Libraries will create for the [University] community a comprehensive digital library program to provide a powerful, useful, and exciting environment for access to digital information and knowledge. The Libraries will catalyze and develop collaborations among the campus' various information and knowledge centers to enhance scholarship and research.

While few mission statements can be lauded for their modesty or understatement, relevant here is the notion of libraries as catalysts, taking an active role in developing collaborations between disparate units of the University. In its original definition, a catalyst increases the rate of a chemical reaction or process, but the word has been extended in common usage to include senses of initiation and transformation more generally (OED, 2003). This gets to the very core of connection work: it is an active, conscious process, an attempt to create beneficial synergies that would otherwise be made less efficiently, or not at all:

> I've been convinced you can use one medium as a way of navigating another, with unanticipated results, which can give you new knowledge. By bringing photos, text, and data from multiple agencies together, you get different views – maybe perspectives is a better word – on the same stuff. Like the fish catch stats in combo with [historical] photos, you can get two senses of the economic history of local tuna fisheries. When you

study the two collections together, you can get there, but if you studied each alone, you couldn't.

University Librarian

Coming up with the initial vision is one challenge, but communicating it effectively is another. Did the other participants buy into this vision?

I don't think we thought we were revolutionizing academic libraries or anything. But there was an excitement then ... this new guy coming in, young and forceful. You wanted to be part of it.

DLIT team member

The paper trail continues with a document from May 2000 which summarizes "discussions to date" and outlines next steps in the digital library effort. It is an informal document in which the University Librarian essentially summarizes and responds to the recommendations of the DLIT:

DL development priorities should be driven by the needs/interests of our primary clientele, initiatives should reflect who we are as a campus and a community, and development should be opportunistic (in the best sense of the word)...So, in my mind our discussions to date argue for a [Research Institute]-based (but including content from other collections as appropriate) content creation project with an environmental focus.

University Librarian

The Research Institute is connected with the university and generates a significant amount of collection items and demand for library services – an important player to include in a project such as this. The University Librarian's goal of content creation can be understood in both a stronger and a weaker sense. The weaker sense is that simply by digitizing print materials, one can be said to be creating digital content. In the stronger sense, digitizing and juxtaposing different forms and types of content can be thought of as the production of hybrid knowledge. However, at this early point in the project, there was little evidence to support one interpretation over another.

The University Librarian's reference to user-driven priorities might be seen as an obligatory statement, so common as to scarcely merit comment. Beneath it, however, is evidence of libraries' longstanding habit of deference to users both real and imagined. One way to interpret this statement is: no digital library initiative will be developed without prior user demand. The danger of taking this posture is that a library or any information organization might, consciously or not, abdicate its expertise and creativity. In this case, however, the University Librarian reclaims some flexibility by including the statement about "opportunistic" development. Library administrators are well positioned to identify opportunities actively, not reactively, and decide how best to act on them.

Certainly not all of the decision-making processes in this project relied on rational debate and abstract visions about the role of the academic library. The development and management of any information system is situated in a social and political context, and these institutional actors shape planning and practice as well. An excerpt from an internal document from the DLIT provides a glimpse of relationship management processes at work:

> Generally, in suggesting a content creation project I am mindful of who we are, where we are, and the value of defining a niche predicated on both. In suggesting a [Research Institute]-based content creation project, I am mindful of [the Research Institute Director] as a powerful political ally .... In suggesting the possible desirability of developing (an) open archive(s), I am mindful of the likely advantages (political, financial, etc.) of aligning ourselves with those.
>
> University Librarian

The concept of aligning the interests of diverse actors in this project appeared again and again, and out of the mouths of many individuals connected with the project. Even when grant funding was being discussed, the idea of interpretation, integration, and synthesis as a means to move the project forward recurred:

> I have a long track record with grants and the State Library, I'm very familiar with the selection process. The [State Library] already features some content from our [Research Institute] archive. That was the first directory using LSTA grant and federal money, a few million over a few years to create an online archive. So we framed it as leveraging that investment that had already been made. Funding agencies like to leverage past work.
>
> University Librarian

One way to think about "leveraging past work" is connecting a proposed project with work that has come before. Having the ability to see and articulate connections across projects provides an advantage when seeking grant funding. A successful grant proposal will link the stated or perceived goals of the funding agency with those of the project as explicitly as possible, even when the connection might be rather tenuous. But merely reciting bullet points is generally not enough. Something surprising or innovative must come out of these goals – a "hook" – to get a funding agency interested.

> Part of the art of grant writing is interpreting vague language in a way that lets you do what you want to do. If we could digitize a chunk of our collections, partner with related institutions and provide Web access, that would make them happy enough. But I knew

what would distinguish our proposal was the integration aspect, bringing together this variety of resources. So we really hung our hat on that.

University Librarian

The University Librarian was the most central individual in the social network during the initial phase of the project. He set the agenda, invited people from various University libraries and community institutions to participate, guided discussions, and evaluated and prioritized the recommendations of the project team. He was also the connector between the DLIT, the Director of the Research Institute, the State Library, and the digital library community in general. However, the importance of staying connected with the larger political and economic environment, and having the ability to see connections and anticipate opportunity, cannot be overstated:

There's a big political angle to this too. There's a budget crisis, and a big boom of 18-year-olds coming into the university system. Priority one is educating these kids, so there's less of an emphasis on preserving these collections that are pretty much just sitting there occupying space and resources. People are freaking out, and this panic has made them more open to the idea of sharing their collections, digitizing them, partnering with libraries, and listening to our ideas. It gives the library more influence, which is a good thing for everyone. Crisis makes people very creative.

University Librarian

Though the University Librarian is the primary focus in this discussion, other project participants also reported doing connection work, in various forms, that they identified collectively as contributing to the success of the project. For example, the environmental scientists and the information specialists participating in the design of the system had vastly different conceptions of the system's goals. The scientists saw the project primarily as the means to digitize environmental data sets and create a database, and thought other collections were "just along for the ride." Though the scientists did participate in conversations outside their domain of expertise, for example about appropriate metadata, they tended to be interested in metadata issues only insofar as they made the environmental data sets accessible. This suggests a difference in the "relative informational value" of different collection items and access points, in terms of Budd's (2002, p. 97) sense of warrant. A common access point in many databases is a statement about an item's form, which sometimes appears as a Resource Type or Document Type field, with a value like text, image, or data set. In a usability study conducted on a beta version of the system, geography students and instructors often suggested that the forms of information are an indicator of whether an item is likely to be useful or not. In contrast, the information specialists who conceived and built the site worked from the assumption that all forms could be equally useful, if they could be presented in an integrated way.

Throughout the project, other examples of connection work included document-related activities such as merging different classification schemes, social processes such as patterns of knowledge sharing and linking otherwise disconnected individuals, and creative acts such as imposing a unifying narrative across merged collections. In the social network analysis, the people who did connection work linked otherwise disconnected individuals, received information from a variety of others, were able to articulate the roles and goals of diverse others, interacted with members of multiple communities, and could perceive connections between disparate information forms. In the eyes of the project participants, what moved the project forward was incidents of connection work, not the application of library management theory or best practices found in a textbook.

General barriers to connection work in this project included contested collaboration, lack of shared vision about the goals of the system, institutional differences, and differences in the prestige of the diverse actors. Though the stage had been set for a collaborative design project, environmental scientists primarily wanted digital access to archival resources, new data sets and to have their work portrayed in historical context. The information specialists wished to use their knowledge of the disparate yet related collections to create a system that could catalyze new knowledge. The grant provided the funding and infrastructure, but opportunities for idea exchange were more and more rarely acted upon as the project moved forward. Interestingly, the fragmentation of the constituent groups in the project increased as the University Librarian's involvement decreased. The University Librarian's initial vision to catalyze new knowledge was implemented in the design phase by someone without as much institutional clout. It is certainly debatable whether research scientists or outside institutions would have responded to the University Librarian's personal influence had he been more involved throughout the project, but his later absence did correlate with a general decline in connection work.

The results suggest that though some of the collaborative and integrative aspirations of the project were not ultimately achieved, evidence of various forms of connection work and integration was found in the project. Interviews with project participants and the results of the usability study support the suggestion that the most successful aspects of the system were those where some connection work took place.

In sum, indicators of connection work during the digital library project's initial phase included:

- The University Librarian's initial vision to connect disparate University libraries via a digital library initiative
- The formation of the DLIT
- The DLIT's stated goal of "catalyzing" research collaborations between disparate University research units via "content creation"
- DLIT brainstorming meetings, where candidate collections for digitization were debated and linked to user needs and University missions
- The linkage of digitization project goals with those of funding agencies
- Targeting a wide audience including researchers and the public
- Collaborating with non-academic institutions.
- Consulting with scientists about content decisions
- Integrating disparate collections in a conscious attempt to create new knowledge

Throughout the project, activities identified by the participants as most effective were those which required the ability to identify and integrate diverse people, organizations and resources, as well as sheer creativity. The results of this case study support the idea that the actual work of library managers and administrators, at least in some environments, does justify an analogy as glamorous and intriguing as agent-provocateur. But what do students think?

LIBRARY MANAGEMENT SKILLS AND INTERESTS SURVEY

To help determine library school student attitudes about various aspects of library operations, a survey was administered to 106 library school students at three different institutions over the course of 3 years. Students were given a list of 40 statements about their work styles, attitudes, and preferences, and were asked to rate each statement on a scale of 1 (strongly disagree) to 5 (strongly agree). The complete instrument can be found in the appendix (and it should be noted that some questions were intentionally poorly worded to serve as a research methods and survey instrument evaluation exercise).

While this research is still ongoing, Table 1 lists the statements that the students to date have most strongly agreed with, while Table 2 lists the statements that students have most strongly disagreed with.

Table 1. Statements that LIS Students have Most Strongly Agreed With
($n = 106$).

Statement	Mean
I enjoy solving problems	4.32
I enjoy the physical atmosphere of libraries	4.27
I'm good at integrating diverse views or conflicting data to arrive at a decision	4.23
I feel more comfortable making a decision when I have data to back it up	4.13
I like being a source of information	4.10
I'm good at collecting, synthesizing, and analyzing information	4.00
I can communicate with a wide variety of people	3.97

Table 2. Statements that LIS Students have Most Strongly Disagreed
With ($n = 106$).

Statement	Mean
I'd like to manage people	2.69
I'm good at giving presentations and public speaking	2.77
I'd like to manage projects	2.81
Analyzing how work is done is as important as doing the work	2.86
I'd like to direct a library someday	2.95
I thrive on change, and am always looking for ways to "shake things up"	3.02

The results summarized in Tables 1 and 2 suggest a fundamental disconnect between what management is, and what students think it is. Any of the seven statements shown in Table 1, those with which students most strongly agreed, could form a significant part of a library manager's job description. However, when you package the same attitudes and activities and call them management, students' interest and confidence wither.

In addition, most management courses include at least a mention of the contingency theory of leadership (Fiedler, 1967), which, briefly stated, posits a dynamic interaction between individual leadership skills and a favorable situation. Some students interpret this as evidence that since management decisions can only be understood in the context of their application, a management course is essentially moot. A passage extracted from one student's library management course evaluation further illustrates the problem:

> I found the case study exercises we did in class useful, but it seemed like most of the discussion had to center around getting a handle on the context of the fictional situation, not the wider issues (much as you tried to steer conversation in that direction).

This student is exactly right. The data from the digital library development project were collected over the course of a 10-month participant observation, and even being present to observe the dynamics of the design process was not sufficient to uncover project success factors until the interview instrument was refined several times, and participants' interview responses were analyzed and compared to one another. Most project participants claimed some conceptual underpinnings to their decision making, but their decisions were always tempered by the messy reality of the situation, where one's skill with people is almost always more important than one's skill with spreadsheets.

Integrating diverse views, communicating with a variety of people, collecting and synthesizing information—following the data analysis method of the digital library study, all of these statements would be coded as instances of connection work, and positively associated with success in a collaborative project. However, the results of the survey also suggest that library management instructors are in the unenviable position of having to "teach uphill" – they must attempt to overcome negative student perceptions of the course content in addition to teaching the content itself. What can be done to demonstrate a clearer connection between management concepts from outside the library with library management in practice, and more importantly, to give students a reason to challenge their own conceptions of what management is?

CONCLUSION

The common themes in the library management literature, case study, and survey results seem somewhat paradoxical. There are calls for more conceptual content in library management courses, and a parallel need for more realistic examples of management concepts in the context of their application. An approach to library management education that takes the middle path, and relies on fictional case studies and teaching best practices for "generic" academic, public, school, or special libraries risks a one-size-fits-all portrayal of library management that students know very well is not realistic.

A library manager is concerned with successful execution of the goals of the organization, but within that apparently narrow charge there is abundant opportunity to manage relationships, integrate diverse people, organizations and information, assess and anticipate environmental factors, and work creatively. In the digital library development study, people who did connection work were identified as more critical to the success of the project than people who had the word "manager" in their title. With sufficient immersion in other library environments, different and even less-obvious success factors could be found, yielding more data with which to support or challenge high-level management concepts.

A hybrid library management course and practicum is proposed here, one that introduces management concepts outside the library, and gives students the opportunity to evaluate for themselves which can be applied to particular library situations. To provide real-world context, students could then be placed in a library for the latter part of the course, with the charge of evaluating how the concepts are being addressed by a particular group or within a particular project. For example, having learned about branding, marketing, and competitive intelligence in the first part of the course, one might investigate how the local public library branch is marketing its storytimes, as more and more diverse organizations are offering similar parent–child experiences, such as "mommy and me" yoga classes. Observing and asking how decisions are made, and juxtaposing how similar issues are treated in non-library organizations, can yield educational benefit for the students, and benefits for the practicum site as well.

The educational infrastructure to pilot this sort of hybrid library management course is already in place. Most library schools have an internship or practicum built into their degree programs, but few link the practicum experience explicitly with management (two notable exceptions are Emporia State, which offers an Information Management practicum, and Pittsburgh's Supervisor of Library Science Certificate program, which has a school library management practicum). There are service learning and community engagement course credit opportunities in many programs that could be extended to support a hybrid management course as well.

At bottom, the means by which students are provided a broader and more realistic picture of the work of library managers is less important than the task itself. This chapter began by reviewing previous work suggesting that the role of a library manager has evolved from passive caretaker to active integrator of diverse people, organizations, and collections, which the results of the digital library development study supported. The skills associated with success – the ability to see connections – are precisely those that students report not just having, but enjoying. All they need is room to run.

NOTES

1. The name and certain details of the system are withheld to protect the privacy of the participants, in accordance with UCLA Office for Protection of Research Subjects policy.

REFERENCES

Agre, P. E. (2000). *Information systems analysis and design*. Available online at: http://pola-ris.gseis.ucla.edu/pagre/240/week6.html.

Bierce, A. (1911). *The devil's dictionary*. Cleveland and New York: World Publishing Co.

Bowker, G. C., & Star, S. L. (1999). *Sorting things out: Classification and its consequences*. Cambridge, MA: MIT Press.

Buckland, M. K. (2003). Five grand challenges for library research. *Library Trends, 51*(4), 675–686.

Budd, J. M. (2002). Jesse Shera, social epistemology and praxis. *Social Epistemology, 16*(1), 93–98 Greenwich, Conn: JAI Press.

Budd, J. M. (2003). Management education for library and information science. In: E. D. Garten & D. E. Williams (Eds), *Advances inlibrary administration and organization*, (Vol. 20, pp. 149–163).

Fiedler, F. E. (1967). *A theory of leadership effectiveness*. New York: McGraw-Hill.

Frye, B. E. (2001). Some reflections on universities, libraries and leadership. In: E. D. Garten & D. E. Williams (Eds), *Advances in library administration and organization*, (Vol. 18, pp. 293–305). Greenwich, Conn: JAI Press.

Gazan, R. (2004). *Creating hybrid knowledge: A role for the professional integrationist*. Ph.D. dissertation, University of California, Los Angeles.

Jacobsen, T. L. (2004). The class of 1988. *Library Journal*. Available online at: http://library-journal.com/article/CA434406.html.

Kingston, D. (2002). Academic library managers at work: Relationships, contacts and foci of attention. In: E. D. Garten & D. E. Williams (Eds), *Advances in library administration and organization*, (Vol. 19, pp. 101–136). Greenwich, Conn: JAI Press.

Klein, J. T. (1990). *Interdisciplinarity: History, theory and practice*. Detroit: Wayne State University Press.

Magretta, J. (2002). *What management is*. New York: Free Press.

Mosher, P. H. (2001). The research library director: From keeper to agent-provocateur. In: E. D. Garten, D. E. Williams & E. Delmus (Eds), *Advances in library administration and organization*, (Vol. 18, pp. 307–316). Greenwich, Conn: JAI Press.

OED. (2003). *Oxford English Dictionary*. Available online at: http://www.oed.com.

Star, S. L., & Griesemer, J. R. (1989). Institutional ecology, "translations," and boundary objects: Amateurs and professionals in Berkeley's Museum of Vertebrate Zoology, 1907–39. *Social Studies of Science, 19*, 387–420.

Stueart, R. D., & Barbara, B. M. (Eds) (2002). *Library and information center management*, (6th ed). Greenwood Village, CO: Libraries Unlimited.

APPENDIX: LIBRARY MANAGEMENT SKILLS AND INTERESTS INSTRUMENT

Circle the number that best corresponds to your opinion about each statement. Take time to consider the implications of your response to each statement, and answer as honestly as you can.

1 – Strongly disagree|2 – Disagree|3 – Neutral or no opinion|4 – Agree|5 – Strongly agree

I'm a "big picture" sort of person; I like generating ideas and strategies	1 2 3 4 5
I'd like to direct a library someday	1 2 3 4 5
I'd like to manage projects	1 2 3 4 5
I'd like to manage people	1 2 3 4 5
I enjoy the technical side of librarianship	1 2 3 4 5
I enjoy the personal/service side of librarianship	1 2 3 4 5
I enjoy the intellectual side of librarianship	1 2 3 4 5
I enjoy the physical atmosphere of libraries	1 2 3 4 5
I like working with people outside my group and/or outside the organization	1 2 3 4 5
My career is only a small part of what makes me happy	1 2 3 4 5
I can communicate with a wide variety of people	1 2 3 4 5
I'm usually aware of how other people are feeling	1 2 3 4 5
I'm usually sensitive to how my words might be received	1 2 3 4 5
I think I'm politically astute; I know when to speak and when to remain silent	1 2 3 4 5

Statement					
I'm somewhat suspicious of "leader types"; sometimes lying is part of their job	1	2	3	4	5
I enjoy solving problems	1	2	3	4	5
Analyzing how work is done is as important as doing the work	1	2	3	4	5
I'm good at collecting, synthesizing, and analyzing information	1	2	3	4	5
I'm good at writing	1	2	3	4	5
I'm good at making charts and graphics	1	2	3	4	5
I'm good at giving presentations and public speaking	1	2	3	4	5
I'm good at planning and time management	1	2	3	4	5
I prefer working alone	1	2	3	4	5
I enjoy interacting with others	1	2	3	4	5
I'd rather work for one boss than have to constantly negotiate among equals	1	2	3	4	5
Meetings and process analysis are a waste of time; just let me do my job!	1	2	3	4	5
I tend to feel more loyalty to co-workers than to the organization	1	2	3	4	5
I thrive on change, and am always looking for ways to "shake things up"	1	2	3	4	5
I like a stable, dependable work environment	1	2	3	4	5
I tend to do things at the last minute	1	2	3	4	5
Working under deadline pressure brings out the best in me	1	2	3	4	5
Co-workers have to earn my respect	1	2	3	4	5
Underperforming co-workers must be confronted	1	2	3	4	5
I'm uncomfortable around conflict	1	2	3	4	5
I actively attempt to resolve conflicts	1	2	3	4	5
I enjoy making decisions	1	2	3	4	5
I like being a source of information	1	2	3	4	5
I tend to follow my intuition when making decisions	1	2	3	4	5
I feel more comfortable making a decision when I have some data to back it up	1	2	3	4	5
I'm good at integrating diverse views or conflicting data to arrive at a decision	1	2	3	4	5

INNOVATIVE LIBRARY PROGRAMS FOR THE HISPANIC POPULATION: OPPORTUNITIES FOR THE PUBLIC LIBRARY ADMINISTRATOR

Anna Maria Guerra

ABSTRACT

For centuries, the Hispanic population has been proving itself as an emerging majority in the United States. The United States census shows that the Hispanic population more than doubled from 1970 to 1980 and from 1980 to 1990. However, despite these data, libraries have not adapted their library services to meet the needs of this population, despite their knowledge that Hispanics do not feel welcome in libraries. Authors from 1970 to 2001 have highlighted the long-standing problem of Hispanic under-utilization of libraries and have provided recommendations for the library community regarding adapting their services in a culturally sensitive manner. Despite these publications, there is still literature in 2001 reporting that Hispanics do not feel welcome in libraries. The purpose of this study is to examine the current status of three facets of librarianship: (1) outreach efforts to Hispanics; (2) specialized training for Hispanics in bibliographic and information literacy; and (3) current attitudes of Hispanics toward public libraries.

Advances in Library Administration and Organization, Volume 24, 249–317
Copyright © 2007 by Elsevier Ltd.
ISSN: 0732-0671/doi:10.1016/S0732-0671(06)24008-2

For centuries, the Hispanic population has been proving itself as an emerging majority in the United States. The United States census showed that the Hispanic population more than doubled from 1970 to 1980 and again from 1980 to 1990. The Census Bureau predicted that the Hispanic population would grow from 22.4 million in 1990 to 59 million in 2030, and to 81 million in 2050. The census also showed that Hispanics were less likely to complete high school and to hold fewer managerial and professional jobs than non-minorities. Seventy-eight percent of the Hispanics who participated in the census reported not speaking English at home, and 2 out of every 10 Hispanics reported an income at or below the poverty level. The data for non-Hispanic respondents indicated that 1 out of every 10 of these respondents reported an income below the poverty level.

However, even given this long-standing growth trend and other demographical attributes of Hispanics, libraries have not adapted their services to meet the needs of this population despite the profession's understanding that Hispanics have not felt welcome in libraries. Authors writing from 1970 to 2001 have commented on the lack of information in the library literature regarding the issue of under-utilization of public libraries by Hispanics. During the same 30-year period, authors have highlighted the long-standing problem of under-representation of minorities in Masters in Information and Library Science (MLIS) programs, and many of them have provided recommendations about adapting their services in a culturally sensitive manner. But, despite these publications spanning three decades, there have still been regular reports that minorities, including Hispanics, have not felt welcome in libraries.

This paper examined under-utilization of public libraries by minorities (including Hispanics) and the limited efforts by libraries to address this problem. Possible explanations and remedies for the minority population's sense of alienation from libraries were explored, with an emphasis placed on the Hispanic population. The author then analyzed the impact of the programs that have developed in response to the scanty literature that has addressed how to provide and market programs as well as how to develop collections which are culturally sensitive to the needs of the Hispanic community. Finally, the author evaluated a community that is 56% Hispanic. Individuals from this community responded to a questionnaire about community members' experiences and perceptions of public libraries. The analysis of these survey results, combined with the overview of library literature, will assist library administrators in the development of programs more closely aligned with the interests and needs of the Hispanic community. Throughout this paper, the terms "Hispanic," "Latino," and the

"Spanish-speaking" were interchanged. "Latino Librarianship" was defined here as library services to users with roots in Hispanic cultures.

MINORITIES AS UNDER-UTILIZERS OF LIBRARIES

This portion of the paper will explore the literature concerning under-utilization of libraries and computer technology by minority groups. The author also examined how libraries have attempted to engage minorities in general, and Hispanics in particular, in order to make them feel more welcome. Typical Foundations of Library and Information Science (LIS) textbooks have taught beginning LIS students that minorities have not felt welcome in libraries and are under-represented in the library workforce (Rubin, 2000; Eberhart, 2000). Multicultural LIS classes have presented the readings of two renowned authors (Haro, 1981; Stern, 1991) who hypothesized that Hispanics recognized the benefits of better education, and saw the library as an avenue to better education, but also saw the library as an institution created by Anglo Americans to serve Anglo Americans, not Hispanics. Stern (1991, p. 96) recommended approaching Hispanics as a population, which is "ethnically enfranchised and as equal partners with non-ethnic residents in the fight to improve the quality of their lives and the communities in which they reside." Stern concluded, therefore, that the Hispanic population needed to be empowered.

Computer literacy has been identified as significantly different for minorities than for non-minorities. Howland (1998) asserted that technological advances were facilitating the social and economic advancement of society members unequally. These technological advances were allegedly contributing to the disparity in society between the "haves" (those who have money and/or socioeconomic status) and the "have-nots." Howland continued by describing America's society as having a "digital divide" or a technological chasm between people with higher socioeconomic status and those with lower socioeconomic status. He reported surveys showing that one out of five renters in South Central Los Angeles did not have a phone and that 60% of the global population did not possess phones; he concluded that Internet access was probably non-existent for the individuals surveyed in these two studies (p. 287).

Venturella (1998) concurred with Howland. She discussed how even library electronic resources were divided along economic lines, arguing that grant money tended to go to libraries that were already wealthy enough to have started purchasing technology, and that this phenomenon replicated the pattern of computers benefiting those who already had socioeconomic

power (the "haves"). She even claimed that, in higher education, "historically Black colleges, institutions serving 'Americans,' and those with large
low-income populations" were the educational programs that "get the benefits of technology last." She proffered a similar argument with regard to
school children. Venturella reported that national studies of access to computers among school children have shown that "the predictable two-tier
pattern" (the "haves" versus the "have-nots") has been found in children's
schools and that this pattern was also divided along racial and ethnic lines
with regard to technological resources in school settings (p. 24).

McCook (1997) reported on a survey of individuals who were over 18 years
of age and lived in an area that included two separate counties. The results
showed that the majority of the citizens surveyed did not have phones, were
Spanish speaking, and lived in poverty. Therefore, according to McCook, the
Internet would not be understandable or accessible to these "have-nots." This
survey included personal interviews conducted at shopping areas, such as
Wal-Mart. A few previous Internet studies, claiming that the "digital divide"
was narrowing, had conducted their surveys by phone, and thus had not
tapped the segment of the population without phones. These surveys were
allegedly performed to justify spending more library funds on technology.
McCook's argument was that, if such spending had occurred, there would be
no funds to perform the community outreach needed to reach the segment of
the population that required other library services before even becoming
technologically literate. She contended that librarians would be cutback in
order to buy computers, and that, as a result, there would not be sufficient
personnel to serve the community. McCook contended that the misplaced
emphasis on funding computers was analogous to library schools changing
their name from Masters in Library Science (MLS) to MLIS programs.
McCook called for rebalancing "information science" and library services.

The United States Department of Commerce performed a study in July
1998, which found that the technological disparity was growing between
minorities and non-minorities in all income groups and that the disparity
had even doubled in some income groups. For details of this study, see the
worldwide web URL presented in the Bibliography section under NTIA
(2001). The San Jose Mercury also reported in 1998 that the "digital divide"
was growing between the "haves" and "have-nots," citing a study under the
Clinton administration which found that Hispanics and African Americans
were even further behind Anglo Americans with regard to owning computers than they had been in 1995 (Plotnikoff, 1998). As a result, the Clinton
administration outlined plans to take the Internet and online knowledge to
inner city and rural schools in an attempt to close the digital divide. The

program involved encouraging online tutoring of students by volunteer "mentors" in the government and the private sector. The National Science Foundation and the Department of Education sponsored a workshop to recruit companies, unions, and other groups for this program (San Jose Mercury Newswire, 1998).

Castillo-Speed (2001) concurred with all of the above theories about the "digital divide." She reported that the gap was only narrowing in research studies where surveys were performed by phone, such as in the Cheskin Research (April 2000–Fall 2002). However, the author contended that these studies did not accurately represent the extent of minority usage of the Internet because they assumed that minorities possessed telephones. She also asserted that the Cheskin Research studied only a group of acculturated minorities, not the entire population (Cheskin, 2000-2002). Bagasao (1999) and Schement (1999) utilized a much more accurate representation of Hispanic access to the Internet because their surveys did not require interviewees to possess phones. Bagasao (1999) warned against assuming a narrowing divide based on the work of researchers like Cheskin because the Hispanic group they interviewed represented a more acculturated segment of Hispanics with a higher income than that of the average Hispanic. Schement (1999) also emphasized that income, or a lack thereof and its relationship to maintaining a phone through harder economic times, was integral to the deepening of the "digital divide". Furthermore, Castillo-Speed stressed that even if Hispanics made progress regarding Internet access, more and better information literacy would become crucial so that Hispanics would know how to evaluate the information they found on the Internet.

Gorski (2002) believed not only that any attempts at showing that the "digital divide" is narrowing were not accurate portrayals of reality, but also that the issue of the "digital divide" needed to be examined as more than just a differential in access to technology. Gorski asserted that there was also a difference in the technological education provided to "have" and "have-nots," that the Internet was not safe for minorities due to the intimidation by White Supremacist performed over the Internet, and that the support and encouragement that the "haves" received regarding technology was much more frequent than for the "have-nots." Gorski's beliefs were based on findings that teachers in schools with a high percentage of White students and a low percentage of "Free Lunch" students, engaged their students in creative thinking activities with technology; while teachers with a high percentage of students of color and of "Free Lunch" students used technology merely for skills and drills. Gorski also contended that capitalists who were trying to hide the fact that the "digital divide" existed did so by donating technological materials to a "have-not" facility without any support to enable the "have-nots" to benefit from that technology.

Many more authors have concurred that the "digital divide" was deepening. Lower income children have had to utilize their school or the library to access the Internet. However, African American and Hispanic children usually have only had access to the Internet through their school. With budget cuts in schools, this has proven to be an unreliable source for access to the Internet. Some research has even shown that school access to the Internet has decreased. Authors also were concerned that, when access did come, minorities were not given appropriate direction regarding the use of the Internet; some times leading to negative consequences when minorities used the Internet in self-destructive ways (McCook, 2002; Buckler, 2001).

LITERATURE ADDRESSING HISPANIC UNDER-UTILIZATION

Duran (1979) proffered one last unique suggestion regarding how to address under-utilization of libraries by Hispanics and other minorities. Duran argued for research regarding library under-utilization by the Hispanic population. Duran asserted that American libraries had a history of poor service to Hispanics as evidenced by the lack of research results available relating to the problem before 1970. Duran stated that the Hispanic population had been proving itself for many centuries to be a developing majority population, yet no library research had addressed the alienation this group felt regarding libraries. Guereña and Erazo (2000) concurred that the lack of publication regarding this issue was significant, pointing specifically to the lack of documentation on efforts made by Latino librarians to improve services to Hispanics. This lack of attention in the literature has caused the works of librarians such as Pura Belpré and Lillian López to go unrecognized even though their work might have provided valuable building blocks for librarians that came later. Pura Belpré provided culturally sensitive children's library services for 60 years to Puerto Rican children in the Bronx and inspired other Hispanics to pursue the library profession. Lillian López, a mentee of Pura Belpré, worked in the South Bronx, providing appropriate library services to Puerto Ricans, including outreach and programming. Little information has been available about these women's efforts. Guereña and Erazo also asserted that, until the establishment of REFORMA in 1971, the issue of services to Hispanics had received little attention, particularly from the American Library Association (ALA). ALA became involved in these issues through REFORMA's efforts to: promote culturally sensitive materials in Spanish and bilingual formats, to celebrate the Latino and Hispanic culture, and to focus attention nationally on Hispanic Librarianship (p. 139).

REFORMA was instrumental in the development of committees at ALA, such as the Social Responsibilities Round Table, the Council's Committee on Minority Concerns (CMC), and the Office of Library Outreach Services (OLOS). ALA then developed the "Guidelines for Library Services to Hispanics" in 1988 (Guereña & Erazo, 2000; ALA, 1988), which recommended that libraries purchase materials written in Spanish, English, and in a bilingual format. The guidelines suggested that these materials be visible and accessible to the public; that library programs reflect the diversity of the Hispanic culture; and that libraries implement outreach and programming ideas obtained through consultation with local Hispanic organizations. They also recommended that libraries offer bibliographic instruction in Spanish; and, further, that library buildings be made accessible to Hispanics whenever possible. The guidelines also suggested that the interior of library buildings be of a décor that was welcoming to Hispanics and that libraries recruit bilingual/bicultural librarians. Finally, ALA recommended that libraries compensate bilingual support staff when their knowledge of Spanish is a requisite of their job (ALA, 1988; Guereña & Erazo, 2000). ALA's momentum did not stop there. About 10 years later, ALA produced recommendations for professional training of librarians that included the promotion of diversity as one of its five major recommendations (ALA, 1999a). Then, in 1996, ALA's Association for Library Services to Children (ALSC), and REFORMA began sponsoring "The Pura Belpré Award" to honor Latino or Latina writers and illustrators whose work portrayed, affirmed, and celebrated the Latino cultural experience in an outstanding work of literature for children or youth (Association for Library Services to Children (ALSC). American Library Association, 1999).

EXPLANATIONS OFFERED FOR UNDER-UTILIZATION

Given the findings regarding Hispanic library use and the CENSUS 2000 (2001) data reporting that California is now 46.7% Whites and 32.4% Hispanics, Hispanic under-utilization of libraries must be addressed now.

Furthermore, Robinson (1998) reported that Hispanics were increasing at almost four times the rate of the rest of the population and would represent one out of every four Americans in 2050. To fully understand the status of library services to Hispanics, the author examined the research on the use of libraries by patrons of other minority groups to see whether their situation was similar to that of Hispanics.

Liu (1993) examined the use of libraries by foreign college students and found that in 1984, 32% of all foreign students attending colleges attended United States' colleges; these students came from 180 different countries; and 60% of the students were non-English speaking. Liu's findings regarding their library usage suggested that these foreign students had difficulty understanding how to use United States libraries unless they were from Western European countries, were students of the natural sciences, or were more acculturated students. Some of the foreign students said they were afraid to check out and return books for fear of being accused of theft. Therefore, it seemed that these students could have benefited from Library Literacy lessons to help them overcome their discomfort with library systems. This discomfort was consistent with the lack of empowerment and comfort which Stern and Haro described as characteristic of the Hispanic population.

Scarborough (1991) presented findings similar to those of Liu. She suggested that patrons defined as ethnic minorities went into a library and found nothing for themselves in the library due to the weak ethnic collections held by most libraries. Scarborough asserted that if minority patrons were to find better ethnic collections, they would feel more welcome and would then make use of other facets of the library. She contended that these patrons have felt that the materials and services were not relevant to them. She also noted that California librarians responded to this dilemma by developing a forum called "Change California's Public Libraries to Address the Information Needs of Multicultural Communities."

D'Aniello (1989) echoed the sentiments of Haro, Stern, and Scarborough. He discussed how reference services could be described as both "elitist and ethnocentric" to Anglo Americans (p. 370), thus rendering its services culturally insensitive to minorities. Haro, Stern, and Scarborough all claimed that minorities did not find library services relevant to them. However, D'Aniello made the argument that minorities should be empowered by making them culturally literate in order to make the reference services more relevant. In considering this point, it was important to explore the literature relating to special programs for Hispanics designed to increase library literacy/information literacy, or as D'Aniello named it, bibliographic literacy.

Rubin (2000) commented that library personnel have been ambivalent regarding recruiting under-utilizers. The trend has been for libraries to expend their resources on the traditional and active/existing patrons. Rubin described this approach as having been perceived as more "cost-efficient" (p. 250). The question had arisen or arose from a lack of a unified definition of the library "community," according to Rubin. Was "service to the community" working with the public who had historically used it? Alternatively, did "service to the community" mean actively seeking out patrons who could benefit from library services, but "for whom the library had been an unwelcome and unresponsive institution? (i.e., the poor, members of minority groups, and the undereducated)" (p. 259). Guereña and Erazo (2000) concurred that libraries had been reluctant to address the issue of Hispanics as under-utilizers. Rubin also asserted that not enough effort had been put into tailoring recruitment approaches to attract minority patrons or librarians.

UNDER-REPRESENTATION OF MINORITIES IN GRADUATE PROGRAMS

Eberhart (2000) also discussed the need for a multicultural workforce to serve the multicultural society of the present and the future. Eberhart stressed that library personnel of diverse racial and cultural backgrounds should be the priority target of recruitment by LIS programs. He reported a survey showing that only 10% of LIS students were minorities and discussed how, with the constant changes in technology, minority students might shy away from a career in librarianship. Eberhart, therefore, contended that minority students who did enroll in LIS programs should receive encouragement throughout their LIS training.

Knowles (1990) concurred with Eberhart and Rubin regarding the need to attract minorities to the library workforce. Knowles also argued that more than just recruiting minorities to jobs was necessary. Helping minorities through school (e.g., through mentorship programs) and buffering minority employees from subtle discrimination at work once they were hired were additional steps that needed to be taken.

Gomez (1994) echoed the sentiments of Knowles and Eberhart that, in order to cultivate a diverse workplace, minority employees would need to be empowered. Her answers mirrored theirs in that she asserted that programs would need to foster mentor–protégé relationships for minorities in the field.

St. Lifer and Rogers (1993) argued that, given the size of the Hispanic population (8.8% of the nation's population at that point in time), the cultivation and hiring of Hispanic librarians needed to be encouraged. They reported that only 1.8% of librarians (faculty, graduate students, and professional librarians were included in this figure) were Hispanic, and that this low figure had been constant for several decades (p. 14).

Proof that this under-representation of minorities in MLIS programs has been long-standing was found in McCook and Geist (1993) and McCook and Lippincott (1997). They reported on rates from surveys performed in the 1980s. Cabello-Argandoña and Haro (1977) reported on surveys performed near the beginning of the 1970s. McCook and Geist (1993) reported on a survey showing that in 1992, 92% of the new MLIS students were Anglo American, an increase of 1% since 1982. Of the 8% minority graduate students, 4.6% were African American, 2% were Hispanic, 0.2% were Native American, and 1.8% were Asian. In 1982, the percentages were 3.2% African American, 1.2% Hispanic, 0.2% Native American students, and 1.8% Asian. McCook and Geist concluded that the increase in minority graduate students over this 10-year period was negligible.

McCook and Lippincott (1997) reported findings from a study showing that minority graduates from LIS programs increased from 6.79% to 10.01% over the 10-year period of 1985–1995. However, according to McCook and Lippincott, all ethnic groups were still under-represented except for Asian/Pacific Islanders. In 1985, the United States minority-student graduation rate resulted in a percentage of minority graduates, in comparison to the minority population, of 30.49%. The percentage ratio in 1995 grew to 37.92%. McCook and Lippincott called for a quintuple increase in the rate of graduation of minority LIS students in order to reach parity with the percentage of minorities in the United States population. ALA responded to this data by creating a series of programs titled "Stop Talking and Start Doing: Recruitment and Retention of People of Color at the State and Local Levels," in an effort to expand the pool of minority graduates (McCook & Lippincott, 1997).

As early as 1977, Cabello-Argandoña and Haro were writing about a lack of minority students in MLS programs, in general, and Hispanics in particular. These earlier studies were performed by Haro and were reported in multiple sources, including Cabello-Argandoña and Haro (1977). This latter article documented a shortage of MLS graduate students (LIS programs were not MLIS programs in the 1960s) indirectly through the findings of studies performed in 1967, 1968, and 1969, which included 600 urban Hispanic residents of Sacramento and East Los Angeles. Haro, who interviewed people walking on the streets, performed these studies personally. Fifty-seven percent of the residents endorsed speaking and reading English although they primarily spoke Spanish at home. Sixty-five percent of the residents had never used a library. Eighty-nine percent stated that they would have used libraries if there had been Spanish-speaking personnel and/or if the library had possessed Spanish materials. Cabello-Argandoña and Haro also developed specific recommendations from Haro's study. For example, they suggested that librarians use Spanish-speaking media to advertise libraries; that mobile units be utilized in Hispanic neighborhoods that were a great distance from any library; and that recruitment strategies focus on obtaining minority library students and personnel. These authors also recommended that non-print materials be available for non-readers and that libraries use subject headings and indexing systems designed for the Spanish-speaking. They also advocated for mini-library centers that could be located at community centers where the Hispanic population could receive employment assistance or medical care, while also being exposed to library materials and services. Finally, they recommended that administrators should support the above-suggested programs, which were adapted to the needs of Spanish-speaking patrons.

McCook and Lippincott (1997) concurred with the above historical presentation of all these theories regarding minority under-representation. They reported that a study by the Association for Library Information Science Education showed a major discrepancy between the number of LIS graduates and the percentage of minorities in the population; only 10.01% of the United States LIS graduates in 1994–1995 were of minority persuasion, while the country's population consisted of 26.4% minority residents. McCook and Lippincott advocated for a 162% increase in minority LIS student graduations in order to meet the diversity needs of the United States. They provided specific recommendations, such as training by minority faculty, mentoring, encouragement of minority paraprofessional staff to pursue the profession, financial support while in graduate school, and targeted recruitment strategies (e.g., advertising in ethnic yellow pages).

At the turn of the century, ALA responded to this long-standing problem by starting a "Spectrum" Program, which provided scholarships and mentoring to minority MLIS students (Watkins, 1999). ALA also developed a recruitment training kit for libraries on how to benefit from minority personnel, rather than acculturating these employees into the library's non-culturally sensitive practices (Watkins & Abif, 1999). A predecessor to the above movements was the HEA Title II-B program, which provided funds for a Graduate Library Fellowship aimed, among other things, at promoting cultural diversity (U.S. Department of Education, 1997). For more information about the HEA Title II-B program, see http://www.ed.gov/pubs/learning/learning.html. For more information on the ALA "Spectrum" program, see http://www.ala.org/spectrum/ (American Library Association, 1999b). It should also be noted that HEA Title II-B also funded the advancement of minority librarians into leadership positions in academic and research libraries through a program that trained them in advanced leadership skills (McCook, 1998).

These authors noted how minorities under-utilized libraries due to various factors, including a lack of minority personnel, and the allegation that minority patrons did not find relevant services at the library. Allen (1987) proffered both of these arguments a decade earlier and even went one step further to advocate for collection development performed in a culturally sensitive manner. Therefore, recruitment of minority personnel should target reference librarians, as well as culturally sensitive technical services librarians.

THE NEED FOR CULTURALLY SENSITIVE COLLECTION DEVELOPMENT

Scarborough (1990) addressed the issue of culturally sensitive collection development by providing a list of guidelines. Librarians should choose items that prevented stereotyping and promoted a positive ethnic image. They should choose items that were relevant to the languages and religions of the minorities in the library's catchment area. Furthermore, items should not be rejected if they did not meet collection development policies regarding formatting and binding, because small or independent presses published many of the culturally relevant items. Selectors should choose items after consulting with community leaders, the user population, staff, faculty, and colleagues. Selectors should also respect the input of these various constituencies, even if that input contradicted the local collection development policy. The author also suggested that community contacts should be encouraged to recommend materials on a regular basis. Selectors should also read review journals, newspapers, and other information resources pertinent to a particular ethnic group before acquiring materials. Scarborough recommended that selectors establish relationships with several vendors, particularly for out-of-print or rare materials, to insure maximum coverage. Selectors should also be aware of cultural resource collections like ethic studies libraries in their geographical areas in order to develop consultation relationships and interlibrary loan possibilities with these resources. Finally, selection criteria should include a focus on oral histories and audiovisual materials for cultures with a strong oral tradition (p. 61).

Moller (2001) concurred with most of Scarborough's ideas about collection development for minorities, but focused her attention on Spanish-speaking minorities. Moller suggested that selectors be sensitive to whether books originated in Spain, South America, or Latin America because monolingual Spanish, Mexican American children might not be able to read items from other Hispanic countries without a dictionary. However, Moller concluded that it would be easier for these Mexican American children to read something from another Hispanic country than to read something in English. Her preference was for children to read books by authors from their native country; however, she maintained that books written or translated in Spain were far superior to books translated from English to Spanish in the United States. Moller asserted that these latter translations often contained improper interpretations, grammar, spelling, flow, and cadence. Moller's other recommendations regarding collection development were: that books that had good cultural content should not be rejected due to their binding quality; that many appropriate books were only distributed in Mexico or Ecuador; and that librarians should read *Publishers Weekly* because it reviewed trends in publishing in Latin America. She also cautioned against building a collection of translated Anglo pop literature because it praised Anglo culture rather than promoting Latino culture. Moller's last general recommendation was that librarians purchase new books on a regular basis just as materials were purchased routinely for non-Spanish-speaking clients. She stated that a good guideline was to use a percentage of the budget for Spanish language materials, which equated with the percentage of Spanish speakers in the population served.

The guidelines developed by Moller (2001) regarding selecting materials for Spanish-speaking children were very similar to Scarborough's guidelines. Moller's recommendations were varied. Books that should be included in a collection should contain characters similar to Hispanic children and who have shared their values. The collection should avoid materials with negative stereotypes and include materials that have demonstrated accurate cultural settings and values. These collections should also possess literature that has included entertaining plots and characters, attractive illustrations, Hispanic heroes/heroines who solved their own problems, and translations by native speakers. Moller asserted that a variety of materials was appropriate for a children's bilingual collection. Such collections should include audiocassettes, beginning reference books, such as almanacs and atlases, and biographies of historical, cultural, and literary figures. She also recommended a children's encyclopedia and materials covering contemporary issues, such as immigration, bilingualism, migrant labor, prejudice/discrimination, intercultural marriage, and intercultural adoption. The collection should include Spanish only and Spanish-English dictionaries, items regarding ESL for children, and items regarding higher education and career opportunities. Moller recommended literature with Hispanic, Latin American, and indigenous content, such as: folklore, legends, mythology, art, and historical accounts reflecting perspectives of the particular culture/peoples discussed. She advocated for collections with "how-to" books in English and Spanish, magazines in both languages, and items by native Spanish-language children's authors, such as picture books, poetry, books depicting positive Hispanic/Latino role models, and materials regarding the sports most popular in the library's community. Moller also recommended supplemental materials for school curricula, translations of classics or favorites that other students were reading in English, wordless books, and materials regarding World Cultures.

An extensive list of national and international publishers and distributors of Spanish-speaking items in all formats for all ages was located in Moller's appendix (2001). However, discussions of trends in publishing and distributing materials for the Spanish-speaking have been very erratic. Prior to Moller's recommendations regarding publishers and distributors, Lodge (1995) had reported that American publishing companies had dabbled in publishing bilingual books, in importing literature in Spanish from Spain, and in commissioning Spanish translations of titles with solid sales histories. Most of these business ventures involved releases in picture-book format. The dabbling ceased in 1995 because publishers had little faith in a Spanish language line and because they did not know how to market their product. Beardon (1995) expressed the same concerns as Lodge: that companies were just dabbling rather than studying the market and its demand for materials other than translated pop-fiction; that these companies, because of their lack of information, were not building the correct alliances; and that these companies were withdrawing too soon from the Spanish language publishing market.

Lodge's ideas for marketing were very specific. Businesses should: build relationships with Spanish wholesalers and distributors; advertise at stores such as Wal-Mart, and Target; publish "stories about the culture by authors and artists from the culture"; work with Hispanic community retailers in areas where there were no bookstores; collaborate with community organizations to arrange for author visits and readings; perform outreach programming to inner city schools; and be able to stay committed through the ups and downs of the market. Lodge also argued that children needed to continue to develop their Spanish-speaking reading skills, even in an English-speaking environment, because this would result in their gaining pride and self-esteem.

Kiser (1999) also expressed a belief in the solidity of the market for Spanish-speaking materials. Kiser's argument was that, as long as college students were still learning Spanish, the Internet was still in existence, and the economy of the United States Latino population was still growing, the Spanish book market would thrive. He asserted that with more than 30 million Hispanics, the United States was already the fifth largest Spanish-speaking nation in the World and that, by 2010, Mexico would be the only nation with more Spanish speakers than the United States. He contended that since 1990, the bilingual buying power of Latinos in the United States had risen 65% to total 348 billion dollars. This was a sum greater than the entire gross national product of Mexico. The buying power of the California Latinos alone increased by 1 billion dollars every six weeks per Kiser. Despite these numbers, Kiser admitted that this market still presented challenges to those who did not understand it.

Milo (1995) discussed the importance of buying Spanish materials despite possible confrontation from non-Spanish-speaking library community members. Milo emphasized the need to follow through with one's library Mission Statement in serving the needs of a culturally diverse community and with the findings of one's current Needs Assessment. Milo's article explained how his public library was not reaching the Hispanic community, which represented 21% of the library's population. His library's Needs Assessment plan called for the development of a collection for any population that represented at least 5% of the community. Milo's answer to challenges when he began spending money on building a collection for the Spanish-speaking was that Spanish speakers were taxpayers who had written important literary works and received Nobel Prizes. Therefore, this underserved population had an equal right to information regarding health, law, parenting, and other areas of interest. Milo also asserted the familiar hypothesis proffered throughout this paper, that literacy in Spanish enhanced English literacy. Milo contended that Spanish-speakers could not learn English, as the law mandated, without ESL materials and that Spanish-speaking community members had proven themselves eager learners as exhibited by their attendance in ESL classes. Despite the fact that his collection of Spanish materials represented only 1% of the library's books,

Milo was attempting to model his library after libraries that had successfully built Spanish book collections in New York, Los Angeles, and Chicago.

Almost 10 years earlier, Taylor (1988) addressed the same issues in the acquisition of materials for the Spanish-speaking population. Taylor felt that the strongest market for obtaining appropriate materials was in Mexico; Mexico was publishing and translating books in Spanish, on self-help, health, child-family issues, and sex education. Taylor also contended that the quality of materials from Latin America was improving because conglomerates were establishing publishing houses dedicated to quality and to public education in Latin American countries. According to Taylor, Mexican publishers had begun competing with Spain and Argentina. Mexico's niche, then, appeared to be in the publication of children's books and nonfiction adult materials.

However, there were realistic threats to publishers and distributors of bilingual materials. There was the constant threat of state budget cuts and the successful elimination of bilingual education (Castillo-Speed, 2001). In addition, libraries had shown little follow-through on utilizing these books, despite the fact that these books were recommended by all authors specializing in Hispanic children's literature (e.g., Moller, 2001). It should be noted that all of the above authors, who had addressed a lack of follow-through on collection development recommendations, had also commented on the lack of follow-through by libraries on recruiting minority library candidates, and on training librarians regarding cultural sensitivity.

Guereña (2000) discussed similar issues as those presented above regarding collection development. Guereña explained that accessing data in retrieval systems was very difficult for Spanish-speaking patrons, particularly when the dominant society developed the system, when the system provided information in a foreign language, and when the system used a technology that was unfamiliar to the patron. Further ideas proffered by Guereña included placing the Spanish materials collection in a visible and separate section, utilizing bilingual catalogers, and providing a bilingual catalog. This author also recommended ensuring that the Spanish materials collection was well labeled to reflect the type of materials available (e.g., bilingual format, Spanish subtitles, Spanish translation of English materials, Spanish materials dubbed in English, materiales bilingüe, materiales en Español, etc.). Libraries should also employ Spanish on-line catalog instructions or Spanish translated subject headings at the library's on-line catalog. Guereña made further suggestions including avoiding Cutter numbers as they would not make sense to Hispanics (using surnames instead), and reworking the Spanish translations of Library of Congress subject headings, utilizing a manner that was more informed and global in expression. He also favored adding bilingual summary or content notes to the bibliographic record, to assist Spanish speakers with understanding the types of materials in the catalog; and finally, Guereña recommended having a readily available dictionary for Spanish-speaking patrons to utilize at the on-line catalogs, such as the Diccionario de literature Española or Hispano-Americana.

ENCOURAGEMENT OF CULTURALLY SENSITIVE PERSONNEL

Allen (1987) attributed the minority patron's sense of alienation from the library culture as more than the result of culturally insensitive collection development, but as also being due to library schools not educating their students regarding cultural sensitivity. Vandala (1970) made this same argument almost 20 years earlier. Vandala asserted that continuing education centers developed cultural diversity programs for librarians, due to the lack of library schools' programming in this area.

Guereña (2000) repeated Vandala's sentiments, 30 years later. Guereña highlighted how no library schools are requiring a second language requisite, despite Bush's campaign of America 2000 and Clinton's campaign of Goals 2000. The emphasis of these campaigns was to encourage secondary high schools and colleges to require their students to learn a second language. The library courses, which have attempted to meet this objective, were courses at University of Texas (an "Information Resources for Hispanics" course), and at UCLA (a "Latin American Research Resources" course). Therefore, without such MLIS training, librarians needed to pursue continuing education in order to learn cultural sensitivity. Guereña recommended programs to prepare librarians to work with Hispanics that involved teaching simple Spanish words, as well as immersing the students in the Hispanic culture. This immersion exercise would consist of assignments to listen to Spanish radio stations, to watch Spanish television, to navigate Spanish websites, and to visit Hispanic community service centers.

A thorough discussion of cultural sensitivity has been presented in Guereña (2000). He defined culture as the accepted and patterned ways of behavior of a given people, both through physical and cognitive manifestations of those patterns. Physical manifestations included diet, dress, costumes, customs, traditions, language, and technology. Cognitive manifestations of culture included ethics, values, religion, and aesthetics.

Guereña asserted that diversity involved recognizing and respecting all these attributes of other cultures, as well as including members of another culture into the structure and institutions of the dominant society. He contrasted diversity with monoculturism, where the dominant society ignored the existence of the values and heritage of other cultural groups. He also contrasted diversity with multiculturism, which he defined as an environment that recognized and valued the importance of ethnic and cultural diversity in shaping lifestyles, social experiences, personal identities, and educational opportunities of individuals from all cultural groups (pp. 50–53).

A commentary on how education and service-oriented institutions usually reflected the norms and values of the dominant culture followed the above discourse. According to Guereña, these institutions failed to recognize cultural differences in verbal communication styles and non-verbal communication. This discussion of communication styles extended into an explanation of proxemics, semifixed space, personal space, the intimacy zone, and high-context versus low-context societies, which are all nonverbal parameters that vary by culture. For an in-depth analysis of these issues, see pp. 54–57 of the Guereña text. The important conclusion to this discourse, however, was how a member from another culture may be discouraged from ever revisiting a library after his or her visit, due to an employee's insensitivity to these non-verbal factors. The example given was that reference librarians would react enthusiastically to a European or French accent, but inadvertently look at an individual with a Spanish accent or an African American dialect of English with disdain.

The United States Task Force on Library and Information Services to Cultural Minorities also concurred with the findings in the above references. In the task force report, the members said that libraries should address under-utilization by recruiting minority library personnel, performing culturally sensitive collection development, and allocating a budget specifically toward improving services to racial minorities (National Commission on Library and Information Sciences, 1983). Moller (2001), almost 20 years later, went one step further by recommending not only the mentoring of potential Hispanic personnel, but also that libraries assist non-Spanish-speaking personnel with tuition at community colleges for Spanish classes. She also proposes giving staff paid time-off to attend community college Spanish classes. Moller cautioned, however, that the professional Spanish-speaking staff at the library might inadvertently promote a division of social class between the patron and the bilingual staff. She provided suggestions to overcome this possible pitfall in her guidelines for welcoming Hispanics to the library, in the next section (not subsection) of this paper.

Guereña (2000) also presented a strong argument for recruitment of Latinos/Hispanics into librarianship, citing the prediction that, in 2050, California would consist of 68% minorities, and the fact that Hispanics were growing at a faster rate than non-minorities or African Americans. Guereña, however, suggested more than just recruitment of Latinos/Hispanics into librarianship. He asserted that these librarians needed to be capable of teaching Hispanic patrons bibliographic and technological instruction tailored to the learning style of Hispanics. Therefore, Guereña contended, Hispanic recruitment of librarians needed to involve librarians and paraprofessionals who were bilingual, bicultural, familiar with Hispanic literature, and who shared the cultural values of the specific Hispanic community represented by their catchment area. The library then needed to recruit minorities as librarians and paraprofessionals, who could meet a diversity of library tasks; these tasks would require employees to perform roles that varied from collection development, to being public service providers, instructors, role models, and administrators with leadership qualities. Guereña asserted that despite the above-described studies showing that less than 12% of library school graduates were minorities in 1994, and that minority graduation only rose by 1.2%, between 1982 and 1992, it appeared that only a few specific library schools in certain regions had attempted to improve the above statistics. As of 1995, MLIS school enrollment had increased to 25% minorities. According to Guereña, it was now incumbent upon MLIS programs to assist these minorities in graduating (e.g., through mentorships), and to attract these graduates into a library career by providing salaries that compete with other professions.

ADDRESSING THE NEED TO WELCOME MINORITIES

Today there are books, articles, and committees that discuss methods for welcoming minorities. An example of a committee developed to address the issue of welcoming minorities was one that formed in Minnesota. This committee, called the "Minnesota Social Responsibilities Round Table," had as its duties drafting policies regarding "direct representation of poor people" and policies regarding "putting low income programs and services into regular library budgets" (Venturella, 1998, p. 20). This committee was relevant to minorities because Venturella defined poor people as those who were economically disadvantaged, such as minorities, women, children, homeless individuals, and displaced workers.

A committee called the "Planning Group for A State of Change" in Stanford, California, undertook a similar study 10 years earlier. This study published its conference and forum proceedings in Jacob (1988). It began with a summary of the findings of a Rand study, which investigated whether public libraries were meeting the needs of racial minorities; the study was undertaken because, statistically, racial minorities were emerging as the population majority in California. The forum began by reviewing the findings of the Rand report. The committee members remarked on the demographical statistics presented by the RAND report (e.g., that in 2000, 92% of Californians would be living in counties where the population of minorities would be more than 30%, and that in 2000, California's population would grow by 5 million, with 61% of those additional 5 million being Hispanic). The committee members also reacted to the reportedly implied expectation in the study that library under-utilizers should adapt to libraries, and not vice versa. A closer examination of this issue showed that the RAND report made a few conclusions; the study found that there was no systematic empirical evidence of barriers preventing public library access to minorities. It also concluded that individuals in minority groups were as likely as non-minorities to find what they wanted from public libraries, "within the libraries' mission." Rand determined that library use was voluntary. Thus, a disparity between the racial demographics of library users and the racial demographics of the general population would not necessarily constitute a cause for concern; and finally, it was concluded that minorities were making an informed decision when not using libraries (Jacob, 1988).

Tarin (1988) shared the Stanford committee members' sentiment that libraries should adapt to the under-utilizers rather than expecting these potential patrons to adapt to the traditions of the library. Tarin objected to the report because it seemed to her that the report was asking minorities to fit into prescribed roles determined by traditional library staff and traditional library patrons. Furthermore, Tarin perceived that the report was implicitly giving libraries an option to adapt to minority needs, despite the fact that minorities, who were emerging as the majority population, had a history of paying taxes to public libraries. Tarin's argument was that these majority taxpayers, even though they were not the majority library clientele, should not have to fit into the roles predetermined by the library's traditional practices. She also interpreted the report to blame the lack of minority access to libraries, on the minorities, and not on the libraries. She argued that the report missed the fact that libraries choose to serve the traditional clientele unless they are pressured to adapt their programs to meet the needs of minorities; libraries needed to be shown how they were the roadblocks to minority usage of libraries. Tarin also took exception, along with other committee members, to what appeared to be an implication by the Rand report that minorities were the roadblocks to library usage, and that minorities were making an "informed choice" not to use libraries. Tarin's argument was that under-utilizers did not even know what the library could provide because the services were not adapted to meet their needs; thus, minorities were not, in Tarin's opinion, informed decision makers.

The Stanford committee concurred with many of Tarin's points but also proposed various solutions to minority under-utilization of libraries. Their recommendations were extensive (Jacob, 1988). Six hundred committee members made 260 recommendations. Some of the recommendations were innovative, while others were so repetitive of other committee recommendations, that there was no excuse for the extant disregard of these suggestions by libraries.

The innovative recommendations were numerous. Librarians should explain to potential funding groups the cost to welfare and corrections departments that could result from the growing majority's illiteracy and increasing school dropout rates (the alleged inevitable outcome of libraries not providing these outreach programs that would allow these individuals to become productive members of society). Libraries should waive the fines for families that were unfamiliar with library practices so that their patronage would not be lost by the imposition of a fine; these families could dramatically misunderstand the fines, until they were more familiar with library practices. Librarians should begin minority, personnel recruitment efforts in high school and college, not just at the graduate level. They should be sensitive to the reluctance of minorities, particularly recent immigrants, with regard to giving their names for library cards, due to their fear of the government and/or immigration. Librarians should attempt alliances with corporations in order to find new sources of funding. They should provide staff with flexible schedules that would allow them to go to the people, to perform their outreach, as well as allow staff to attend training. Libraries should provide monetary incentives for minority graduates to work in public libraries rather than at higher paying corporate positions. Catalog information and library signs should exist in the dominant minority language of the community. Librarians should have exhibits of materials in this language in an attractive and visible layout. Mission statements should address cultural diversity programs that reallocate resources from "dinosaur" programs to the outreach programs. Librarians should seek pro bono work from professional marketing and public relations companies. They should evaluate effectiveness of libraries in ways other than circulation figures.

Librarians should possess a familiarity with the political process in order to lobby for the rights and resources of libraries. They should forge a link between education departments and libraries because each of these parties is just as needy of the resources that the other party has to offer. Librarians should join community ethnic boards in their efforts to collaborate with community groups.

The committee also recommended that at times of budget cuts, libraries should form "county systems," take their libraries out of sinking county systems, or join special districts. Special districts were defined as groups of up to five library service providers who could join forces; eligible partic- ipants could be county service areas, community service districts, library districts in unincorporated towns, library districts, and union high school library districts. Libraries should build business advisory councils that have knowledge regarding how to promote the library, as well as how to elicit the financial and marketing aid of businesses in the community. Librarians should welcome Hispanic children rather than treating them like "illegal aliens." It was also recommended that the term "undocumented persons" be utilized in place of "illegal aliens." Libraries should stage mock voting booths in the library so that non-voters could familiarize themselves with this process and desensitize themselves with regard to fears about voting. Finally, librarians should incorporate the research, which showed that Hispanics read for religious or educational reasons, not for recreational purposes, into their collection development efforts.

There were suggestions by the committee that were not novel. For ex- ample, libraries should adjust their hours to meet the community's needs; community playgrounds were open until 10:30 p.m. while their local librar- ies closed at 5:00 or 6:00 p.m. This was not a culturally sensitive public policy. Furthermore, librarians should avoid books with ethnic biases and stereotypes and should arrange free local transportation to the library for those without transportation. They should provide legal and survival information in Spanish, hold programs targeted at preschool children, and use non-traditional publishers. Librarians should purchase non-print ma- terials, provide materials that account for differences in cultural heritage and acculturation, and place posters on the wall of famous minorities. Libraries should recruit at community centers such as church parking lots or GED programs, and have librarians teach parents the value of reading to children even if the parents do not speak English or own books. Parents could learn how to pretend that they are reading a story, while making up a story, as they leaf through the yellow pages in Spanish. Librarians should provide a creative/welcoming/supportive library environment and network with the appropriate publishers to obtain materials for the library that would be attractive to minority cultures. They should help celebrate cultural differences rather than allowing society to fear immigrants, as they did years ago when Polish and Irish immigrants infiltrated the East Coast. Librarians should emphasize, during outreach efforts, that the library services would not cost money. The committee also recommended investing in research regarding these issues, and providing cultural sensitivity training at all levels (including directors and board members). Librarians should market the library as a place that is reaching out to the members of the community, hire staff at all levels that are bicultural/bilingual, and develop more YA programs for at-risk youth. Librarians should teach information literacy to Youth Authority inmates so that they will use libraries when released. Finally, the committee recommended creating short-term and long-term objectives, and holding family nights that did not just interest children, but engaged parents in programs regarding cooking, sewing, sports, and home repair.

Committee and forums continued their efforts in order to keep attention focused on the above issues. A committee formed 20 years before the Stanford committee is the Border Regional Library Association (BRLA) (2003). This organization lobbied for the promotion of library services and librarianship in the El Paso/Las Cruces/Juárez metroplex. Membership prior to 2003 included over 100 librarians, paraprofessionals, media specialists, library friends, and trustees from all types of libraries in the tri-state area of Trans-Pecos Texas, southern New Mexico, and northern Chihuahua. This committee held continuing education classes, annual workshops, and award banquets for books, employees, and scholarship recipients. The committee also published a newsletter to discuss the above issues, as well as issues of interest to local librarians and information specialists. The committee described itself as "a support group to promote libraries as important education and cultural institutions, which have a direct impact on communities and democratic action." For more information regarding this committee, see http://libraryweb.utep.edu/brla/default.html.

In 1993, librarians from the United States and Mexico held a forum regarding improving library services to Spanish-speaking patrons on both sides of the border. They discussed resource sharing, collection development, and literacy programs, as well as exchanging information and cultural insights about Latino-Hispanic Librarianship. The result of the forum was the development of plans to set up interlibrary loans and internet networking between the two countries, particularly given the budget cuts that the United States librarians were anticipating (Hoffert, 1993).

This forum occurred again in Mexico in March 1999, among the United States, Mexican, and Canadian librarians. The forum discussed the importance of the following: creating, publishing, and acquiring bi-national and bilingual literature; preparing librarians and information professionals in management strategies; the effects of political, economic, and techno-logical changes of the 21st century on libraries; collaboration and interli-brary loans; and successfully engaging Hispanic children in reading (McPhail, 1999). The forum participants scheduled another "transborder" forum for 2001 in Sonora, Mexico. This forum would address already set objectives. The issues for the agenda included professional development, new ideas and abilities to improve library collections and services, copy-rights, and border affairs. The forum would explore techniques for infor-mation searches, computer resources, and methods to enhance relationships between Mexican and Northern American librarians. Other issues on the agenda included extending the knowledge of Mexico's and the United States' information resources, planning and implementing cooperative projects between libraries across geographical borders, and sharing each other's cultural heritage. The forum would also address educating librarians about current products and services, and the development of resource net-works beyond the boundaries that separate libraries (U.S. National Council on Library Services, 1995). For more details about this forum, see http://www.ciad.mx/biblioteca/eventos/foro_xi.htm.

The findings from a task force developed to address the minority patron's sense of alienation were contained in "A summary report of the 1996 Forum on Library and Information Services Policy." This report focused on the topic of special programming by library services to special populations, and could be found on the World Wide Web at http://www.nclis.gov/libraries/forum96.html. The report discussed barriers to library use by special populations such as "Asian mothers being afraid that filling out library cards is part of a government plot to obtain information about them" (p. 18). The report listed many examples of steps that libraries all over the country have taken to engage special populations.

A few of the project descriptions from the report described in the previous paragraph follow. In Washington, D.C., the staff of the Martin Luther King library provided literacy training and family materials for incarcerated par-ents in local jails. In Fort Worth, Texas, there were gang-prevention pro-grams directed at teens in housing projects. Massachusetts' Lawrence Library provided a Family Science Program for families of "Spanish and Southeast" persuasion; in some southwestern states, "Fotonovelas" in Spanish were used to instruct families on how to use public libraries; and finally, in Decatur, Georgia, there was a project, which provided gift books, storytelling, and computer access, to homeless shelters (p. 18).

In March 1999, the Trejo Foster Foundation for Hispanic Library Education – Fourth National Institute held a forum on the topic of Library Services to Youth of Hispanic Heritage. This forum addressed delivery of services, collection development, and staff education. Tips from participants such as REFORMA discussed how to perform these aforementioned library services with sensitivity to youth and to cultural diversity (Trejo Foster Foundation for Hispanic Library Education-Fourth National Institute, 1999). For more information on this conference, see http://www.cas.usf.edu/lis/hispanic/index.html.

Lynn, O'Connell, and Phalen (2003) reported on libraries, which had tried some of the suggestions from the various forums and task forces. This article described libraries, which had been set up in hotels, at restaurants along highways, and at hair salons. These libraries, centered outside the walls of the library, would go far in providing a new image for libraries. The article also described an innovative program in Berkeley, California, that lent gardening tools using a library card. All of these strategies would spread the word that public libraries had much to offer and that they were willing to go to the people.

The above-described programs were not borne from new ideology. In 1988, Jacob described a library program in Brooklyn where librarians would take their wares to bars, barbershops, and beauty salons. They would pass out kits with about 10 paperback books, including information about settling disputes, about life insurance, and about names for babies, as well as biblical resources, and a world almanac.

In February 2002, the *Teacher Librarian* presented innovative projects addressed at narrowing the "Digital Divide." The article discussed how libraries throughout the country had used "cybermobiles" to take computer equipment to neighborhoods where the residents would otherwise not have had access to computers, and to residents for whom the distances they would have to travel to get to the library would be an obstacle to library use. Other libraries have put their computers in high-traffic areas, such as children's museums and shopping malls. The article also discussed attempts at providing computer literacy to minorities. Libraries have expanded their Internet training programs to involve bilingual classes and to involve physical accommodations for the health impairments of senior citizens. Libraries have targeted summer, Community Park, day-camp participants, as a recruitment priority, and have provided these children with technological instruction. The article also described the ALA's technology program geared toward families; the program provided five workshops with lessons covering child safety, the history of the internet, homework assistance, and website evaluation (Teacher Librarian, 2002).

McCook (1998) described a taskforce similar to the ALA technology program. This taskforce gathered information specialists who would meet monthly to customize programs regarding digital age resources for economically and ethnically deprived youth in Tallahassee, Orlando, Fort Lauderdale, and Miami. The taskforce set up a website for librarians to utilize in order to customize their own programs.

HOW LIBRARIES HAVE ATTEMPTED TO RECRUIT AND ENGAGE HISPANICS

REFORMA has been one group that has provided tips for library programming, which was culturally sensitive to Hispanics, such as holding events involving Hispanic arts and crafts, dance groups, magicians, and musicians, as well as providing patrons with pan dulce (sweet bread) from local Hispanic bakeries, during library programs (see http://clnet.ucr.edu/library/reforma/). In addition, REFORMA recommended that librarians invite parents and grandparents to participate during their children's activities. As Hispanics felt unwelcome in libraries, the extended invitation would represent a gesture honoring the Hispanic value of family, and possibly a step in breaking that discomfort barrier. REFORMA has had an extremely active chapter in Orange County and in Northern California. Information about the Orange County chapter was found at the URL address provided earlier in this paragraph (Bibliotecas Para la Gente, 2003). To learn more about the work of the Northern California Chapter, called "Bibliotecas para La Gente," see http://clnet.ucr.edu/library/bplg/about.htm.

REFORMA held its first annual conference in 1996 to honor its 25th anniversary. The group praised the inroads they had made into ALA, into helping increase Hispanic graduates from library schools, and into promoting Hispanic Librarianship; they were instrumental in creating the California State Fullerton, "Mexican American Institute for Library Science" and the Tucson, Arizona University program called the "Graduate Library Institute for Spanish-Speaking Americans." However, the group also lamented the common trend in libraries throughout the United States to avoid purchasing Spanish-language materials. REFORMA attributed part of the avoidance, to the growing sentiment across the United States, against bilingualism (Guereña & Erazo, 1996). Therefore, a second REFORMA conference was held in 2000 that dedicated itself to the Spanish language issue and the committee published a book from this second conference entitled "El Poder del Palabra/The Power of the Language" (Castillo-Speed, 2001).

Cuesta and Tarin (1978), like REFORMA, addressed the issue of welcoming Hispanics to libraries. Cuesta and Tarin outlined guidelines for a library program that was culturally sensitive to Hispanics. They recommended bilingual story hours, puppet shows, films, and arts and crafts events, as well as reserving a budget that specifically funded these events. Another one of their guidelines was to commemorate Hispanic holidays as well as American holidays. These authors provided as examples, celebrating well-known holidays, such as Cinco de Mayo, as well as less-known holidays, such as the official Hispanic Mother's Day, Día de las Madres (May 10th). Their outreach suggestions involved utilizing neighborhood bilingual fliers, as well as advertisement through bilingual newspapers and news media.

Villagran (2001) incorporated the guidelines outlined in Cuesta and Tarin (1978). Villagran described in her article, an event she held for two consecutive years called "Día de Los Niños." Her library in Multnomah County, Oregon, dedicated one day to celebrating children and bilingual literacy. Volunteers served refreshments. All the children who attended the event received books and T-shirts. Hispanic performers from different fields danced, held art workshops, and read stories. There was a clown named Cha Cha who did magic tricks. The city offered free transportation for the day, while the newspapers and radio stations provided free advertisement before the event. The library held the event in a library branch near the residences of the majority of the Hispanic population, as opposed to the year before, when the event occurred in a location distant from the Hispanic neighborhood. As a result, their attendance increased to around 3,500 from 750, the prior year.

The San Jose Public Library system also continually provided a culturally sensitive program for Hispanics at a branch called la Bibliotheca Latino Americana. This city branch has maintained a collection that contained 80% of its materials in Spanish. The library had to eliminate a senior librarian position in order to create a librarian position that focused on multicultural services. The "Bibliotheca" has had committees dedicated to staff awareness, cultural responsiveness, outreach, program services, recruitment, and collection development. The library hired outside consultants to perform a community need assessment, followed up with focus groups. This "Bibliotheca" has even succeeded at acquiring higher pay for bilingual staff, which facilitated the hiring of bilingual staff, which in turn allowed minority patrons to feel more comfortable in asking for assistance, or perhaps in participating in general, at the library (Fish, 1992).

Alire and Archibeque (1988) are authors of a book that discussed not only programming tips, but also how to justify funding for the above-mentioned programs. The authors argued that funding of Hispanic recruitment leads to two major, eventual benefits for libraries. They discussed how outreach literacy programs with adults would promote Hispanic student achievement, because the parents would be able to assist their children with schoolwork once they were literate; furthermore, the parents would value reading once they were literate. This would result in the parents passing that value onto their children.

The second benefit to outreach literary programs for Hispanic adults was that it served a majority population in society that represented an untapped resource for library advocacy. Through recruiting Hispanics to the library, the library gained a large segment of the population who would learn to vote and who could physically contribute to libraries. Alire and Archibeque claimed that Hispanics tended to become library advocates once recruited; they claimed that these new library patrons tended to become Friends of the Library, library board members, and other types of volunteers. Furthermore, these new patrons, with their fresh appreciation of the library, tended to vote on measures that would support libraries. According to Alire and Archibeque, Hispanics represented, therefore, an untapped majority in society that could benefit libraries in many capacities.

Specific guidelines for developing collections and programs were also proffered by Alire and Archibeque. They recommended performing a need assessment of the Hispanic community by performing surveys to determine the language level, income level, education level, and culture of the neighborhood that the library served. The bilingual surveys could include a $1.00 bill with the questionnaire; this has proven to be a successful marketing strategy. The surveys could be sent in the mail with ALA bookmarks that read "Celebrate Latino Heritage." Surveyors could go door to door, and/or utilize phone interviews for families with phones. These authors also stressed that local Spanish-speaking media should publicize the survey results in order to show the library's sincere concern regarding the needs of the persons who completed the surveys.

Once the library has determined the needs of their Hispanic community, then it should perform collection development in accordance with the results of the survey. Perhaps, the community consisted of Puerto Ricans, Mexican Americans, and Cubans; this would mean that the books acquired should represent all three cultures. The collection should be relevant and culturally sensitive to the educational and recreational needs of the community, and should be available in various language formats; this would mean the books should accommodate English-speaking Hispanics, Spanish-speaking Hispanics, and bilingual Hispanics. Cuesta (1990) also emphasized the need for the collection to match the diversity of the Hispanic population it serves with regard to factors, such as language preference/facility, the length of residency in the United States, and the specific Hispanic cultural group that the patrons represented. Cuesta asserted that these factors would determine whether patrons required survival information, "high-end" materials, or materials of varying levels of sophistication. She discussed how the reading interests of recent immigrants would vary from settled immigrants, and that major Hispanic groups have demonstrated a very high interest in reading materials about political systems.

Alire and Archibeque also provided specific guidelines for programming. They asserted that programs should involve: local Hispanic artists or musicians; food donated from local stores; art displays from the Hispanic culture; events that involve grandparents; events utilizing bilingual puppeteers, clowns, and finger-players; and, bilingual signs and directions throughout the library. These authors stressed the importance of obtaining décor and graphics that conformed to the culture of the community, for both the exterior and interior of the library. Whenever possible, they also advocated for placing libraries in visible and accessible sections of the Hispanic neighborhood.

These authors provided tips for making the library more welcoming to Hispanics. One idea was to obtain from the various Hispanic country embassies flags for display. They advocated for providing personnel or volunteers that could translate if Hispanic personnel were not available. They suggested holding the events on days that were special to the culture (Alire and Archibeque provided a list of holidays for Argentina, Bolivia, Colombia, Cuba, Chile, the Dominican Republican, Ecuador, Guatemala, Honduras, Mexico, Nicaragua, Panama, Paraguay, Peru, El Salvador, Spain, Uruguay, and Venezuela, p. 111) and exhibiting artwork by Hispanic children who were patrons of the library. Their ideas for topics of events were programs that would be fun for children, as well as programs that children's parents would view as valuable; two such examples were programs that addressed bilingual etiquette classes and shark safety. These programs were great recruitment opportunities for handing out library cards to the children's parents. These authors also recommended various topics for adult programs, to include information regarding literacy, ESL programs, immigration, CPR, and drug prevention. Programs could also address health issues, such as education for pregnant mothers, nutrition, and vaccinations, as well as coping with Alzheimer's disease and AIDS. Other suggested topics included: household lead poisoning; starting one's own business; minority contracts with the government; paying for college; applying for small business loans; how to write a resume; how to dress for success; building a neighborhood watch group; obtaining a GED; and finally, dealing with divorce, drug abuse, and domestic violence.

Moller (2001) represented another comprehensive book, like Alire and Archibeque, which detailed guidelines for providing welcoming services for Hispanics. She began with a history of the various Spanish-speaking populations who had migrated to the United States. She then provided tips for welcoming Spanish-speaking populations to libraries. Specifically, Moller recommended holding events (such as a day of films from Hispanic countries) for the Hispanic population, as well as for the non-Hispanic population, to "inspire and promote the love of Latino-Hispanic culture." She also recommended chatting lessons (i.e., informal-conversation training events) where Hispanic and non-Hispanic individuals could meet to practice becoming bilingual. Each participant could take turns "making small talk" in the language, she or he was trying to learn (p. 32). It should be noted that these were the first recommendations proffered which suggested mixing cultures.

Cultural sensitivity training to all library staff, from paraprofessionals to board members, was also emphasized; Moller's argument was that a patron could be deterred from returning to the library if any library affiliate inadvertently made an insensitive remark or used the wrong body language. Moller included in her request for culturally sensitive behavior by library staff behaviors such as calling patrons by titles instead of first names (e.g., Senor, Senorita, Senora, etc.); she discussed that such actions would imply respect and would make the patrons feel more welcome. Moller also contended that Spanish-speaking patrons would feel more welcomed by attempts to eliminate language barriers in the library; that is, an English-speaking librarian could make it seem as if it was the librarian's fault that he or she did not understand a question. The librarian could have the patron write down his/her question for the librarian, confidentially, so that the non-Spanish-speaking librarian could find the answer later by consulting with a Spanish-speaking staff member. Another welcoming tip that Moller suggested was to have all the library forms available in Spanish, including interloan library forms, suggested purchases forms, etc.

Moller proffered the following programming tips. Libraries should hold events on Hispanic holidays for the specific population in the library's catchment area. They should have a bilingual answering machine on the library's voice mail, have bilingual personnel wear nametags that say "Hablo Español" at the bottom, and invite Hispanics as well as non-Hispanic patrons to events in order to build cultural awareness. Moller further suggested holding exhibitions of children patrons' artwork and celebrating Spain's holiday on April 23 called "Book Day and Lover's Day"; this is a day in Spain where corner-stands stock books and flowers throughout its cities. The men give women a flower and, in return, the women give the men a book. Moller also recommended having a good video collection since this has proven to serve as a good recruiting device to attract the Hispanic population; she asserted that the checking out of videos has generalized to Hispanics using other parts of the library. Other recommendations included events aimed at intergenerational families to show respect for Hispanic values, and encouraging Hispanic patrons to lead library events on popular topics, such as Hispanic cooking or Hispanic arts and crafts. This, in theory, would help banish the potential sense of inferiority to higher class Hispanics that Hispanic patrons could perceive when they were always the recipients of services from Spanish-speaking staff. This author also suggested holding workshops with topics such as immigration, legal and consumer issues, and how to start one's own in-home child-care center for mothers who did not want to work outside of the home (due to having their own children to baby-sit). Librarians could also hold programs on job searching tips, income taxes, citizenship, how to qualify for the low-income Energy Resource programs, literacy, ESL, child/prenatal/neonatal care, and pesticide treatment (pp. 30–32).

Marketing strategies were also very important (Moller, 2001). Librarians should: advertise with public announcements through Spanish local radio and TV; place bilingual flyers at grocery stores, self-service laundry mats, bus stops, video rental stores, and hair salons; attend health fairs, community celebrations/festivals, little league parks, and parent/school conference night; and finally emphasize that library services are free. At the aforementioned events, the recruiters should hand out library cards without asking for a Hispanic individual's identification; recruiters should ask for only an address. Moller also recommended providing library services at churches and community centers to ease the transition of the Hispanic population into librarianship.

WORKING WITH HISPANIC CHILDREN AND YOUNG PEOPLE

Guereña (1990) also authored a comprehensive book regarding providing culturally sensitive services to Hispanics. He covered similar topics as Alire

and Archibeque (1998) and Moller (2001). Guereña recommended collection
development (including attending the Guadalajara book fair), as well as
reference services to the Spanish-speaking, including utilization of bibliographies, indexes, biographies, genealogical resources, and referral systems
such as Info-line and Community Access Library Line (CALL). He discussed acquisitions (including utilizing knowledgeable members of the community who were proficient in Spanish, to review books), evaluation of
vendors, short- and long-term objectives, a community need analysis, the
politics of the bilingual language and education issue, and finally programming in public libraries. However, Guereña (1990) did not address services
to Hispanic children. His follow-up volume (Guereña, 2000) and sections of
Moller (2001) have provided substantial tips on programming for children.

Guereña (2000) discussed many topics relating to children's services. For
example, how librarians had historically opted to use the "excuse" that
they did not have funding to purchase materials for a Spanish Children's
Literature collection when, in reality, according to Guereña, they did not
purchase items because it was very difficult to build an adequate collection.
He noted that it took almost 20 years for librarians to respond to the 1968
Bilingual Education Act with regard to taking collection development in
this arena seriously. He contended that, even after librarians began to
collect materials in this area, they chose the easy way, by only purchasing
materials from United States publishers. Although these purchases resulted
in what the Guereña text terms "inadequate" collections, books from these
publishers allowed the librarians to acquire items that were easily accessible, easy to review, and easy to catalog (p. 77). However, United States
publications were primarily Spanish translations of American best sellers
and award winners. Adequate collections should contain bilingual books
and Spanish books published from all the different Spanish-speaking
countries that represent the Hispanic-American population (Mexico, Central America, South America, the Spanish-speaking Caribbean islands, and
Spain). He feared that with books published in the United States, Hispanic
children would see Anglo Americans as the heroes and would then seek to
replicate the American culture. Hispanic children needed to read books
that contained heroes that resembled them; from such books, children
would learn about their cultural and literary heritage. These books would
provide Hispanic children with strong roots to face the new world into
which they were attempting to integrate. As a result, these Hispanic children would be armed with a thorough knowledge of, and pride in their own
heritage. Research has also shown that students, who use schoolbooks in
their native language, have been more likely to develop high levels of

English proficiency and that bilingual and Spanish materials would enhance the learning of bilingual and LEP students. According to Guereña, in the 1990s, United States publishers began to realize the importance of producing materials that provided an authentic presentation of the experience of a Hispanic child in America, but he still contended that the United States productions alone were not sufficient to build an adequate Spanish children's literature collection. The collection also needed to contain books from the Guadalajara book fair (an annual event that is the World's largest gathering of books for the Spanish-speaking) and other foreign markets. When building these collections, librarians should anticipate attending book fairs in other countries and establishing networks with new vendors who specialized in keeping current with the trends in Spanish language literature.

Another of Guerena's recommendations was that librarians make written policies about establishing and maintaining a Spanish Children's Literature collection and hire qualified personnel who can carry out the specified procedures. These personnel should be capable of evaluating the political perspectives in books (e.g., did the material reflect the Spanish or American, versus the Mexican and Latin American version of events?) They should assess the language dialects utilized in books, evaluate the publication dates, and determine whether the translated version of a book retained the spirit of the original work. These qualified personnel should assess whether the chosen material appropriately reflected the Hispanic culture's contribution to America's society and history. Evaluations of translations for misspellings or misplaced accents also should occur, as should a determination as to whether the collection contained writings by authors from various Hispanic countries. This was important because Hispanics of different cultures would have difficulty understanding the variations in language grammar and vocabulary of a Hispanic country that was not their native country; a task that could be easily ascertained by looking at the first two or three numbers of the ISBN that reflect the country of origin. According to Guereña, librarians also need to evaluate the authenticity of the cultural portrayal in their collections (e.g., are the chosen materials reflective of the specifics of the culture and the contemporary Hispanic lifestyle, without distortion or stereotyping?).

The collections should consist of books in all subject areas and reading formats. They should include picture books, beginning reader books, concept books (such as, those that cover the ABCs and 123s), small books, board books, fiction, non-fiction, poetry, historical pieces, biographies, videos, read-alongs, magazines, and "Big Books." There should also be an appropriate reference section. This section should support the research needs of elementary school children, their teachers, their parents, and other librarians who need to learn about the "vast world" of Spanish materials. Such a section should include dictionaries, almanacs, encyclopedias, atlases, and thesauri (Guereña, 2000. p. 78).

Guereña also provided a list of various types of resources that librarians could utilize in acquiring materials. Two United States companies were named that were good distributors to use because "they understand the politics of how publicly-funded institutions are regulated with regard to acquisitions; these companies work with libraries given those constraints." Guereña described a tool called "Libros en Venta," which is equivalent to "Books in Print." This tool would provide annotated catalogs from three foreign companies to facilitate book selection. Another tool cited as useful for librarians was a listing of the books that should be included in an "adequate" collection. Various institutions, including the Los Angeles Office of Bilingual-ESL Instruction, the Los Angeles Unified School District, the California State Department of Education, and the New York Public Library, have produced these lists.

Moller's chapters on children's services provided a discourse regarding collection development, which is similar to that presented by Guereña. However, Moller covered many areas regarding Hispanic children's services. For example, Moller contended that collaboration with community members for children's programming was just as important as the collaboration recommended for adult programming. She promoted networking with public television stations, the Mexican Embassy, local high school, college/ literacy or GED programs, Latino newspapers, and even specialized associations. She even provided examples of collaboration with specific associations.

Moller also discussed how one should deliver children's programming. She emphasized that in developing an infant and toddler program, it was important to involve the mothers, whether at the library or at an outreach site in order to model storytelling and reading. By participating, mothers would learn the importance of reading, how to read to their children, and the value of actively participating in their children's learning rather than just viewing it as the school's responsibility. Moller explained that sometimes the storytelling programs were slow to form. Hispanic mothers often had pressing concerns about jobs and health assistance, which could prevent them from seeing the value of spending time at storytelling programs. However, Moller asserted that, through innovative strategies such as using "lead moms" to start programs at apartment complexes, storytelling programs could blossom in these mothers' homes. She contended that once the mothers understood these programs' value, the storyteller could model taking the bus to the library, and then eventually move the storytelling groups to the library (pp. 50–58).

A variety of other strategies were recommended by Moller, such as having volunteers do the storytelling if there were not sufficient bilingual staff members. High school teachers or teaching assistants who were off for the summer, grandmothers, or even participants could lead the groups. Mothers who did not know how to read could learn how to narrate books that just contained numbers and pictures. Libraries could recruit local television or radio stations as well as the telephone company to provide story hours. Children could call the "Tele Cuento"/"Dial a Story" number to hear stories or they could listen to story hours on the radio. Audio participation in storytelling was just as effective as visual participation because children needed to learn the music of their language. Therefore, Moller argued that audio programs or story hours that contained poems, rhymes, and songs were valuable to the toddler's language development.

Moller also discussed the importance of dolls, toys, puppets, and illustrations in books that exhibited characters of different skin colors and different ethnicities. She contended that Spanish-speaking children would be facing culture shock when they entered school, particularly if their mothers believed in keeping them at home and not in day care; librarians could help these children acculturate while they retained pride in their heritage and their cultural values. Librarians could reinforce children's skills by teaching them to tell stories to their dolls and stuffed animals. Librarians could also reinforce storytelling skills in children by holding events such as "Meet the Author" where parents would come and see displays of stories that their children had written.

Moller also provided tips for Spanish-speaking students in middle school. She asserted that if middle school children had not learned the fundamentals of speaking and reading in Spanish, they would not have developed a good foundation to learn more than superficial English skills. As the academic demands increased in higher grades, this superficial foundation would not prove to be sufficient. Therefore, she contended that it was important for Spanish-speaking students to continue developing their Spanish skills. By continuing to read in Spanish, they would have the cognitive skills to handle middle school academics. These students should be encouraged to read books in Spanish to their parents at night; and the parents needed to learn how reading in Spanish could promote their children's English skills.

Immroth and McCook (2000), as well as earlier works by Duran (1979) and Ramirez and Ramirez (1994), addressed the issue of providing services to Hispanic youth. These texts contained information very similar to the recommendations made by Moller (2001), Guereña (2000), and Alire and Archibeque (1998). However, they added additional insights into how these programs could be delivered. The fact that many of their suggestions were similar to those cited above indicated how librarians possessed, but did not utilize, this information over the past 20 years.

The Immroth and McCook text emphasized that children's cultural heritage was a major part of their identity and that this identity was constantly seeking self-expression. These authors believed that libraries were responsible for helping develop culturally integrated children through children's programming that included Hispanic history, art, music, and folklore. In addition, the books chosen for the collection should reflect the Hispanic experience of urban, rural/migrant, and working class members of the community. These programs should be long-term and continuous programs rather than short-term programs funded by grants. Children's programmers should also create short- and long-term, as well as general and specific, objectives. As an example, Immroth and McCook cited a program called "Homework and Reading Partners." This program would recruit bilingual high school students to serve as "partners" for younger children who may not have had any homework assistance at home in tackling difficult school assignments. Before beginning such a program, however, the library would need to perform a community analysis to determine the linguistic and academic skills of the children who would be participating in this program; librarians would also need to identify objectives and consistent funding for the program. This would ensure that these types of program were not fleeting, as well as assuring the Hispanic community that the library was dedicated to meeting its needs, rather than as an institution, that served Hispanics on an inconsistent basis.

Guidelines for developing programs for children were also provided by Immroth and McCook. They recommended involving the entire extended family and always providing refreshments for the families. With regard to toddler and preschool programs, they recommended rhymes, chants, and songs from the Hispanic oral culture. These authors also suggested slowly introducing the American culture into the program, in order to expose children at an early age to other cultural perspectives. Using finger-puppet and flannel board stories, having age-appropriate bilingual books available, and limiting the presentations to 15 min in order to maintain the children's attention span (p. 20), were also suggested.

These authors discussed programs for older children as well. These are discussed in the later section of this paper entitled "Specific Programs designed to welcome Hispanic patrons," presenting descriptions of programs for older children. These authors also provided an extensive bibliography of outstanding Spanish or bilingual materials for children of all ages. They cautioned, however, that librarians should be very aware of the cultural differences between the various Hispanic cultures, and that materials purchased should represent this diversity; they provided the example that some Spanish-speaking countries use the word "librería" for libraries, while other cultures used the word "bibliotheca." Immroth and McCook also discussed how most of the literature for older children was non-fictional because Hispanic parents associated reading with education, not recreation (pp. 21–23).

Ramirez and Ramirez (1994) provided a list of children's books for Hispanics, African Americans, Asian Americans, and Native Americans. These authors asserted that multiethnic literature would help minority children better understand who they were while simultaneously teaching the Anglo American majority children, to respect the contributions and life styles of the minority cultures. Ramirez and Ramirez also contended that a minority child's sense of self would improve by seeing books with characters like him or herself, in the books. Although their perception was that there were not many books to choose from, Ramirez and Ramirez asserted that librarians should utilize the books available. Ramirez and Ramirez envisioned that the books on their list would instill in minority children a sense of value regarding their diversity and would promote a multicultural and multiethnic society.

Duran's work, produced 15–20 years prior to the above works, espoused the same philosophy as the above authors. Duran (1979) described the "Chicano" and "Puerto Rican" literature that existed at that time, as published for the good of children. He described a movement in which poets, anthropologists, sociologists, and educators were all joining in the new trend to have children's literature be a way to make Hispanic and non-Hispanic children alike aware of the history and contributions of Hispanics and to combat the Americanization of Hispanic children. He also asserted that Hispanic books should be multiformatted; presenting texts that were English-only, Spanish-only, or bilingual, to their public simultaneously. He described how the bilingual formats could have the English and Spanish versions on the same page, separated as two parts within the same book, or as a two-book set. Duran pointed out that some of the existing bilingual books even included word glossaries, pronunciation instructions, or other educational features.

He also discussed the utility of bibliographies, as well as the formatting of books. According to Duran, librarians could look to the compilation of books provided by authors such as Trejo, Woods, Barrios, Vivo, Cabello-Argandoña, and Padilla, in order to know which books to select for their collections. Furthermore, with what Duran described as a growth in the past 20 years, of "Latino-owned or oriented, publishers, producers or distributors of Latino materials," librarians had access to a wider selection of materials. Duran also proffered his belief that "Latino" writers presented a much more favorable view of the Hispanic culture than the "non-Latino" authors who wrote in the 1960 (Duran, p. 12).

SPECIFIC PROGRAMS THAT ARE WELCOMING TO HISPANICS

Now, actual library programs that have attempted to institute some of the culturally sensitive approaches discussed above will be listed. Café Libros, sponsored by the Nevada County (2003) Public Library system, has presented appealing multicultural events, such as Open Mike Nite, where teens at the library can read poetry, sing, or read books in Spanish while the library provides free pizza and free access to the Internet during the program (see http://www.cafelibros.net).

The San Ysidro Branch of the San Diego Public Library has developed a small Legal Resource Center in the library, which contracts with various law groups to do programming in Spanish on immigration law, landlord/neighborhood/tenant law, employee rights, medical patient rights, citizenship, wills, living wills, and estate planning (Alire & Archibeque, 1990, p. 106).

The San Jose Public Library (2002) website, in its Teen section, has sponsored ongoing events for Hispanic youth in their teen groups. Such events have included tarot readings, meditation lessons, and book readings in Spanish, translated for the non-Spanish-speaking members of the group. These activities were chosen because they appeared to be culturally sensitive activities that would be welcoming to Hispanic youth (see http://www.sjpl.lib.ca.us/events/monthly.htm).

The El Paso Public Library has been offering more than just a bilingual "Read to Babies" program for Hispanic parents. Their program also addressed the prevention of teenage pregnancy; drug abuse prevention; CPR for infants; prenatal care; and parent education (Alire & Archibeque, 1990, p. 106).

Alire and Archibeque also described a literacy and ESL program hosted by the New York Public Library called "Familias con Libros." This program involved four workshops with daycare for young children, and reading and writing lessons for their parents and older siblings. The families made a photo album at the end of the program, which included home photographs, as well as photographs taken at the library. The program, however, did more than address literacy; the parents participated in groups regarding parenting issues, while children's books were distributed, and families received an almanac to start their own home library. This program proved very effective at promoting future library use by the participants, once the program ended (p. 107).

The Houston Public Library also started a creative program. They held a Spanish-oriented poetry and music program for four consecutive Valentine's days. Poetry reading occurred in two different rooms, one with bilingual poetry, and one with poetry in Spanish only. Children were entertained with an arts and crafts program while their parents listened to the poetry and music. It was a festive time for all as a local company donated snacks for the gatherings (Moller, 2001, p. 32).

The Newark Public Library started a program for Hispanic young adults called "Gente Y Cuentos" (People and Stories). This program involved inviting both Hispanic young adults and Hispanic senior citizens, to joint book reading and discussion sessions. Hispanic authors wrote the books selected. The program served to demonstrate the library's cultural understanding of the importance of grandparents to Hispanics, and it served as a good advertising avenue for the library's bilingual homework hotline for young adults (Alire & Archibeque, 1990, p. 104).

Other public library systems have been just as creative as the library systems described above. The New York and Queen's Public Library systems offered young adult programming for Hispanic youth, which involved events that included theatre, rap music, and creative writing. The El Paso Public Library used special events to recruit Hispanic young adults to the library, such as art workshops and martial arts demonstrations. The library also recruited Hispanic young adults to their teen group by holding a Mardi Gras celebration. At this event, the teenagers were encouraged to decorate their bikes and wear costumes of their cultural preference (Alire & Archibeque, 1990, p. 104).

The Tucson-Pima library offered varied young adult programs for Hispanic youth. The program for the urban youth included a bilingual homework-help center, and for rural Hispanic youth, there was a program called "Burgers and Books." The "Burgers and Books" program involved bilingual book readings, as well as discussions regarding careers, peer pressure, and drugs. During the young adult group meetings, hamburgers contributed by Burger King were available (Alire & Archibeque, 1990, p. 104).

Moller (2001) described a storytelling project conducted in South Central Colorado in a rural area dominated by Hispanic residents. A school district librarian joined with a public school librarian to acquire a grant to teach storytelling skills to Hispanic grandparents. The workshops, which covered how to choose appropriate materials, how to read aloud, how to tell someone else's story, and how to tell your own story, cost students (grandmothers) $25. The librarians gave scholarships to the grandparents who could not afford the $25. Any grandparents who finished the training and performed three storytelling events were refunded their $25. The grant was funded by the Colorado State Library system in an effort to foster intergenerational communication. The goal was for students to gain an understanding from their grandparents, of the way things were and of the Hispanic traditions.

The Queen's Public Library provided programming for Hispanics that included music and dance performances, festivals, poetry readings, bilingual storytelling, author talks, and craft demonstrations. However, the most popular programs were the cultural arts programs. The library system assembled cultural arts performers from almost every country in Latin America and Spain. These events were well attended by Hispanic and non-Hispanic members of the community. The library system also provided bilingual lectures and workshops in the cultural dialect of the intended audience. The workshops and lectures covered topics, such as immigrant law, parenting, continuing education, careers, health, family relationships, and other topics related to coping with moving to a new country. The neighborhood libraries even presented workshops on topics as specific as dealing with ADHD or cancer, becoming a home health aide, starting a childcare business, prenatal care, changes in welfare laws, and dealing with depression.

These programs were advertised with attractive bilingual flyers (English was always on one side of the flyer in order to not alienate English-speaking patrons). The flyers were mailed to cultural and immigrant oriented service agencies, while press coverage was solicited from the local ethnic media. The workshops also provided exposure to the "Say Sí" collection. The Queens Library system maintained a collection called "Diga sí a tu bibliotheca" or "Say Sí" for short. This collection consisted of over 96,000 items in Spanish, covering the following range of topics: cooking, politics, history, parenting, the occult, computer programming, classics by Spanish-speaking authors,

American classics translated into Spanish, and American pop fiction translated into Spanish. Music, videocassettes, and audio books were also a part of this successful collection (Guereña, 2000, pp. 137–138).

The Miami Dade Public Library system provided two programs for children over five, which were extremely popular. The programs, called "La Hora de Cuentos" and "Colorín Colorado," were so popular that Hispanic members of other demographic areas attended, as did non-Spanish speaking families. The programs were aimed at promoting the Hispanic heritage through various presentations styles. The programs utilized finger puppet, regular puppet, oral storytelling, flannel board stories, drama, games, songs, music, bilingual counting games, poems, parent presentations of favorite rhymes and riddles, and game songs like "Ring around the roses" in a Spanish version. The attendees of these programs represented various Hispanic cultures. They shared their various cultural versions of songs and rhymes with one another. Parents reported that the programs motivated their children to use their Spanish more and to learn more about their culture because they enjoyed playing games and listening to stories in Spanish with their parents (Immroth & McCook, 2000, pp. 21–23).

The following section will describe programs that utilized efforts or strategies, which seemed to go over and beyond the norm with regard to engaging the Hispanic population. Colley (1998) wrote about a progressive Young Adult Teen Library Program in Phoenix, Arizona, which served youth "ranging from gang members to student council officers." The Phoenix Parks, Recreation, and Libraries Department sponsored the program. Services were delivered to approximately 35,000 Phoenix youths through collaboration with other youth-servicing agencies, and with businesses. The catchment area of the program had a high percentage of Hispanic residents. This program offered many activities in order to match the diversity of interests represented in the targeted population. The philosophy of the program was to challenge the whole individual, not just the intellect of the program participant. As a result, the program provided program participants with physical activities, such as the opportunity to go white-water rafting, as well as providing library services, such as bookmobiles in Hispanic neighborhoods that provided tutoring and career counseling during school hours for suspended students. The program also provided opportunities, such as free tattoo removal by volunteers who are local businesspersons in the neighborhood.

The Lake County Public Library in Colorado attempted a unique outreach program. It placed parts of its Hispanic collection at a Catholic church, a public health office, and a community day care center, to be checked out based upon an honor system. The library also sent bilingual bookmobiles to neighborhoods with isolated families, such as stay-at-home women who lived in outlying trailer courts and who had no access to public transportation. Before the bookmobile began traveling to these areas, however, bilingual staff went door to door, publicizing the advent of the bookmobile service (Moller, 2001, p. 30).

There were also many innovative programs targeted at Hispanic mothers. The American Academy of Pediatrics started a program at medical clinics in Colorado for Hispanic children, 6 weeks to 5 years of age. The physicians would provide medical care to the Hispanic children and then write prescriptions to the mothers on how to read to their children and how often they should do so. The Carnegie Library of Pittsburg, in conjunction with the ALA program called "Born to Read," had a program of outreach to pregnant adolescents. These mothers received not only prenatal checkups and parenting classes, but also instruction on the value and the "How-to" aspects of reading to their babies once they were born. The Aurora, Illinois Public Library worked with the Visiting Nurse Association to locate mothers with infants; these mothers received free books to promote reading, in addition to medical assistance with their infants (Moller, 2001).

The Forsythe County Public Library system in North Carolina puts tremendous effort into outreach services and discovered that generalization to the library did not result from their outreach efforts. This library system began tailoring their services toward their Hispanic immigrants in 1996 after performing a special Hispanic census in 1996 to determine the demographics of their immigrant Hispanic residents. The census discovered that 71% of the Hispanic residents had been in the country less than 3 years. Furthermore, the census showed that public libraries were an unfamiliar concept to these residents; that 75% of the residents wanted further education as over half of them of them had the functional literacy level of a second grade student; and that 89% of the Hispanics had jobs (the County's employment rate was 79%). These residents spent 65% of their free time in church and said they wanted to learn English. The survey also led the library to conclude that their libraries were inaccessible to their Hispanic population because: (1) the population was so new to the country; (2) transportation to the library was a major obstacle for this population; and (3) the immigrants mistrusted the government.

Therefore, the seven libraries in which the resulting programs were housed built their collections by placing all Spanish materials, whether in print, audio-visual, or E-book formats, in one central and visible location, with a large red sign with white letters. Before acquiring Spanish language materials, a Hispanic librarian who was fluent in Spanish interviewed a group of Hispanics who were receiving tax assistance on a Saturday at a local high school to find out what materials they would want in a collection. The survey indicated that the Hispanic population, which was primarily immigrants, wanted magazines, romance novels, novelas, Western bolsili-bros, and music of all types (from ranchero to classical). The print materials included text with large font, written at an easy-reading level, and enhanced with illustrations. A "Gift book" program, similar to the "Mail a Book" program in Queens, was the main marketing strategy for the library system; Hispanic residents received a certificate good for 12 books delivered by mail. The families could use the certificates to acquire free books in exchange for filling out a library card application. This activity would represent that Hispanic family's first interaction at the public library; Spanish and English dictionaries, as well as books for every age member of the family, were available through the "Gift Book Program."

The library system also had a staff member join the board of the Hispanic Service Coalition and visit various locations, such as churches, the YMCA, the Boys and Girls Club, the Visual Art Center, and a local community college. Staff members also affiliated with various public school committees in order to encourage collaboration. The libraries set up collections or made presentations at all of these centers, as well as at sites with nutritionists or other health care providers. The library also held functions and festivals featuring popular local bands. They advertised their functions and resources through local media outlets. However, none of these efforts was successful in drawing much response from the immigrant Hispanic population. After a couple years of extraordinary attempts at serving this population, the library system concluded that services for this community needed to occur only in the community. It was decided that, given the population's commitment to work and church (leaving them little free time), transportation barriers, and mistrust of the unknown, the Hispanic immigrant population was not going to generalize from attending the programs in their community to visiting public libraries. The Forsythe County Public Library system decided to apply for grants that would only sponsor services in the community (e.g., at local churches or apartment complexes) or that would sponsor radio educational programs, which the population could learn from in the comfort of their home. The library system also received feedback that this immigrant population: (1) did not see the library as a place to spend their free time; (2) was resistant to commit to certain times; and (3) considered education as the school's responsibility, not theirs (Guereña, 2000, p. 143).

The Monrovia Public Library (2003) in California had a fine outreach program called "Road to Reading/El Camino a la Lectura." The librarians held bilingual classes for mothers and toddlers at a church and a Boys and Girl's club in the Hispanic neighborhoods that the librarians were trying to reach. The program occurred 2 days per week in the morning. The children and parents participated in a story time program for toddlers ages 2–5. The classes included 60 min of stories, songs, fingerplays, and creative activities. The library also had a bilingual class for parents to learn how to read to their children. This program was co-operated by the Monrovia library and two neighboring city libraries. The $1\frac{1}{2}$ hour classes rotated through the three different libraries on different weeks. Information regarding this program, called the SPARC Families for Literacy Reading Club, was found at http:// ci.monrovia.ca.us.

The above listed programs were presented because they either used innovative outreach techniques or exhibited sheer tenacity in their attempts to make the Hispanic population feel welcome. The next section will describe programs that attempted to engage the Hispanic population in bibliographic or technological instruction.

Specialized Training Programs

A program in Boulder, Colorado, was an example of a program that performed exceptional outreach regarding technological and bibliographic literacy. This program used volunteers from the Hispanic community extensively and handled these volunteers in a culturally sensitive manner. The program did not have them follow the standard volunteer procedures, such as turning in hours on a certain schedule, because it was felt that they were not congruent with the volunteers' cultural values. Staff often even drove volunteers to the library. These cultural accommodations were considered useful as these volunteers were integral contributors to the development of the Spanish-language collection.

This collaborative effort resulted in a collection of Spanish materials that included books, magazines, audiotapes, videotapes, and arts and crafts items. These materials were not only made available at the library but also provided at designated "community houses." Materials for adults and children were available at these homes/centers in the community, along with homework help, assistance with filling out library card applications, and storytelling instruction. Staff also developed Spanish brochures that advertised classes on how to understand the Dewey Decimal system and regarding how to use the library. The library's assessment efforts also determined that the Hispanic community wanted technological instruction. The library staff, however, felt that one-on-one sessions were more culturally sensitive than services where the Hispanic individuals would participate in a group workshop regarding using computers and the Internet. The individual lessons began with sessions on how to use the OPAC, and proceeded to topics that were more difficult. It should be noted that many of the OPAC students went on to be volunteers who taught other Spanish-speaking members in their community about how to use the library's OPAC system.

Members of the Boulder Hispanic community asked that staff translate the library's Calendar of Events into Spanish. The library also responded to the community's desire for an international, family-memory, storytelling program. The library developed a program where Hispanics of different countries shared their cultural and historical experiences with other members in the program of different ethnicities. These program volunteers also organized events where the different ethnic members of the Hispanic community could share their individual cultural traditions and celebrations. Furthermore, the library, in conjunction with these Hispanic community volunteers, began an Oral Latina/Chicano History Project. The Boulder Library system attributed its success with Hispanic populations to many factors, to include support from the administration and collaboration with community agencies. These two specific factors enabled librarians to focus on outreach work rather than on constantly justifying their effort to reach the Hispanic population. Furthermore, the librarians were able to spend their time obtaining assistance from community agencies for activities, such as transporting materials to the community and/or putting together culturally sensitive and appropriate programs (Guereña, 2000, pp. 194–203).

Moller (2001) described successful computer training programs provided by libraries aimed at preschoolers and their parents. The libraries used preschool-oriented materials so that the bright animation would attract the preschoolers and so that the computers would not intimidate the parents. The curriculum software-selected curriculum was found to be non-threatening to the adults due to its basic/elementary demand level.

In Philadelphia, the Ramonita G. de Rodriguez branch library was conducting an outreach program with a $50 million technology grant for the disadvantaged in the branch's catchment area. The library provided free computer training ranging from the use of the Internet to the use of software, such as Microsoft Word, Access, PowerPoint, Desktop Publishing, etc. The branch's service area, called the "American Street Empowerment Zone," according to the 1990 Census, included a population of 15,486 residents, which was 61% Hispanic, 20% White, and 18% Black. The Census also indicated that 53% of the residents in this area had incomes below the poverty level (Venturella, 1998).

The Tucson-Pima Public Library delivered bilingual literacy services and GED programs outside of the library, at community agencies frequented by Hispanics. Books were checked out on an honor system basis at these community agencies. For mothers who were in this program and had children in Head Start, the library hosted story time at their children's respective Head Start programs. Meanwhile, the mothers received more than GED and literacy assistance; they were given an introduction to library literacy, as well as an invitation to the "Parents as Publishers" program. In this program, the mothers wrote short stories for their children and for the grandmothers in their extended family. The library then bound the stories in a professional book format and handed the graduating mothers diplomas that included both the mothers' books of short stories and bilingual booklets called "Let's Read Together." These booklets contained a reading guide and a bibliography of books for Hispanic parents to read to children of all ages (Alire & Archibeque, 1998, p. 107).

The Pasadena Public Library (2003) system not only provides quarterly bilingual Internet classes, but it also devoted 1 of its 10 branches completely to the Hispanic community. The outstanding feature of this library branch was that it was part of a community center, which combined a library with a computer center, a basketball auditorium, and a softball field (see http://ci.pasadena.ca.us/library/ for more information).

The Oxnard Public Library had a research skills program targeted at Hispanic children. They called the program for children in grades 3–5, the "Junior Information Professional" program, while the program for children in grades 6–8 was the "Junior Information Specialist" program. The participants graduated after 10 consecutive weeks of 45-min classes that addressed utilizing references. The program culminated with a graduation ceremony where staff awarded the participants with diplomas. This technological literacy program performed its marketing through a partnership between the library system and the school district (Alire & Archibeque, 1998, p. 103).

Venturella (1998) also described the teen programs at the Ramonita G. de Rodriguez branch of Philadelphia. One program called the Internet Mentoring Program for Teens linked Hispanic neighborhood teens with community organizations. The teens volunteered their time helping an organization in exchange for learning skills about HTML coding, graphics, and creating personal websites. The library branch also had an after-school program to assist teens with homework.

The Queens Public Library system averaged 3,000 students in various ESL programs. About half of the participants were Hispanic. There were 73 classes between the central branch and the other 62 branches. The participants not only learned how to read and write in English, but also received instruction that addressed how to use libraries, self-help skills, coping skills, and technological skills. There were three levels of ESL classes to address the needs of both beginning students and ones that were more advanced. The beginning classes helped patrons become literate in their own language. The intermediate classes received bibliographic instruction along with their ESL training, and the advanced classes addressed technological literacy along with their ESL training. Staff marketed this bilingual program through flyers to over 350 city agencies in Queens.

The Queen's Library system also used the STF3 (U.S. Census Summary Tape File 3) to identify the nationality of their Spanish-speaking residents in different boroughs. The library system then tailored programs and book collections to those specific populations. It then followed up with a "Books-by-Mail" program in seven languages that identified the demographics of block groups or zip codes and then mailed out lists of free books from which non-English speakers could order four free books. Staff sent the books in reusable bags with postage paid and self-addressed return labels. Hispanic circulation was second among the various ethnic groups using the reusable mailbag exchange (Alire & Archibeque, 1990, pp. 106–107; Guereña, 2000, pp. 135–137).

Alire and Archibeque (1990) also described a program provided by the Santa Monica City Public Library system in California. The library held a series of bilingual programs addressing self-esteem, assertiveness training, preparation for college, Internet training, and health issues. The library also hosted career exploration days where Hispanic professionals shared their histories and provided career tips for the Hispanic young adults in attendance. There was also a young adult program at the Oxnard Public Library in California called "Teens and Tots." Within this young adult program, the library joined forces with a local health clinic to develop a program for teen mothers. This program hosted events regarding reading to children, self-help skills, and an introduction to library literacy (p. 104).

The Public Library for Charlotte and Mecklenburg Counties in North Carolina offered year-round training that involved four, 2-h bilingual computer sessions with 10 people in each class. This program reportedly had a long waiting list of Hispanic individuals who were interested in participating in these Internet classes. Graduates from the program received a diploma and tended to volunteer as assistants in future classes (Moller, 2001, p. 30).

This library also offered, for \$25, access to many databases including Spanish encyclopedias and a preschool website (Jasco, 2002).

The Institute on Library Services to Migrant and Seasonal Farm Workers in Florida held a workshop in June 1998 for 40 school, public, and community college librarians from 14 Florida counties and 2 Texas cities. The training addressed how to increase and improve library services to families of migrant and seasonal farm workers. The trainees received instructions regarding the daily language and culture of these farm workers. Trainers had the trainees make posters and flyers in Spanish for their libraries. Trainers held planning and evaluation sessions. The trainers gave trainees a tour of farms and the local Mission and introduced them to a migrant worker program that had already been established by one of the county school library systems. At this workshop, the trainees learned about programming tips, marketing tactics, and collection development policies for Spanish-language materials. The training ended with a performance by a bilingual storyteller. The trainees were all eager to attend a follow-up workshop scheduled for the following year (McCook, 1998).

The University of California at Riverside developed a Virtual Resources center through an initiative called the Riverside Community Digital Initiative. This initiative funded a computer laboratory and computer education center for the Hispanic population. The center was located at the Cesar Chavez Community Center, which served the east side of Riverside and which targeted youth between the ages of 12 and 23. Meanwhile, the Chicano Studies Research Library at the University of California, Los Angeles, developed a training program that taught technological literacy and informed the Hispanic population about the importance of not being "left out" of the technological revolution. The library's efforts were motivated by 1992 studies showing that, nationwide, the average Hispanic student's school had 19% fewer computers per capita than the average non-Hispanic student's school. Studies also showed that the average Hispanic student's elementary school used advanced tools 40% less than the average non-Hispanic student's elementary school (Guereña, 2000, pp. 190–191, 237–238).

The Northern Manhattan Library district established an outreach and bibliographic instruction program, which was very successful. This program, called Connecting Libraries and Schools Project(CLASP), was originally sponsored by the DeWitt Wallace Reader's Digest Fund in an attempt to bring Hispanic readers into the library. It recognized that its majority population (67% of the Northern Manhattan district's residents were Hispanic) was underutilizing their library services. The outreach librarians decided to go into schools at hours when parents would be receptive. They made entertaining presentations about how important it was to read to children even if a parent could not read. The outreach librarians would bring books with pictures so that they could explain to parents who could not read, how they could make up stories based on the picture books. They would also bring non-picture books, written in Spanish, to teach literate parents how to read to their children.

The librarians also stressed to the parents the importance of teaching their children Spanish. The librarians explained that the children would learn English better if they learned Spanish thoroughly and that their children should learn about Hispanic culture from their parents. These parent workshops at the school also contained lessons regarding all types of storytelling, such as stories with finger puppets, flannel boards, and origami. The workshops did not last more than 30 min in order to maintain the parents' attention. Interwoven into the storytelling presentations were promotions of the library's ESL materials and Spanish books for adults, as well as bibliographic instruction (Immroth & McCook, 2000, pp. 41–44).

In Santa Ana, California, the Adelphia cable company volunteered to provide broadband access to an adult-education program aimed at teaching Mexican Americans how to access the Internet. The National Association for Minorities in Cable, and the Mexican American Opportunity Foundations, sponsored this program. The program was an effort between Adelphia and its sponsors to bridge the digital divide for Hispanics (Hogan, 2002).

Evidence has been presented showing the existence of literature regarding the under-utilization of libraries by minorities, as well as literature regarding addressing the problem through solutions, such as recruitment of minority library personnel and educating library students. Even literature regarding strategies to make libraries more welcoming to minorities, including specific strategies for the Hispanics population, has been presented. However, the literature has also shown that few libraries have followed through on the suggestions offered (Tarin, 1988; Guereña & Erazo, 2000). From 1970 to 2001, authors published guidance regarding marketing library programs, collection development, and actual programming for the Hispanic population. Training programs were strongest in two areas – exemplary programs of outreach to Hispanics (e.g., where the services left the walls of the library), and special training programs (e.g., efforts to make a library's neighboring community technologically literate or library/information literate). However, the number of programs listed was too small in relation to the size of the Hispanic population.

HISPANIC OPINIONS OF LIBRARIES

Finally, this paper examines the opinions of the Hispanic population regarding libraries and library services, using an English and Spanish version of a survey regarding these issues.

The Population Surveyed

The questionnaires were offered to individuals in front of the "Ranch Market" in downtown Monrovia, California. The city of Monrovia consists of 32% Hispanics according to the 2000 Census, but the downtown district of Monrovia is 56% Hispanic. Participants had to be at least 18 years old. Volunteers received $5 gift certificates for the market, for their participation.

The Instrument

It should be noted that this survey was an attempt to replicate Haro's "one man" surveys of the late 1960s, which were described earlier in this paper. Some of the same questions from Haro's survey were included, along with other questions that have proven valuable in later surveys. Therefore, the survey was developed to address the recurring themes in research regarding Hispanics' under-utilization of public libraries. The following were proposed as explanations for Hispanics feeling unwelcome in libraries and as possible solutions to remedy this situation:

(1) The presence or absence of Spanish-speaking personnel
(2) The presence or absence of Spanish-speaking materials
(3) The presence or absence of materials of interest to Hispanics

The above issues were addressed by the survey located in the Appendices A and B of this paper. Furthermore, the aim of this survey was to obtain answers from patrons and non-patrons, as in the Haro survey. The hope was to eliminate any bias introduced by interviews conducted at libraries with existing patrons or by using phone interviews. Those methodologies discriminated against under-utilizers and families without phones.

Procedure

The survey was offered to non-Hispanic individuals as well as Hispanics. The volunteers were asked if they preferred to speak in English or Spanish.

The surveys were conducted in whichever language the volunteer chose. The interviewer was present at the market from 3:00 to 7:00 p.m. on a weekday, in order to obtain input from families after school or individuals after work. The interviewer was also present at the market on a Sunday from 1:00 to 5:00 p.m.; allowing for the inclusion of participants who went to church in the morning but who had Sunday evening family gatherings.

The responses of the Monrovia Hispanic residents to the library survey were evaluated to determine if there had been any improvement in attitudes toward libraries over the past few decades. The answers from the Hispanic patrons were compared to answers from non-Hispanic patrons, as well as to answers from subjects in previous studies. The limitation of this research design, however, was that the survey was not administered to a captive audience; therefore, the population size was relatively small. However, this research design allowed opinions to be gathered from both patrons and non-users. If the survey had been administered at a library, which is a captive audience, then the responses would only have been from existing patrons, excluding non-patrons of the library.

Another limitation of this survey was that there might have been a bias toward families who shopped at the hours when the survey was administered and toward families who shopped at that market. However, prior to administration of the surveys, the market was observed for a 30-min period at 10:00 a.m. on a weekday. It was determined that the sample of market users observed accurately reflected the demographics of the community. Five Hispanic men in their 30s or 40s, 13 Hispanic women in their 30s or 40s, and 4 Hispanic individuals over the age of 55, were present at the market during the observation period. Furthermore, the market was located two blocks from a park and an elementary school and across the street from a Home Depot parking lot, which was often a heavily populated location for male Hispanics seeking work. A hair salon, video store, Viva Discount Toy Store, Pronto Income Taxes, Casa Dental Clinic, a Burger King, Popeye's, Radio Shack, discount clothes store, and a store called Aqua Fresca were located in the same mini-mall as the market. Therefore, this market, which contained a carnicería and was adjacent to shops of the kind recommended in the literature as optimal locations for recruiting Hispanics, seemed to be the best option for sampling the actual residents of downtown Monrovia.

Survey Instrument and Findings

Sixty-four subjects agreed to fill out a survey regarding public libraries. Fifty-six of the subjects were Hispanic (83%) and eight were not. The survey consisted of nine questions grouped into four main categories: (1) library usage; (2) language usage patterns; (3) demographic information; and (4) an evaluation of public libraries. The 11 subjects who had never been to a public library only had to answer the five questions that pertained to the first three categories. The remaining 53 subjects answered all nine questions, including items addressing the subjects' opinions regarding public libraries. It should be noted that the 11 subjects who had never been to a public library were all Hispanic.

Non-Users

The 11 non-users were asked to indicate why they had never been to a public library. Three explanations for this lack of usage were listed for the subjects to accept or reject. Respondents were asked to choose all that applied. A fourth option read "Another reason _____." The first three possible responses were: (1) "There is nothing interesting or useful in the public library"; (2) "There are not enough items in Spanish in the library"; and (3) "There is no one to help me because most of the public library workers do not speak a language other than English." Six of the non-"library-goers" elected to use the "other response" option. They filled in the blank with the following statements: (1) "I do not have time"; (2) "I do not know where the nearest library is"; (3) "There are no Spanish-speaking workers"; (4) "There are not enough Spanish materials"; and (5) "My family brings me things so I do not have to go."

The answers to the first three options of Question #3 followed a specific pattern. Five of the subjects endorsed option #1 ("There is nothing interesting or useful in the public library") as the reason they had never been to the library. Seven of the subjects selected option #2 ("There are not enough items in Spanish in the library"); and eight of the subjects chose option #3 ("There is no one to help me because most of the public library workers do not speak a language other than English"). Given these results, it was concluded that the two major reasons the subjects had not been to a public library were that they believed that there was a lack of Spanish materials and Spanish-speaking workers there. As only 19% of the subjects endorsed option #1, this author did not conclude that the lack of interesting or useful items was a major obstacle to these Hispanic subjects' use of the library. These conclusions were reinforced because a number of the subjects endorsed both options #2 and #3, and also spontaneously stated in option #4, (the "other response" option), that they felt there was a shortage of Spanish materials and Spanish-speaking personnel at public libraries.

After answering question #3, the 11 non-"library-goers" were also prompted to skip questions 4–7 and proceed to questions 8 and 9. Question #8 addressed demographical information. Question #9 was another "other response" option, where the subjects were given the option to "add any additional comments." The 53 "library-goers" were also prompted to answer question #9. Seventeen subjects in total answered this ninth question. Hispanic subjects provided 15 of the 17 responses, and non-Hispanic subjects provided the other 2 responses.

Library Users

Question #4 was only applicable to the 53 "library goers." The subjects were asked to indicate what items they were looking for the last time they went to a public library and whether the items they sought were for adults, teens, or children. Fourteen types of materials were listed in an "accept" or "reject" format, and an opportunity was offered for subjects to provide an "other response." The "other response" asked the subjects to list "Other types of materials, information, and services _____" that they were seeking during their last visit to the public library. Nine of the 53 subjects answered the "other response" to question #4. Six of the responses were from Hispanic subjects while three of the responses were from non-Hispanic subjects. Questions #5–7 also only applied to the 53 "library-goers." Question #5 addressed whether the subjects had asked for help and whether they had received sufficient help during their last visit to the public library. Question #6 asked them if they had found what they were looking for during their last visit to a public library. Question #7 instructed the 53 subjects to make qualitative evaluations of 16 different library collections at the library they last visited, if they were familiar with those collections. See the appendices for the 16 collections included in the survey.

Although questions #3–7 addressed opinions regarding public libraries, questions #1 and 2, addressed library usage and language usage patterns. Question #8 gathered the subjects' demographical data. These three questions were relevant to all 64 subjects. Question #1 asked whether the subject had ever been to a public library. Questions #2 addressed language usage in terms of (1) What was the language spoken most often in the subject's home; (2) How often does the subject speak English; and (3) How often does the subject read English? Question #8 addressed the demographics of the surveyed population, asking (1) What is your zip code; (2) Do you work in Monrovia; (3) How old are you (within age ranges); and (4) What is your race?

The trends in the answers of the Hispanic subjects matched the trends found in the literature, with the one exception – only 20% (11/56) of the Hispanic subjects had never been to the public library. Haro's surveys in the late 1960s indicated a higher percentage of Hispanic individuals who had never used a public library (65%). However, the major reasons given for not going to the library were the same as presented in the literature. The 11 subjects espoused the belief that there were no Spanish materials and no Spanish-speaking personnel in the library. Even some of the Hispanic subjects who had been to the library spontaneously voiced these two beliefs. Thirteen of the 56 Hispanic "library-goers" spontaneously wrote in the "additional comments" section that libraries needed more Spanish materials and/or Spanish-speaking personnel. Hispanic subjects offered only two other "additional comments." One subject wrote that he did not know where the nearest library was, while another praised both the Monrovia city library and the library of an adjacent city. These were the only "additional comments" provided by the Hispanic subjects (15/56).

Of the 56 Hispanic subjects, 50 (89%) endorsed Spanish as their predominant language as opposed to six (11%) who primarily used English. This pattern held true with the Hispanic subjects' reading and conversational approach to the survey. Only six of the Hispanic subjects chose to use an English version of the questionnaire. Those same six subjects were the only subjects who spoke to the researcher in English; the other subjects spoke to this researcher in Spanish. The Hispanic subjects who had never attended a library all endorsed Spanish as the major language spoken in their home. These subjects gave responses indicating that they either "never or sometimes" spoke English at home and "never" read English at home. Most of the Spanish speakers who had been to a library said that they "sometimes" or "always" spoke English at home, and "sometimes" or "always" read English at home. Only 4 of the 45 Spanish speakers who had been to the library said that they "never" read English at home; none said that they "never" spoke English at home.

Another trend noted in the literature and confirmed by this study involved the types of library materials used by Hispanic subjects. In this survey, adults tended to utilize the library to obtain books, English-literacy materials, Spanish materials, and newspapers. Some adults also used the library as a source for obtaining magazines, videos, and computer-related items. This pattern of library usage was consistent with the findings presented in the literature review. However, Hispanic subjects, in contrast to the non-Hispanic subjects, said they often used the library to obtain materials for their children. Forty percent of the Hispanic subjects endorsed seeking out materials for their children while only 20% of the non-Hispanic subjects marked that they had done so.

The literature review discussed how Hispanics saw the library as an educational avenue for their children. Hispanic adults tended to visit the library to find books for their children to use in the library, and to check out books and Spanish materials for them. Some adults also acknowledged checking out children's videos and English literacy materials. Non-Hispanic adults tended to utilize the library for all types of materials, except for Spanish materials and CDs. The 20% of the non-Hispanic subjects who checked out items for their children checked out a variety of items without a clear pattern. The "other response" option for this question, about what items the subjects were looking for the last time they went to the library, was answered by three Hispanic subjects and two non-Hispanic subjects. The Hispanic subjects' answers to the "other response" option were "educational materials," "history books," and an "American history book for a school project." The non-Hispanic subjects' answers to the "other response" option were "large print books" and "adult fiction."

The Hispanic subjects also differed from the non-Hispanic subjects in terms of how they evaluated the collections at the last library they attended. The subjects were asked to rate different collections, ranging from career materials, to encyclopedias, to English literacy materials. The ratings were placed on a Likert scale, which had options that ranged between a "1" if the collection was considered poor and needed a lot of improvement, and a "5" if the collection was excellent and not in need of any improvement. Subjects were instructed to mark N/A (not applicable) if he or she did not have knowledge of one of the listed collections of the library. If an item received 80% or more of the possible points it could have received from everyone who graded that collection, the collection was rated as "excellent" (N/A scores were disregarded). If a collection received 70% or more, it received a "good" rating. Sixty percent or more equaled an "OK" rating; 50% or more equaled a "weak" rating, and any percentage under 50 was considered "poor."

The Hispanic subjects only rated one collection as "weak" – the Spanish materials collection. All the other collections were rated "OK" or higher. The non-Hispanic population rated two collections as "weak" (immigration materials and parenting materials) and one collection as "poor" (homework help). It was interesting that the non-Hispanic population marked the Spanish materials collection as "excellent," even though only one of the non-Hispanic subjects marked having used the library for Spanish materials. Under "additional comments," one non-Hispanic Monrovia resident spontaneously wrote "good work." One other non-Hispanic subject made an "additional comment." That subject was not a Monrovia resident and wrote, "Libraries need more materials regarding special needs children like the Autistic Spectrum Disorder, teen parents, parenting, and career training." The 15 "additional comments" made by the Hispanic subjects were described earlier in this section.

The Hispanic subjects, however, did not differ much from the non-Hispanic subjects with regard to their brief evaluations of their last experiences at the library. Seventy-eight percent of the Hispanic subjects asked for help during their last visit, and 86% of those who asked for help received the help they needed. Sixty-three percent of the non-Hispanic subjects asked for help during their last visit, and 100% of those who asked for help said they received it. Eighty-two percent of the Hispanic subjects marked that they found the items they were looking for during their last visit to the library, while 88% of the non-Hispanic subjects marked that they found the items they sought.

The Hispanic and non-Hispanic subjects also had similar residential and occupational demographics. Slightly over half of the Hispanic subjects lived in Monrovia, with 51 of the 56 Hispanics living in Monrovia or two adjacent cities. Half of the non-Hispanic subjects lived in Monrovia, and 7/8 of the non-Hispanic subjects lived in Monrovia or two adjacent cities. Forty-two of the 47 Hispanic subjects who did not work in Monrovia lived in Monrovia or in two adjacent cities. All six of the non-Hispanic subjects who did not work in Monrovia lived in Monrovia or two adjacent cities. Age demographics for the two groups differed. As many census reports have shown, the Hispanic population appears to be younger than the majority population, and this was reflected by the survey. Forty-three percent of the Hispanic subjects were under the age of 45, whereas only 13% of the non-Hispanic subjects were under 45.

CONCLUSIONS

Literature has been presented that discussed the under-utilization of libraries by minorities. Some of that literature addressed the need to recruit multicultural library personnel and better educate graduate library science students. There was also a small body of literature regarding strategies to make libraries more welcoming to minorities, as well as handbooks on working with Hispanics in particular. This study concluded, however, that despite reports in the literature, there were still too few libraries following through with the recommendations in the literature.

Articles published from 1970 to 2001 presented strategies regarding marketing library programs, collection development, children and family-based programming, innovative outreach programs, and specialized trainings in areas like information literacy and technological instruction. Libraries were identified that have used mailbag programs, kiosks in community centers/ malls/apartment complexes, collaboration with Latino agencies/other libraries/businesses, targeted programs/materials to the different ethnic cultures that make up the Hispanic population, and many other strategies. However, the number of programs listed was small in relation to the size of the United States Hispanic population.

Nevertheless, it should be noted that the survey administered in this study showed a significant increase in Hispanic patronage as well as satisfaction with public libraries since the late 1960s when Haro performed his studies. Haro found that 65% of his Hispanic subjects had never been to the public library while this study found that only 20% of the Hispanic subjects had never been to the public library. Therefore, outreach efforts and specialized training efforts, like those cited in the research "Findings" section of this paper, could be contributing factors to the improved relationships between Hispanics and public libraries demonstrated in this study, at least within the community studied.

Although the suggestions presented throughout this paper have been followed to some degree, the majority of the follow-through seems to have been limited to certain geographical areas – California, North Carolina, New York, Arizona, Minnesota, Pennsylvania, Florida, Colorado, Texas, New Jersey, and Illinois. It is possible, however, that the findings were an artifact of the research method employed by this researcher. Perhaps, there were more efforts occurring in other geographical areas, but there was little in the literature to document such efforts if they existed. For instance, the author would never have known about the program in Pasadena, California, if she had not done an internship at that library. Similarly, this author would never have known about work done at the Monrovia Library, if Monrovia had not been chosen as the site for her survey.

Artifacts of the research method may also have affected the survey results. The Hispanic population studied was a relatively acculturated group. This would tend to bias the findings in favor of libraries because few recent Hispanic immigrants were included. However, when the sample in this study was compared to the sample in Haro's study of East Los Angeles and Sacramento residents, the demographics were very similar. Fifty-six percent of Haro's subjects endorsed reading and speaking English, but speaking primarily Spanish in the home. Seventy-three percent of the subjects in this study said they read and spoke English, but primarily used Spanish at home. Therefore, the samples in these two studies were similar; the subjects in both studies were randomly selected from the sidewalk rather than from a population of library users, and they were solicited in a city rather than in a rural setting.

Furthermore, it is possible that more libraries might have developed similar programs but have not been able to implement them due to the drastic budget cuts faced by libraries. Some libraries may even have acquired a designated budget, but have encountered a shrinking market from which to acquire bilingual materials. As described earlier in this paper, this shrinkage has been the result of state budget cuts and the elimination of bilingual education. These two factors have resulted in publishers being hesitant to invest in bilingual materials. However, a couple of authors were cited who provided lists for anyone interested in finding publishers, distributors, and vendors of bilingual materials and/or materials written in Spanish.

Since the review has not provided evidence that enough programs are being implemented to recruit Hispanics to libraries, perhaps the ALA or the California Library Association could conduct surveys; these surveys could assess whether libraries in geographical regions that have a heavy Hispanic population, have programs targeted at the Hispanic community. This could serve to motivate libraries to implement programs or to identify libraries that need training in this area. Furthermore, future research could measure the variables of acculturation and income level in order to study their effects on Hispanic patronage and opinions of public libraries. The income-level was not included in this study because it was felt that the topic might alienate subjects. However, it is an important variable and should be included in future library-satisfaction studies, particularly in geographical areas where large immigrant populations reside.

In conclusion, this study has presented some library program that should be lauded for their innovative attempts at engaging the Hispanic population. As has been stated throughout this paper, however, there are too few of these programs, relative to the percentage of Hispanics in the population. Nevertheless, this study does note that some progress is being made and provides suggestions that can assist library administrators in their planning of outreach and collection development.

REFERENCES

Alire, C., & Archibeque, O. (1998). *Serving Latino communities: A how-to-do-it manual.* New York: Neal Schumann Publishers, Inc.

Allen, A. A. (1987). *Library services for Hispanic children: A guide for public and school librarians.* Phoenix, AZ: The Oryx Press.

American Library Association. (1999a). *Recommendations: Congress for professional education.* Retrieved on 3/15/03, from http://www.ala.org/congress/recommendations.html# diversity#diversity.

American Library Association. (1999b). *Spectrum initiative mission.* Retrieved on 3/15/03, from http://www.ala.org/spectrum/.

American Library Association (ALA). (1988). *Guidelines for library services to Hispanics.* Reference and Adult Services Division. Retrieved on 1/3/03 from, http://www.ala.org/RUSA/stnd_hispanic.html.

Association for Library Services to Children (ALSC). American Library Association. (1999). *The Pura Belpré Award.* Retrieved on 1/2/03, from http:www.ala.org/alsc/Belpre.html.

Bagasao, P. (1999). Knowing about who has access: A matter of strategy. *Information Magazines Impacts.* Retrieved on 1/03/03, from http://www.cisp.org/imp/december_99/12_99bagasao.htm.

Beardon, M. (1995). Buenos dias, U.S.A. *Publishers Weekly, 242*(35), 77–83.

Bibliotecas para La Gente. (unknown date). *Bibliotecas para la gente: The Northern chapter of Reforma.* Retrieved on 3/14/03, from http://clnet.ucr.edu/library/bplg/about.htm.

Border Regional Library Association. (2003). *BRLA.* Retrieved on 3/15/03, from http://libraryweb.utep.edu/brla/default.html.

Buckler, G. (2001). Digital divide creates haves and have nots. *Computing Canada, 27*(24), 21.

Cabello-Argandoña, R., & Haro, R. P. (1977). *System analysis of library and information services to the Spanish speaking community of the United States.* Los Angeles: Bibliographic Research and Collection Development Unit of the Chicano Studies Center at University of California, Los Angeles.

Castillo-Speed, L. (Ed.) (2001). *The power of language/El poder de la palabra.* Englewood, CO: Libraries Unlimited.

CENSUS 2000. (March 30, 2001). Who We Are. *San Francisco Chronicle,* p. A15.

Cheskin Research. (April 2000–Fall 2002). The digital world of the U.S. Hispanics. *Cheskin: Strategic consulting and management research.* Retrieved on 1/03/03, from http://www.cheskin.com/think/studies/ushisp.htm.

Colley, J. A. (1998). Youth development-risky business: Innovative at-risk programming. *The Journal of Physical Education, Recreation, and Dance, 69,* 39–43.

Cuesta, Y. (1990). From survival to sophistication: Hispanic needs = library needs. *Library Journal, 115*(9), 26–28.

Cuesta, Y., & Tarin, P. (1978). Guidelines for library services to Spanish-speaking Americans. *Library Journal, 103*(13), 1350–1355.

D'Aniello, C. A. (1989). Cultural literacy and reference services. *RQ, 28*(3), 370–381.

Duran, F. (1979). *Library services to Latinos.* Santa Barbara, CA: American Bibliographic Center in association with Neal-Schuman Publishers Inc.

Eberhart, G. (2000). The whole library handbook: Current data, professional advice and curiosa about libraries and library services (pp. 71–72, 364–370). Chicago: American Library Association.

Fish, J. (1992, February). Responding to cultural diversity: A library in transition. *Wilson Library Bulletin, 66*(6), 34–37.

Gomez, C. (1994). *Cultivating workplace diversity and empowering minorities. Diversity and multiculturism in libraries.* Greenwich, CT: JAI Press.

Gorski, P. (2002). Dismantling the "Digital Divide": A multicultural education framework. *Multicultural Education, 10*(1), 28–30.

Guereña, S. (Ed.) (1990). *Latino librarianship: A handbook for professionals*. Jefferson, NC: Mac Farland.

Guereña, S. (Ed.) (2000). *Library services to Latinos: An anthology*. Jefferson, NC: Mac Farland.

Guereña, S., & Erazo, E. (1996). Hispanic librarians celebrate 25 years with renewed commitment to diversity. *American Libraries, 27*(6), 77–79.

Guereña, S., & Erazo, E. (2000). Latinos and librarianship. *Library Trends, 49*(1), 131–181.

Haro, R. P. (1981). *Mexican Americans: Developing library and information services for Americans of Latino origin*. Meinchen, NJ: Scarecrow.

Hoffert, B. (1993). Crossing borders: U.S./Mexican forum tackles common concerns. *Library Journal, 118*(12), 32–35.

Hogan, M. (2002). Online en Español = Operator opportunity: Hispanic market poised for Internet explosion. *Multichannel News, 23*(12) 14A (3).

Howland, J. S. (1998). The 'Digital Divide': Are we becoming a world of technological 'haves' and 'have-nots? ' *The Electronic Library, 16*(5), 287–288.

Immroth, B., & McCook, K. (Eds) (2000). *Library services to youth of Hispanic heritage*. Jefferson, NC: McFarland & Company Inc.

Jacob, N. (Ed.). (1988). *A state of change: California's ethnic future and libraries* (Conference and awareness forum proceedings). Stanford, CA: Planning Group for "A State of Change".

Jasco, P. (2002). PLCMC – A very Public Library: This institution's online presence is a great role model for others to follow. *Information Today, 22*(1), 7–19.

Kiser, K. (1999). Selling to the Spanish-Language market in the U.S.. *Publishers Weekly, 246*(37), 35–38.

Knowles, E. C. (1990). How to attract ethnic minorities to the profession. *Special Libraries, 81*(2), 141–145.

Liu, Z. (1993). Difficulties and characteristics of students from developing countries in using American libraries. *College & Research Libraries, 54*(1), 25–31.

Lodge, S. A. (1995). Speaking their language. *Publishers Weekly, 242*(35), 86–87.

Lynn, V., O'Connell, B. O., & Phalen, K. (2003). *USA Weekend, January 31–February 2*.

McCook, K. d. l. p. (2002). Rocks in the whirlpool: equity of access and the American Library Association. Notes: Submitted to the Executive Board of the American Library Association at its annual conference, June 14, 2002. Can be accessed as ERIC document #ED462981 at: http://eric.ed.gov/ERICWebPortal/Home.portal?

McCook, K. d. l. p. (1997). The search for new metaphors. *Library Trends, 46*(1), 117–128.

McCook, K. d. l. p. (1998). National leadership grants fund innovative institutes. *American Libraries, 29*(11), 54–57.

McCook, K. d. l. p., & Geist, P. (1993). Diversity deferred: Where are the minority librarians? *Library Journal, 118*(18), 35–38.

McCook, K. d. l. p., & Lippincott, K. (1997). Library schools and diversity: Who makes the grade? *Library Journal, 122*(7), 30–32.

McPhail, M. (1999). Mexicali hosts Foro Conference. *American Libraries, 30*(5), 31–32.

Milo, A. (1995). Ten reasons why we buy Spanish books. *California Libraries, 5*(10), 1.

Moller, S. C. (2001). *Library services to Spanish Speaking patrons: A practical guide*. Englewood, Co: Libraries Unlimited Inc.

Monrovia Public Library. (2003). *Welcome to Monrovia*. Retrieved on 3/2/03, from http://www.ci.monrovia.ca.us.

National Commission on Library and Information Sciences. (1983). *Report of the task force on library and information services to cultural minorities.* Washington, D.C.: National Commission on LIS. (Su Docs No. Y3 61/2 61/4).

Nevada County. (2003). *Nevada County Library Teens.* Retrieved on 1/03/03, from http://www.cafelibros.net.

NTIA. (2001). Falling through the net. *A NATION ONLINE: How Americans are expanding their use of the Internet.* Retrieved on 1/03/03, from http://www.digitaldivide.gov/.

Pasadena Public Library. (2003). *Pasadena Public Library.* Retrieved on 1/03/03, from http://www.ci.pasadena.ca.us/library/.

Plotnikoff, D. (1998). 'Digital divide' growing wider: Computer Internet use spreads, but so do gaps between haves, have-nots. *San Jose Mercury News,* July 28, p. 1A.

Ramirez, G., & Ramirez, J. L. (1994). *Multiethnic children's literature.* New York: Delmar Publishers.

Robinson, L. (1998). Hispanics don't exist. *U.S. News.* Retrieved on 1/03/03, from http://www.usnews.com/usnews/issue/980511/11hisp.htm.

Rubin, R. E. (2000). *Foundations of library and information science* (pp. 246, 249–250, 258–259, 313–314). New York: Neal Shuman.

San Jose Mercury Newswire. (1998). Program planned to take Internet to poor schools. *San Jose Mercury News,* July 30, p. 8B.

San Jose Public Library. (2002). Retrieved on 1/3/03, from http://www.sjpl.lib.ca.us/events/monthly.htm.

Scarborough, K. (1990). *Developing library collections for California's emerging majority: A manual of resources for ethnic collection development.* Berkeley, CA: Bay Area Library and Information System.

Scarborough, K. (1991). Collections for the emerging majority. *Library Journal, 116*(11), 44–47.

Schement, J. R. (1999). Of gaps by which democracy we measure. *Information Impacts Magazine.* Retrieved on 1/3/03, from http://www.cisp.org/imp/december_99/12_99schement.htm.

St. Lifer, E., & Rogers, M. (1993). Hispanic librarians debate issues at the first Latino summit. *Library Journal, 118*(15), 14–15.

Stern, S. (1991). Ethnic libraries and librarianship in the United States: Models and prospects. *Advances in Librarianship, 15,* 96.

Tarin, P. A. (1988). Rand misses the point: A "minority report". *Library Journal, 113*(18), 31–34.

Taylor, S. A. (1998). Mexico: A growing book industry in search of readers. *Publishers Weekly, 245*(37), S10.

Teacher Librarian. (2002). Libraries in the digital age: Bridging the gap between information haves and have-nots. *Teacher Librarian, 29*(3), 62–66.

Trejo Foster Foundation for Hispanic Library Education-Fourth National Institute. (1999). *Library service to youth of Hispanic heritage: March 12–13, 1999.* Retrieved on 3/15/03, from http://www.cas.usf.edu/lis/hispanic/index.html.

U.S. Department of Education. (1997). Analysis of HEA-Title II-B library education and human resource development program: Fiscal years 1985–1991 funding results. Retrieved on 3/16/93, from http://www.ed.gov/pubs/learning/learning.html.

U.S. National Council on Library Services. (1995). Summary report of the 1996 Forum on Library and Information Services Policy: On *impact of information technology and special programming on library services to special populations.* Retrieved on 1/3/03, from http://www.nclis.gov/libraries/forum96.html.

Vandala, J. (Ed.) (1970). *Hispano library services for Arizona, Colorado, and New Mexico: A workshop held in Santa Fe, New Mexico*. Boulder, CO: Western Interstate Commission for Higher Education.

Venturella, K .M. (Ed.). (1998). *Poor people and library services* (pp. 16–34, 80–90). Jefferson, NC: McFarland & Company.

Villagran, M. (2001). Community building and Latino families. *Reference & User Service Quarterly, 40*, 224–227.

Watkins, C. (1999). Chapter report: Libraries, communities, and diversity. *American Libraries, 30*(7), 12.

Watkins, C., & Abif, K. (1999). Can librarians play basketball? *American Libraries, 30*(3), 58–61.

APPENDIX A: UN CUESTIONARIO SOBRE LAS BIBLIOTECAS PÚBLICAS

1.¿Hace usted utilizado siempre una biblioteca pública? Sí_____ No_____

2a.¿Cual lengua usa Ud. la mayoría del tiempo en la casa?_____   2b.¿Ud. habla Inglés cómo a menudo?
Nunca____ A veces____ Con frecuencia____

2c.¿Ud. lee Inglés cómo a menudo? Nunca____ A veces____ Con frecuencia____

3. Si su respuesta a número 1 era "sí," sigua Ud. a número cuatro. Si su respuesta a número 1 era "No," por favor
marque el razón ó los razones para que no haya ido Ud. a la biblioteca pública.

a) No hay cosas de interés ó utilidad en la biblioteca pública._____

b) No hay suficientes materiales in Español._____

c) No hay alguien en la biblioteca pública con quién puedo pedir ayuda porque la mayoría de la gente que
trabajan allí no hablan español._____

d) Por otra razón _____.

Si Ud. contestó esta pregunta, vaya por favor a número 8 y 9.

Nos gustaría saber sus opiniones al respeto de la colección de la biblioteca que Ud. usó lo más recientemente
posible y de su experiencia ese día. Aplica sus opiniones a preguntas 4–7.

4.¿Ud. estaba buscando materiales en cuales áreas? Círculo todos los que aplican.

Libros para usar en la casa	Para Adultos	Para Adolescentes	Para Ninos (0–12)
Libros para usar en la biblioteca	Para Adultos	Para Adolescentes	Para Ninos (0–12)
Libros de casete	Para Adultos	Para Adolescentes	Para Ninos (0–12)
Libros de disco compacto	Para Adultos	Para Adolescentes	Para Ninos (0–12)
Videos	Para Adultos	Para Adolescentes	Para Ninos (0–12)

DVD	Para Adultos	Para Adolescentes	Para Niños (0–12)
Música de disco compacto	Para Adultos	Para Adolescentes	Para Niños (0–12)
Música de casete	Para Adultos	Para Adolescentes	Para Niños (0–12)
Revistas	Para Adultos	Para Adolescentes	Para Niños (0–12)
Periódicos	Para Adultos	Para Adolescentes	Para Niños (0–12)
Información de la Internet	Para Adultos	Para Adolescentes	Para Niños (0–12)
Información de recursos electrónicos	Para Adultos	Para Adolescentes	Para Niños (0–12)
Materiales en Español	Para Adultos	Para Adolescentes	Para Niños (0–12)
Materiales en Inglés	Para Adultos	Para Adolescentes	Para Niños (0–12)
Otra tipa de información, materiales, ó servicios ___	Para Adultos	Para Adolescentes	Para Niños (0–12)

5. ¿Ud. tenía que pedir ayuda durante su última visita para encontrar información ó servicios? Sí___ No___
   ¿Encontró Ud. ayuda suficiente? Sí___ No___
6. ¿Durante su última visita, Ud. encontró lo que buscaba? Sí___ No___
7. Por favor indique la puntuación más adecuada entre "1" y "5," ó "no aplicable" para evaluar la calidad de las materiales en las siguientes colecciones de la última biblioteca que Ud. usó:

	Deben Mejorarla → Excelente					(No Aplicable)
Negocios/Carreras	1	2	3	4	5	N/A
Materiales para cuidar a niños	1	2	3	4	5	N/A
Materiales de ayuda con tarea	1	2	3	4	5	N/A
Libros de esfuerzos personal	1	2	3	4	5	N/A
Libros de poesía	1	2	3	4	5	N/A
Diccionarios/enciclopedias, etc.	1	2	3	4	5	N/A

	1	2	3	4	5	N/A
Libros de historia mundial ó local	1	2	3	4	5	N/A
"Cómo-a" libros de la manía	1	2	3	4	5	N/A
Materiales sobre emigración	1	2	3	4	5	N/A
Materiales sobre el gobierno	1	2	3	4	5	N/A
Salud física ó mental	1	2	3	4	5	N/A
Tecnológica computerizada	1	2	3	4	5	N/A
Libros en letra grande	1	2	3	4	5	N/A
Materiales en Español	1	2	3	4	5	N/A
Libros sin palabras para niños	1	2	3	4	5	N/A
Materiales para aprender Inglés	1	2	3	4	5	N/A

8. Favor de llenar la siguiente sección, solamente para ayudarnos en obtener información demográfica. La información es completamente confidencial.

Acerca de Ud.:

1. ¿Cuál es su zona postal? _____

2. ¿Trabaja Ud. en Monrovia? Si____ No____

3. ¿Asiste Ud. a una escuela en Monrovia? Si____ No____

4. ¿Cuál es su edad 17–22____ 25–34____ 35–44____ 45–54____ 55 y mayor____

5. ¿Cuál es su raza____?

9. Favor de utilizar la parte abajo de esta forma para comentarios adicionales.

Gracias:

APPENDIX B: A SURVEY REGARDING PUBLIC LIBRARIES

1. Have you ever used a public library? Yes_____ No_____

2a. What language do you speak most of the time, at home?

2b. How often do you speak English? Never_____ Sometimes_____ Always_____

2c. How often do you read English? Never_____ Sometimes_____ Always_____

3. If your answer to number 1 was "yes," go on to question number 4. If your answer to number 1 was "no," please mark the reason or reasons why you have never used a public library.

a. There is nothing interesting or useful in the public library_____.

b. There are not enough items in Spanish in the public library_____.

c. There is no one to help me because most of the public library workers do not speak a language other than English_____.

d. For another reason _____

If you answered this question, please go to numbers 8 and 9.

We would like to know about your experience at the last public library you used and your opinions about that library's different collections. Please use your opinions to answer questions 4-7.

4. Circle the types of information from the areas listed below, that you went looking for when you last went to the library.

Books to use at home	For Adults	For Teens	For Children (0–12)
Books to use in the library	For Adults	For Teens	For Children (0–12)
Videocassette books	For Adults	For Teens	For Children (0–12)
Books in CD format	For Adults	For Teens	For Children (0–12)
Videos	For Adults	For Teens	For Children (0–12)
DVD	For Adults	For Teens	For Children (0–12)
Music on CDs	For Adults	For Teens	For Children (0–12)
Music on videocassettes	For Adults	For Teens	For Children (0–12
Magazines	For Adults	For Teens	For Children (0–12)
Newspapers	For Adults	For Teens	For Children (0–12)
Information about the Internet	For Adults	For Teens	For Children (0–12)
Information about computers	For Adults	For Teens	For Children (0–12)
Materials in Spanish	For Adults	For Teens	For Children (0–12)
Materials in English	For Adults	For Teens	For Children (0–12)
Other types of materials, information or services	For Adults	For Teens	For Children (0–12)

5. Did you have to ask for help during your last visit in order to find the information or service you were looking for? Yes ____ No ____ Did you get the help you needed? Yes ____ No ____

6. During your last visit to the library, did you find what you were looking for? Yes ____ No ____

7. Please rate the following collections at the library that you last visited, on a scale of "1" y "5." You can also mark, not applicable:

	Needs Improvement			Excellent		(Not Applicable)
Business/Career Development	1	2	3	4	5	N/A
Children's materials	1	2	3	4	5	N/A
Materials on Homework Help	1	2	3	4	5	N/A
Self-help books	1	2	3	4	5	N/A
Poetry books	1	2	3	4	5	N/A
Dictionaries/Encyclopedias, etc.	1	2	3	4	5	N/A
World and Local History books	1	2	3	4	5	N/A
"How-to" hobby books	1	2	3	4	5	N/A
Materials on Immigration	1	2	3	4	5	N/A
Government Information	1	2	3	4	5	N/A
Physical or Mental Health	1	2	3	4	5	N/A
Computer Technology	1	2	3	4	5	N/A
Large Print books	1	2	3	4	5	N/A
Materials in Spanish	1	2	3	4	5	N/A
Picture books for children	1	2	3	4	5	N/A
Materials for learning English	1	2	3	4	5	N/A

8. Please fill out the following section, to help us obtain demographical information. This information is completely confidential.

Mark whichever of the following are applicable to you:

a) What is your zip code? _____

b) Do you work in Monrovia? Yes____ No____

c) Do you go to a school in Monrovia? Yes____ No____
d) What age range describes you? 17-24____ 25-34____ 35-44____ 45-54____ 55 +____
e) Are you Latino?____

9. Please feel free to use the blank space below for any additional comments you would like to make.
Thank you:

LANDSCAPES OF INFORMATION AND CONSUMPTION: A LOCATION ANALYSIS OF PUBLIC LIBRARIES IN CALCUTTA

Zohra Calcuttawala

ABSTRACT

Investigations of urban public services remain confined to western settings while research on urban public services in non-western cities focuses mainly on the availability and delivery of basic services. Using the case study of Calcutta, this study is an empirical investigation of the evolution, spatial distribution, and changes in spatial patterns of public libraries for the period 1850–1991. It seeks to demonstrate the provision and accessibility to public libraries at the intraurban scale thereby extending research of urban service delivery to a non-western city. Within the context of urban service delivery – who benefits and why, the location of libraries in three time periods are analyzed. The study finds that the urban morphology of the colonial city continues to exert a strong influence on the growth and spatial distribution of public libraries. Empirical evidence suggests that there is no locational bias based on physical accessibility in the distribution of public libraries. No progressive or regressive spatial arrangement based on socioeconomic variables is indicated.

Advances in Library Administration and Organization, Volume 24, 319–388
Copyright © 2007 by Elsevier Ltd.
All rights of reproduction in any form reserved
ISSN: 0732-0671/doi:10.1016/S0732-0671(06)24009-4

INTRODUCTION

Beginning in the late 1960s, information and knowledge have acquired a new centrality in advanced economies with ramifications on all aspects of life – economic, social, cultural, political (Kellerman, 1984; Hepworth, 1987). Various terms used to summarize the growing importance of knowledge in contemporary economies include "knowledge-based capitalism," the "network society," and the "information city" (Knox & Pinch, 2000). Cities are promoted as knowledge-based centers where economic development is fostered by the collaborative involvement of research institutions, universities, and high-technology industries (Kellerman, 1984). Libraries, traditionally the repositories of information and knowledge and the primary participants in their production and dissemination are acquiring renewed importance in post-industrial western cities as an essential part of this knowledge infrastructure, contributing to the intellectual and cultural milieu of the city and towards attracting business, investment, and a professional work force.

In the wave of technological changes wrought by the information age, the library's traditional role of "warehouses of information" is evolving to that of "providers of access to information." Moreover, the principles of equalizing access to information in an electronic age are becoming increasingly relevant in the presence of a digital gap at many different scales – between rich and poor nations, rural and urban communities, or at an intraurban level. Libraries in their mission to provide universal information access are uniquely positioned to bridge this gulf.

Developing countries are, in general, information poor when compared to information-rich advanced industrial economies. Development studies have argued that education has a direct relationship with economic development and an educated population is one of the preconditions for a country's rapid economic growth and development (Gould, 1993). Libraries assume a pivotal role in the social and economic infrastructure because in an information age, education along with quick and reliable information is vital – in business, industry and commerce, in the modernization of an economy, and in fostering socioeconomic transformation.

Statement of the Problem

The main purpose of this study is to examine the growth, spatial distribution, and spatial changes in patterns of information provision, accessibility, and consumption as represented by public libraries in Calcutta, India. As an empirical case study it is also intended to provide some insight into the evolution of these libraries, and examine the social, economic, and political patterns and processes that have shaped the temporal and spatial variation in library distribution. The study spans the time period from 1850 to 1991.

The specific questions, and thus the investigative core of the study, are the following:

(a) How did the public library system evolve in the study area?
(b) What is the spatial distribution of public libraries in the time periods 1900, 1961, 1991? Is the city well served, adequately served, or poorly served?
(c) What are the spatial use patterns of the patrons of public libraries in the study area?

Significance of the Study

The significance of the study and its contributions to the body of knowledge on urban service delivery is as follows:

(a) It provides an understanding about the evolution of public libraries in a large urban setting with a diverse economy and population.
(b) By studying the spatial distribution and changing spatiotemporal patterns of public libraries in Calcutta, it extends the investigation of the provision of basic and non-basic service delivery in a developing country.
(c) It contributes to an understanding of the spatial interaction between patrons and libraries in a city of the developing world where socioeconomic differentiation is conspicuous and service provision may be more varied.
(d) It provides a basis for cross-cultural comparisons about some aspects of urban services facilities and their delivery.

Operational Definitions

Public libraries in Calcutta require a nominal subscription rate from their members to borrow books unlike the West where public libraries are free and open to all. However, they are open to all who can pay the subscription rate. The definition of public libraries adopted in this study is based on inclusion not exclusion. All libraries that comprise the 1961 Bengal Library Association (BLA) survey of public libraries were used for that year. A similar criterion was employed for 1991 for a list of government-sponsored libraries and private libraries obtained from the DLO. No official list exists for *all* public libraries in the city. It is possible that all libraries that are public were not included in the lists but it is not possible to ascertain how many that may be.

The Study Area
Calcutta, India's largest metropolis, is a major port and the capital of the state of West Bengal. The study area is the Calcutta Municipal Corporation (CMC) area. The CMC area or "proper" Calcutta is the center of the Calcutta Urban Agglomeration (CUA), the collection of towns centered upon Calcutta along both banks of the Hooghly, and the Calcutta Metropolitan District (CMD), the entire region that includes a rural as well as an urban component. The whole area depends on the center city for its economic life, and there is a large flow of population between the center and the periphery.

Situated on the eastern bank of the Hooghly, a distributary of the Ganges, it developed as a colonial port city and was entirely the creation of British colonialism (Dutt, 1983; Murphey, 1964). It became the capital of British India in 1772. The locational advantage of Calcutta stemmed from the fact that, situated 60 miles (97 km) upstream from the Bay of Bengal, it could be reached by the ocean going ships of the 19th century. Moreover, it commanded a huge and densely populated hinterland with a very rich agricultural and mineral-based economy (Dutt, 1983). The hinterland was connected to Calcutta by an extensive river and canal system and later by an efficient railroad and road system. In the 19th century, the most significant industrial activity was the jute industry with a chain of mills stretching along both banks of the Hooghly River.

In the post-independence period, colonial cities evolved into commercial/industrial cities to serve the expanding economies and national development plans of the governments of the region (Dutt, 1983). Calcutta contained the largest manufacturing capacity as well as the second largest engineering industry. Other important industries are paper, pharmaceuticals, and synthetic fabrics. As an important commercial center since colonial times, Calcutta had the largest concentration of commercial establishments, including the headquarters of many native business firms and banks. Since the mid-1960s, the manufacturing sector has been passing through a phase of recession. This has meant the relative ascendancy of trade and commerce in the city and, in the late 20th century, Calcutta has once again become a major commercial city of India. In 1991, the city of Calcutta had 40.51% of the total population of the urban agglomeration, occupying an area of 187.33 km^2 with 141 wards and over 5 million people. The average population density was 148,558.48 persons per square mile (57,358.43 km^{-2}) (Fig. 1).

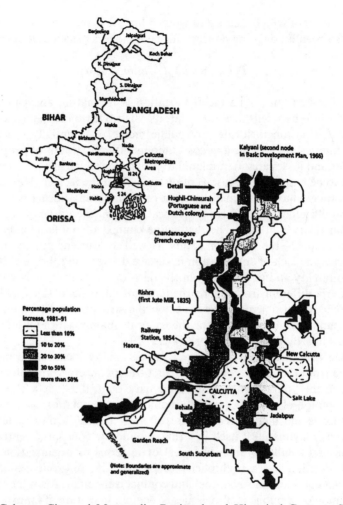

Fig. 1. Calcutta City and Metropolis: Regional and Historical Context. *Source*:
Sanjoy Chakravorty (2005).

LITERATURE REVIEW

There are several research approaches adopted to study urban service delivery. One dimension involves public facility location theory and optimization models in the location of urban public facilities. Another addresses the question of who benefits and why within the context of territorial justice has also been an ongoing concern for geographers (Talen & Anselin, 1998).

Public Sector Location Theory

The basic issue in public facility location is the nature and causes of the relationship between location and its distributive consequences (Dear, 1974). A decision to locate any public facility is essentially a decision to distribute certain benefits and costs among different groups of people. These benefits and losses are often related to proximity, which allows the gains and losses to be treated as functions of distance from the facility (Harvey, 1973). Geographers have examined location problems using normative tools that rely on efficiency derived from classical location theory which are Pareto-optimal (Harvey, 1973). The distinctive context of public facility location models, namely the need for equity as well as efficiency in the locational outcome, the lack of competition in service delivery and the need for public accountability and public input in the decision requires that they be judged by criteria different from their private sector equivalents (Dear, 1974). The private sector problem concentrates on the structure and location of individual units, while public sector theory deals mainly with multiple location systems in a dynamic framework (Dear, 1974).

Some common characteristics of public facility location problems that emerge from the above context are, first, their concern with public goods – either in the "pure" sense of a public park or in the "welfare" sense of a redistribution of resources towards some target population. A second characteristic is the hierarchical nature of most public facility systems. This hierarchy may manifest itself in terms of buildings (one large central library and several smaller branch libraries) or in terms of organization. The location decision has a multiplicity of inputs (diverse groups interact with differing goals and motivations) and conflict is inherent. Also, the "voicing" of opinion over public facility issues is a common feature of many locational decisions, as, for instance, in the construction of controversial expressway access roads (Dear, 1974).

The majority of the private sector location models are programmed to minimize the total cost of transportation and facilities (Dear, 1974) as efficiency and profit are its goals. Efficiency amounts to minimizing the aggregate costs of movement within a particular spatial system (Harvey, 1973). Accessibility enhances efficiency and is a powerful notion to create a system of decentralized facilities (Truelove, 1993). While they may maximize benefits to builders, models of this type do not consider the consequences of location decisions for the distribution of income. Also, to base the public facility location question on the notion of maximum accessibility of service is too simple as the meaning of "accessibility" is different for different people. Accessibility in terms of physical proximity may be a major concern for relatives of mentally retarded children either because they wish to visit frequently or because they do not want their child to travel far. For the drug addict seeking treatment, "psychological accessibility" to sympathetic service may be much more important than physical proximity (Dear, 1974). It is further argued that the notion of "demand" for public facilities is fuzzy, and it is more appropriate to speak of "need."

Equity and efficiency as goals of a system of public facilities are often in conflict (Truelove, 1993). Efficiency is concerned with the aggregate quantity of services provided and consumed whereas equity is concerned with who benefits from the services. Efficiency refers to the distribution of services among the population, and equity refers to the distribution of the effects of these services (Truelove, 1993). Some inequality in access is inevitable as some people will always be nearer the service node than others (Hodgart, 1978). To minimize this inequality, a location which minimizes the longest journey of any consumer may be considered. Optimal location of an extra facility from an efficiency perspective is likely to be different from the optimal location of an additional facility from an equity viewpoint. Where efficiency is the goal, an additional facility in an area of high population density which minimizes average travel cost is considered optimal; where equity is the objective, an additional facility might be located in a distant low-density area so as to minimize the maximum distance that people must travel.

A more flexible method of incorporating an element of spatial equity into the solution of an optimizing model is through the use of covering models (Hodgart, 1978; Toregas & ReVelle, 1972). For certain services, particularly emergency fire and medical services, the quality of service or its value to the user declines with distance from the supply point. A desirable standard of service is defined in terms of a certain maximum time or distance, S, and the facilities are located to ensure that the whole population is within S units from a center.

In the case of library facility location problems, it is argued that drawing an analogy of libraries with retail stores is justified as consumers or patrons visit them to obtain a commodity that is useful to them. Demographic characteristics that influence consumer behavior such as age, sex, income, education, occupation, lifestyle also influence library use patterns (Koontz, 1997). Library visits are also thought to exhibit a pattern of multipurpose trips. Many of the library facility location problems have found solutions from retail location theory. In addition, the locational pattern of a library system significantly affects library use (Koontz, 1997; Coughlin, 1972).

The analogy with the retail environment cannot be stretched too far as there are some fundamental differences between a retail store and a library. The former is distinguished by private ownership and profit motivation, and it exists in a highly competitive environment, while the latter is a public, non-profit-making establishment with little competition. However, research reveals that the spacing between libraries is important as the location of each library relative to others may influence use (Getz, 1978). The proliferating use of the Internet and digital technologies may also be changing this status quo. The resulting spatial patterns and processes in either case are influenced by these factors.

Urban Service Delivery – Accessibility and Use

The question of who gets what, why, and how is a central concern of urban service delivery (Antunes & Plumlee, 1978; Hero, 1986; Talen & Anselin, 1998) and has been an ongoing concern in geographical and political research. Research on urban service delivery within the context of territorial justice (the relationship between provision and need) embraces a wide range of research dimensions. One facet is the empirical inquiry of the geographic distribution of public services, another seeks to determine the underlying causal factors in the distribution of service or distribution inequities, while others probes methodologies for defining and measuring equity.

Geographical Distribution of Public Services
Studies along the first dimension include evaluations of the geographic distribution of subsidies or public services (Cox, 1973; Kirby, Knox, & Pinch, 1984; Pacione, 1989). The goal of the analyses is to assess underlying causal factors that can be shown to account for distributional inequities. In research along this dimension, very few studies correlate accessibility patterns with socioeconomic characteristics. Factors that have been explored in the search for why certain distributional patterns exist include politics (Meier, Stewart, & England, 1991; Miranda & Tunyavong, 1994), urban form (Hodge & Gatrell, 1976; McLafferty, 1982), organizational rules (Lineberry, 1977; Rich, 1982), citizen contacts (Mladenka, 1980, 1989), and race (Cingranelli, 1981; Mladenka & Hill, 1977). Antunes and Plumlee (1978) concluded that the distribution of local street quality was independent of socioeconomic and ethnic biases and was best attributed to random causal factors. Studies by Knox (1978) provide one example of how mapped

distribution systems (in the form of accessibility patterns) could be used in the assessment of resource equity. Utilizing gravity-based measures of proximity to primary medical care, Knox demonstrated how such measures could be used as indicators of social well being in cities. In another instance, a gravity-based model was used to examine differential access to secondary schools by compiling mapped indices of accessibility (Pacione, 1989). Truelove (1993) analyzed access to day care facilities in Toronto by producing various types of accessibility maps and comparing the characteristics of areas with divergent spatial proximities. A longitudinal study employing multiple indicators of the distributional pattern of park and recreation facilities in Chicago revealed that a redistribution of resources between white and black wards had occurred leading to the conclusion that class had replaced race as the primary determinant of service distribution pattern (Mladenka, 1989).

Defining and Measuring Equity

Along the second dimension, the multitude of concepts involved in equity issues and the normative aspects of equity and fairness were explored by Hay (1995). The various meanings of equity for planning purposes were explored by Lucy (1981) who differentiated between equity as equality and equity predicated on the basis of need. Equality assumes that everyone receives the same public benefit, regardless of socioeconomic status, willingness to pay, or other criteria. Alternatively, equity can be defined on the basis of demand (Crompton & Lue, 1992) or market considerations (willingness to pay). Various meanings of spatial equity and its measurement has been systematically treated by Truelove (1993) and empirically applied in a case study of the distribution of day care centers in Toronto. Normative studies of equity preferences (Wicks & Backman, 1994) or formal definitions of equity (Marsh & Schilling, 1994) have also been conducted. Five contending hypotheses have been outlined by Lineberry (1977) that may be used to measure service distribution and explain service patterns in an area. These include (1) the race preference hypothesis, (2) the class preference hypothesis, (3) the power elite hypothesis, (4) the underclass hypothesis, and (5) the ecological hypothesis. An alternative method to measure differential access to public services employs a relative index that incorporates the limits to a correlation coefficient in an area (McLafferty & Ghosh, 1982). It was found that the distribution of r-values for any number of facilities in a particular study was unique, and may have a range of r-values narrower than the range from -1.0 to 1.0. Thus, few empirical studies have found highly progressive or regressive location patterns because a range of r-values of -1.0 to 1.0 was used. For example, an r-value of 0.20 may appear to be quite low but may be near the maximum possible r-value in that case. Major shortcomings in urban service delivery literature are theoretical and normative in nature and other problems derive from it (Hero, 1986). Decisions made before the service delivery stage are very significant and research focused solely on service distribution to different sociospatial groups within a city that leaves the question of the choice of services provided un-addressed affords a limited basis for judging equity in service distribution. Problems in methodological rigor arise from the fact that resource allocation to areas is measured but not benefits and/or accomplishments. The policy or political context with which to assess what such deployment means is scarcely indicated.

Geographical Studies of Libraries

Libraries constitute one of several public services incorporated within geographical research on urban service delivery in the recent past. The library siting problem within the context of public service facility location theory has been an important topic of research during the 1970s and 1980s (Coughlin, 1972; Koontz, 1997). Distance and its effects on library use as well as the market area distance range have been an important focus (Coughlin, 1972; Bennett & Smith, 1975; Shaughnessy, 1970). Patterns of use have also been analyzed using demographic and socioeconomic correlates of library users revealing characteristics such as education (Kronus, 1973), income (Coughlin, 1972), occupation (Shaughnessy, 1970), and gender (Zweizig, 1973). Distributional impacts of libraries have been assessed by Cole and Gatrell (1986) in terms of existing provisions and access to public libraries. By and large such studies are undertaken in a western setting.

Geographical Studies of Libraries in Non-Western Countries

The geographical analysis of urban public services in developing countries has been limited to the distribution and provision of basic services such as housing, water supply, sanitary provision, and the like. A systematic treatment of the spatial patterns and processes of library distribution and provision over time and as part of the social and economic infrastructure are scarce. Relatively little is known of the nature and extent of local inequalities in accessibility to information services, and even less about their relationship with other aspects of social deprivation (education, employment) (Knox, 1978).

User patterns with reference to the location of a public library were influenced by transportation cost and travel time, which increased with distance (Obokoh & Arokoyu, 1991). The development of the spatial structure of the Tel Aviv public library system revealed a spatial gap in the distribution of libraries as a result of "positive discrimination" by the municipality (Herskovitz et al., 1991).

Geography of Urban Public Services in Calcutta

In urban areas in the developing world, research on urban service delivery of non-basic services such as parks and playgrounds, outdoor recreation, and libraries has received scant attention from scholars. Yet, such facilities may be of critical importance for the residents of the predominantly poor and over crowded cities whose mobility and purchasing power are low and for whom alternative sources are minimal (Joardar, 1993). An empirical investigation of the use and perception of residential parks in Calcutta concludes that the potential of public open spaces within the residential areas of cities such as Calcutta may not be realized (Joardar, 1993). The issue of mobilization of scare resources towards the development and maintenance of urban parks receives less priority from overstretched budgets not withstanding their long-term social and environmental significance.

METHODOLOGY

A total of six months was spent in Calcutta for the collection of primary and secondary data and information. The first phase of fieldwork was completed in Autumn 1999 with a second field trip in Winter 2002. During the initial field expedition, census data, library data, and digital as well as non-digital maps were obtained. Key sources such as the District Library Officer (DLO) and the BLA were identified, and informal interviews and conversations with officers and leaders of these bodies were undertaken. A socioeconomic and demographic survey of library users was completed. The survey included a questionnaire designed to ascertain who and where library patrons came from and their social and economic backgrounds (Appendix A).

A postal survey of all public libraries in the final compiled list was also completed (Appendix B). The goal of the postal survey was to ascertain the name of the library, hours of operation, year of establishment, total book stock, and total number of male, female, and child members. The surveys were mailed to approximately 300 libraries. The total number of libraries that responded was 55 (18.3%), 12 (4%) surveys were returned undelivered, while 245 (81.6%) did not respond. It has been assumed for data analysis that those libraries where surveys were returned undelivered have relocated or are no longer operating.

An Autocad drawing of Calcutta streets based on a 1981 street map was converted to an ArcView shapefile (or map) with the help of a conversion module in MapInfo. The resultant digital map is that of Calcutta streets with limited GIS use because it has no database associated with it owing to its source from an Autocad drawing. The lack of a database made the application of a geocoding module, an inherent component of popular GIS software, impossible. Hence, manual geocoding of approximately 300 libraries, a highly time-consuming process, was undertaken. A postal beat directory and the researcher's knowledge of streets aided the effort to accurately locate the libraries. Other maps such as historical maps and census ward maps were hand digitized.

HISTORY AND GROWTH OF LIBRARIES

To understand the wider social, economic, and political context of the distribution of public libraries and library service provision in Calcutta today and posit it in the historical and cultural matrix wherein it emerged a historical perspective is necessary. The genesis of public libraries in the period 1850–1991 is outlined along with a brief history of libraries in the century preceding the study period (circa 1750–1850) to provide continuity of the generative processes.

Early 18th Century

Proprietary Subscription Circulating Libraries
After 1757, when the East India Company consolidated its rule over the Indian subcontinent and metropolitan Calcutta began to flourish as the new hub of trade and commerce, the era of church-based libraries was over (Kabir, 1987). A new type of library emerged in the 1800s called the proprietary subscription circulating library to meet the reading requirements of the public alongside the book trade, as the sale of books was no substitute for a circulating library. The tradition of the proprietary subscription circulating library continued in vogue until the mid-1830s.

Several factors helped promote the establishment and growth of the proprietary subscription circulating library. Chief among these was the introduction of English education (Ohdedar, 1966). As the East India Trading Company strengthened its rule, efficiency in administration demanded a regular supply of learned Indians who were conversant with the laws and customs of the country. This led to the establishment of madrassahs and colleges as early as 1781 (Mukherjee, 1969). Affluent families and leaders of the community who wanted to bring themselves into contact with the new rulers also prized the knowledge of the language (Ohdedar, 1966). The cause of the new education was also advanced by missionary activities in Bengal after 1790 with the commencement of organized missions (Ohdedar, 1966; Mukherjee, 1969).

The early introduction of the printing press in eastern India resulted in the growth of printed books and increased demand for reading material by a burgeoning population in the city. After the first printing shop opened in 1772, Calcutta rapidly developed into the largest center of printing in the subcontinent during the last two decades of the 18th century. The full range of printing included the proliferation of commercial printing shops and newspaper offices as well as missionary and government (Shaw, 1981). The concomitant growth of educational institutions and literary and learned societies encouraged the growth of institutional libraries. Special libraries formed valuable adjuncts to learned societies. The Asiatic Society (1784) was the first and foremost of such libraries, followed by the various other survey libraries under the government of India.

A by-product of the book trade, the proprietary subscription circulating libraries generated a sense of library awareness. However, lacking widespread participation and involvement of the local population, they often remained exclusionary, and their life spans varied greatly.

By 1830, awareness that participation by the European and Indian communities at all levels was essential for sustaining a social library built a momentum that manifested itself in the founding of the Calcutta Public Library in 1836. The Freedom of the Indian Press Act and the Anglicization of Indian education in 1835 (Chaudhuri, 1990) also shaped its founding. In its wake, many more public libraries came into existence. The Calcutta Public Library experienced a slow start but was successful over time as it expanded its services, collections, and number of patrons. However, recurrent financial difficulties hampered its functioning.

Mid-18th to Late 19th Century

With the passage of the Library Act in England in 1850, the library movement received impetus in Bengal and Calcutta in particular. Different localities founded their own public libraries and, between 1850 and 1900, at least 20 libraries were established; many in existence today. The need for libraries appeared greater in cities where English education spread and many neo English speakers became the early subscribers to local libraries. Enthusiastic local young men in their zeal to spread knowledge and information formed groups to establish small subscription libraries in urban and suburban towns (Mukherjee, 1969).

By the turn of the century, Calcutta as the nerve center of the British colonial empire was at its peak. However, many of the proprietary circulating libraries as well as the Calcutta Public Library were moribund. In the vacuum created by the absence of a fine library, the Government of Bengal provided Calcutta with the Imperial Library in 1902. In the late 1930s, its collection stood at 290,000 volumes, and, by the early 1940s, its total collection comprised 390,449 items, of which more than half came as gifts over the span of one and a half century (Kabir, 1987). The historical significance of the Imperial Library lies in the fact that it was accorded the status of National Library following India's independence in 1947 (Kabir, 1987).

Early 20th Century

During the early 20th century not for profit subscription libraries became commonplace, motivated by the principle of free public service. They required a deposit from members and books were not issued free of charge (Dutt & Ghosh, 1934). These libraries played a very important role in the sociopolitical life of a city swept away by a tide of nationalistic fervor. The enthusiasm of the local public was buttressed by donations to these libraries by affluent families sympathetic to the nationalistic cause (Mukherjee, 1969).

The popularity of establishing locally managed not for profit subscription lending library continued unabated for the next few decades. While the zeal with which they were established is unquestioned, a series of articles in *The Calcutta Municipal Gazette* between 1934 and 1938 present a dismal picture of the state of "public libraries" in the city and lament the Corporation's lack of a definite library policy.

Chief among the difficulties encountered by subscription libraries was their financial condition. Periodic reductions of the Corporation library grant further exacerbated their financial difficulties. For instance, the library grant dwindled by Rs. 18,000 in a period of 2 years (circa 1932) (Dutt & Ghosh, 1934). The lack of a good representational collection of books was also an acute problem further accentuated by the fact that neither the Imperial Library nor the various college libraries were willing to loan books to the public libraries. The Imperial Library was already a specialized library and was proving small for the burgeoning community of patrons. The Calcutta University Library was, by its very nature, restricted.

That the Corporation lacked a definite library policy was evident. The Mayor's response to the lack of a municipal library system in Calcutta was that the citizens had never demanded one (Wordsworth, 1937). Several proposals for a citywide library system were put forth (Ray, 1938) including a regional system of libraries cooperating in the areas of book loans, cataloging, and user information services (Dutt & Ghosh, 1934). The Municipal Public Library proposal included a tiered system of libraries with a free Central Municipal Library at its apex, followed by 4 district libraries and 27 municipal libraries in each of Calcutta's wards. Interlibrary loans, library extension work for the illiterate, and children's libraries were also proposed. The perennial problem of lack of space was to be solved by "the workshop idea of libraries as opposed to the museum idea where nothing is discarded" and an open access system was advocated (Dutt & Ghosh, 1934). However, such a system never saw the light of day.

The imperative for a citywide library system was further buttressed by the BLA's survey of 1937. It reported the utter inadequacy of library provisions in the city and the half-hearted recognition by the Corporation of the establishment and maintenance of free public libraries as a primary duty and liability (Ray, 1938). The survey further revealed the unsatisfactory state of libraries that lacked an enlightened policy, improperly organized collections, absence of trained personnel, and inadequate financial support (Kabir, 1987). Of 181 libraries distributed over 27 wards and receiving grants from the Corporation only 13 were free libraries; the rest were subscription libraries with free reading rooms, in most cases only for dailies and other periodicals (Ray, 1938). Other specific problems related to a small stock of books, non-existent cataloging or classification, no library extension or information service, irregular hours of opening and closing, no trained librarian, and no scrutiny of the wants of its clientele.

Nearly half a century later, in 1975, a similar suggestion for a citywide public library system was made to the Calcutta Corporation by the BLA. The Calcutta Corporation again maintained that though aware of the need for public library facilities, financial constraints prevented it from addressing the problem.

Not-for-profit public libraries remained popular institutions within the community, and they continued to grow in the following decades up to 1960. After 1960, a steady decline in establishment of public libraries began, and the trend has not reversed despite the participation of the State government in maintaining a system of public libraries since 1979.

The Bengal Library Movement

A new phase towards a systematic library movement in Bengal began during the 1920s and 1930s from the experience gained and lessons learned from two centuries of library history. Librarians in British Bengal realized that, for achieving all round professional objectives in librarianship, a stable forum for the library movement was essential. The big strides in professional training and the progress in library organization made in the western world had profound effects on Indian librarianship and influenced the shaping of its library movement (Kabir, 1987).

Meetings of librarians in Lahore and Calcutta in 1918 and 1919, respectively, paved the way for the formation of the All Bengal Library Association in 1925. Within a short time the Association was able to generate considerate interest and awareness about libraries. The second All Bengal Library Conference in January 1928 re-emphasized the association's aims, calling upon wealthy citizens to found and support public libraries as part of their philanthropic activities. Establishment of textbook collections was encouraged in libraries to meet the academic requirements of student patrons. Legislation for the development of libraries was called for and universities were requested to provide courses to facilitate training in library administration, which was subsequently started in 1937 at Calcutta University. The institution of popular lectures on libraries in and around Calcutta, creation of public demand for better arrangements in the reading rooms, starting new library centers, and radio talks (Mukherjee, 1969) were some of its strategies to pursue the propagation of libraries. Its main work has been to provide active help to the numerous subscription public libraries in the country and advice—both technical and otherwise, and in preparing groundwork for library growth through lectures and public movements. The Association issues a monthly newsletter – "The Granthagar" in Bangla and has conducted training classes in librarianship for library workers and interested students since 1938 (Mukherjee, 1969).

Post-Independence Period

It was expected that with independence the government and the BLA would work in tandem. Avoiding cooperation with the association, the Department of Education organized District Libraries and District Library Associations under official patronage, ignoring the rich experience of the former in matters such as training workers. The association's call for free book service for all through an organized library system was met by the government's proposal of a library tax to meet the costs of such a system, thus allowing the government to circumvent the issue. It does not seek public approval to increase taxes in other areas, but posed the question to the electorate in the case of library taxes.

The development of libraries under the first two Five-Year Plans in West Bengal was not spectacular nor were details provided to the public about it. The State Central Library was opened (circa 1960) in the northern outskirts of Calcutta on Barrackpur Trunk Road. The site has proved unsuitable as it is far from the population of library users. Four Assistant Librarians were appointed and books were purchased with no readers to use them (Mukherjee, 1969). The report published by the Director of Public Instruction in 1958 states that public libraries received a non-recurring grant ranging from Rs 200 to Rs 600, with the object of improving their book stock, furniture, etc. One of the conditions of the grants was that libraries maintain free reading rooms and offer special reading facilities to groups of neo-literates, women, and children (Mukherjee, 1969).

Recent History

Libraries received scant attention from the government in the decades after independence. Government patronage of libraries was resurrected with the passage of the Bengal Public Libraries Act (1979), enacted "to provide for the establishment of Public Libraries in the State and to regulate, guide, control, supervise and grant recognition to the existing libraries in the state as also to provide for a comprehensive rural and urban library service in the state." Classification of public libraries is now based on the type of sponsorship received, government-sponsored libraries, private Libraries, and recognized libraries. The State has constituted a State Library Council to advise the State Government on the management of the State Central Library and matters of the Public Library system (Bhatt, 1995).

According to the Act, a Local Library Authority (LLA) is constituted for each revenue district. Its Chairman is the District Magistrate and the Secretary is the District library officer. The LLA employs officers and staff in the prescribed manner, if sanctioned by the Government. It has the power to close or discontinue any library. The government is empowered to appoint District library officers and District Librarians in a district. The Government, after consultation with the Authority, may place the District Libraries in charge of the District Librarian. He may manage library affairs subject to the control of the Authority. The financial management of the local libraries is handled by the LLA. The following are the means for augmenting funds:

(a) contributions, gifts, and income from endowments; (b) grants from the Government for general maintenance of libraries or for any specific purpose; and (c) the amount collected by the LLA under the Act or the rules. The Act provides funds from the State Government in the form of Annual Grants. No library tax is provided for in the Act (Bhatt, 1995).

The administration of the Directorate of Library Services falls under the Mass Education Extension Department at present. The Directorate of Library Services is charged with the administration of government libraries and government-sponsored public libraries. Government-sponsored libraries are typically assisted by an annual maintenance grant of Rs. 25,000 (US$ 500). This is used for books, furniture, binding and preservation, and other contingencies. The annual state budget of the Directorate during 1998–1999 was Rs. 327,662,100 (US$ 6,553,242).

SOCIAL, POLITICAL, AND ECONOMIC PROCESSES

Large-scale urban processes, including social, economic, and political, have shaped the spatial and temporal variations in public library growth and distribution. To aid the understanding of such urban processes and study the spatial and temporal variation in library distribution, it is necessary to understand the urban morphology of Calcutta as a colonial port city marked by the twin legacies of mercantile capitalism and imperialism.

The Internal Form of the South Asian City

The urban form of South Asia cities whose historical evolution, cultural connections, and political–economic structures differ from western experiences (Chakravorty, 2005; Dutt, 1993; Noble, 1998) is not explained by urban morphology models such as Burgess' concentric zone (1925), Hoyt's (1939) wedge or sector, or Harris and Ullman's (1945) multiple nuclei. The distinctive type of city that developed in South Asia was the colonial administrative city (Fig. 2) (Dutt, 1983, 1993). The internal morphology was a hybrid, consisting of a large native population and bazaar economy, and a small European population and a firm-based economy. This racial, cultural, and economic division in land use created a native or "black" town and a European or "white" town (Dutt, 1983; Hornsby, 1997; Munshi, 1981).

The distinctive feature of the colonial city is a waterfront location with port facilities forming the nucleus. In the first stage, a walled fort with barracks, officer's residences, church, and educational facilities adjacent to

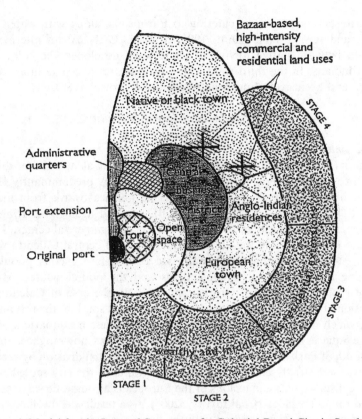

Fig. 2. A Model for the Internal Structure of a Colonial-Based City in South Asia. *Source*: Ashok Dutt (2003).

the port became indispensable elements of the colonial city. Surrounding the fort was the maidan (or extensive open space) reserved for military parade and facilities for western recreation – races, polo, golf, soccer, and cricket. In the second stage, as European power extended inland it allowed for a more spacious and functionally differentiated European settlement. Beyond the fort and maidan developed a "native town," characterized by overcrowding, unsanitary conditions, and unplanned settlements. A western style Central Business District (CBD) grew adjacent to the fort and native town with a high concentration of mercantile office functions, and retail trade, and a low density of residential houses. There were also hotels, churches, banks, and museums. The European town grew in a different direction from the native town. It had spacious bungalows, elegant apartment houses, planned tree lined streets, and amenities catering to Europeans, along with water, electricity, and sewage links (Dutt, 1993; Munshi, 1981). At an intermediate location between native town and white town developed the colonies of Anglo-Indians. In the third stage, these various areas become more clearly defined and exclusively European (Kosambi & Brush, 1988).

The Spatial Structure of Calcutta

The Colonial City
Based on the colonial city morphology 19th century Calcutta can be divided into three zones along a rough north–south axis. A predominantly Hindu "native or Indian town" stretched north and northeastwards from the fort and CBD. The northern edge of the CBD abutted against the fringes of Burrabazar, the pan-Indian traditional bazaar or commercial center. To the south of Burrabazar lay the "intermediate zone" of central Calcutta with a northwest–southeast alignment comprised of a heterogeneous population including the quarters of Anglo-Indians and the poorer whites, Muslim service groups, Armenians, Greeks, and Jews. In the case of Calcutta, the expansion of the European town took place east and south of the fort and the CBD, which included the British official cum business headquarters of Dalhousie Square, the sahib-para (or master locality) or Chowranghee, and the area south of Park Street (Chaudhuri, 1990). The spatial division by race and class was not strictly enforced, for poor migrants to the city settled within walking distance of the mansions of the Europeans as domestic services were needed round the clock (Chakravorty, 2005). As a result, the dwellings of the poorest were always juxtaposed with the luxurious areas of the city.

The Post-Colonial City
After independence, the urban morphology of the city remained unaltered and the spatial divisions of the colonial city (demarcated by class and race barriers) were largely retained. It was not that the "native town" continued to exist or that a European town was maintained. It was the definition of white and native that changed. The "whites" were replaced by a native upper class comprised of Bengali aristocrats, rich corporate officials, and political leaders who now occupied the privileged space once reserved for the colonizers. The natives were not merely dark-skinned Indians but included the less affluent sections of society. The servant enclaves of the colonial times have degenerated into slums, which became interspersed all over the city. In addition, the location of Calcutta's poorest, its pavement dwellers (or homeless population) was concentrated in the CBD in the north and also

in the high-income areas of Park Street and Alipore (Chakravorty, 2005). It will be shown later that the geography of poverty and affluence in Calcutta has important consequences for the question of equity in library service delivery. The presence of an educated middle class, the principal users of libraries, provided a strong buffer between these social groups (Fig. 3).

Urban Processes

Calcutta's Social Environment and Public Libraries

The specific social and cultural milieu of the second half of the 19th century was the Bengal Renaissance which is associated with various forms of bhadralok activism: education, social and religious reform, philanthropy, and patriotic politics (Chaudhuri, 1990). The bhadralok, a broad social category of Bengal, emerged during the 19th century as a result of the colonial situation (McGuire, 1983), and, in the first three decades of the 19th century, no other Indian elite group was so active in public affairs and in such numbers as the elites of the this class in Calcutta (Banerjee, 1987). The term bhadralok is primarily applicable to Hindu Bengalis, and their origins remained firmly rooted in the northern section of the city. They were a powerful political interest group whose social, ideological, and political relationship were molded by formal and informal agencies of the state such as the education system, the printing press, hospitals and law courts, voluntary associations, political pressure groups, and the new kind of government and business offices (McGuire, 1983). As a non-productive class of big rentiers, they assumed many of the characteristics of the British aristocracy. For example, they lived in lavish rajbaris (mansions), had country houses, and educated their sons at the exclusive Hindu College. They patronized literary journals, prestigious European voluntary associations, founded their own newspaper, and organized their own political pressure group in 1851 – the British India Association (McGuire, 1983).

The impetus for the evolution of the earliest libraries in the second half of the 19th century owes its existence to the presence and influence of the bhadralok. Lending their patronage and vast wealth in building libraries was one form of bhadralok participation in 19th century Calcutta society. The spatial linkages between the bhadralok and libraries is evident in the locational decisions of the earliest subscription lending libraries which show a close juxtaposition with the residences of the prominent bhadralok families in the northern part of the city or the "Indian" town (Fig. 4). The formation of libraries as vehicles of social reform, literary activities, political participation, and cultural interpretation was commonplace. Libraries open

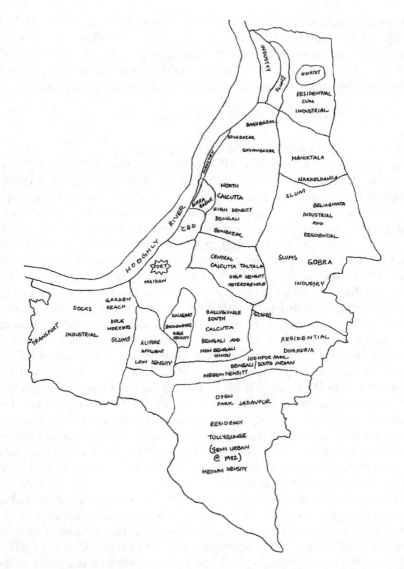

Fig. 3. Some Neighborhoods and Broad Patterns of Land Use in Calcutta, 1981.
Source: Author.

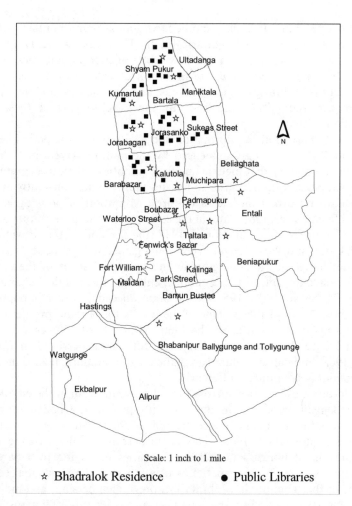

Fig. 4. Spatial Linkages Between Residences of Bhadralok and Public Libraries Location (1850–1900).

to the public from all strata of society became symbols of a progressive spirit and liberal cosmopolitanism.

By the end of the 19th century, the traditional bhadralok class or the literati-cum-gentry had transmuted into another segment of the urban community in Calcutta – the upper middle class professionals, and the culture of subordination of a subject race was giving way to the assertion of a new state of mind which embodied freedom of opinion, racial equality, and constitutionalism (Chaudhuri, 1990). This was the early phase of nationalism and the situation was favorable for literary activities oriented towards nationalism and the interpretation of culture as a basis for national identity. Libraries, reading rooms, printing presses, and newspapers all provided the initial seed bed for the development of these ideas (Chaudhuri, 1990).

The next phase in library formation and location, i.e., the period between 1900 and 1960, is strongly influenced by the multiple layers of Calcutta's very complex society that include linguistic affinities, religious communities, and geographical origins, class, and castes that interact constantly and create an intricate urban mosaic of cultures. Migration of poor agricultural laborers from its vast hinterland in the early part of the 20th century and the influx of refugees after Partition in 1947 (the division of the province into East Pakistan and West Bengal) when India gained independence wrought a dramatic change in the demographic and territorial space of the city that had a massive impact on the economic, cultural, and political character of the city. The period 1931–1950 saw the largest decadal growth in population (Chaudhuri, 1990) (Table 5). One of the results was a rapid proliferation of slums throughout Calcutta. By the 1960s, after almost 300 years of urbanizing influence, languages and language differences persisted in Calcutta (Bose, 1968) and cultural pluralism in the civic community helped indirectly in maintaining communal differences.

The location of libraries mirrors the cultural pluralism in the city. Except for the Bengali, various communities living in Calcutta had more or less built up separate residential concentrations of their own based primarily on language groups (Bose, 1968). This in turn strongly influenced the spatial configuration of libraries in the city. Libraries belonging to a particular community showed a close spatial association with the residential concentrations of that community. Library locations, membership, and individual collections strongly reflect the language and religious affiliations of the neighborhood and community wherein they are established. A preliminary examination of the names of libraries attests to the fact that the predominant community groups active in library establishment were Bengali Hindus, Hindi-speaking groups, and Muslims. For example, north Calcutta is predominantly a Bengali Hindu sector, and libraries in the north cater mainly to them as do most in the south of the city. Concentrations of Muslims in central Calcutta (Mohammed Ali Library), Kidderpore (Islamia Library) in the west, and Entally (Edara Talim O Tabrish) in the eastern sector of the city have resulted in libraries with Muslim names that cater to a predominantly Muslim clientele. Most libraries have managing committees formed of a particular linguistic group.

In addition to maintaining residential concentrations, different language groups are by and large engaged in different kinds of occupations (Bose, 1968). Occupational differentiation of various communities has an impact on library formation because of the differential economic and organizing power of the community. One instance of this is the Oriya community. The majority of Oriya residents of the city are laborers; therefore, the number of institutions run by them is small in comparison to their population. Also, the Oriya community is weakly organized as it has many points of similarity and contact with the Bengali residents of the neighborhood and therefore participates in many of the latter's institutions (Bose, 1968). Communities such as the Gujaratis, Sindhis, Punjabis engaged in commerce have more influence and have built up their own institutions including libraries.

The Bengalis have a strong sense of local patriotism (Bose, 1968). Small combinations take place easily among them for building up a library, a club for physical culture, a sports or a social service organization. Consequently, Bengali institutions are numerous. This is evident in the vast number of small libraries (book stock less than 1,000) that proliferated throughout the city.

Libraries are embedded in the social and cultural life of the immediate neighborhood. The large number of very small libraries may be attributed to the fact that many of the Bengalis' social needs are fulfilled by these organizations. This fact is borne out by the variety of additional functions that are often added to libraries. For instance, libraries have facilities for games and physical culture, children's section, dramatic or literary wing with arrangements for theatrical performances. Libraries also perform communal pujas, like those of Saraswati or Durga.

Calcutta's Political Culture; Economy, and Public Libraries
It is a widely held impression that Calcutta and politics go hand in hand. An important facet of the city's political culture has been its reputation for political volatility that was in turn related to the economic expansion of the city under British colonial rule. In the 1960s and 1970s, Calcutta's reputation as a center of political militancy was cemented as a culmination of increasingly violent political agitations. However, the character of the city's politics changed enormously between the periods before and after 1947 when India won independence. This change in character of the city's politics had important implications for the establishment and growth of libraries in the two periods.

Public libraries were part of the sphere of cultural and social organizations that incorporated political action, from the early decades of the 20th century when revolutionary nationalism emerged. The rallying cry of the times was Mens Sana in Corpore Sano (A healthy mind in a healthy body), the advice of Swami Vivekananda (Mukherjee, 1969). The founding of gymnasiums for physical development and public libraries for mental growth caught the imagination of the people and they became the two arenas where the new ideology was spread and members recruited. Libraries also provided the setting where social activism and reform espoused by the bhadralok were undertaken and adult education in the form of free night schools were begun. However, the growing tide of nationalistic fervor invited suspicion by the colonial rulers, and many of these libraries came under attack and either had to close down or had to curb their activities.

But the trend of establishing small local libraries as cultural, social, and political organizations did not fade. The highest number of libraries was founded during the 1920s, 1930s, and 1940s (Fig. 5), a period of intense political, economic, and social upheaval. And this trend continued past independence into the 1950s, surviving mainstream nationalism, militancy of subordinate social groups, and communal animosities.

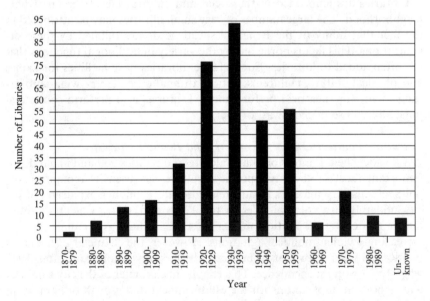

Fig. 5. Number of Libraries by Year of Establishment.

In the 1960s and 1970s, library establishment and growth suffered a general decline (Fig. 5). In the post-independence era, a decade or so of peace and relative prosperity was followed by another period of unrest. The economic problems that threatened the city were tied up with the growing crisis of the Indian economy whose full repercussions were to be felt in the mid-1960s. By the late 1960s when the economic crisis was at its worst, an uprising called the Naxalite movement which sought to bring about an armed revolution proved abortive. However, before it was spent, it had drawn thousands of unemployed urban youth facing a bleak future into active politics. Calcutta became a city of siege and bloodshed, divided into hostile neighborhoods with different political loyalties (Chaudhuri, 1990).

A summary of some of the important differences in political factors influencing library development before and after independence follows:

(1) During the struggle for liberation, libraries played an important role in the sociopolitical field. Libraries often provided the setting for secret revolutionary societies to flourish and were active participants in the political struggle leading to independence. In the post-independence era of the 1950s, libraries ceased to constitute an answer to the socioeconomic political problems of the times and their relative importance declined.

(2) Political volatility was a common element in the city's political culture before and after independence. The crucial difference was that in the former period, militancy was aimed at an imperial power that united people from different backgrounds while from the 1960s onwards Calcutta's politics reflected a class struggle as well as a political power struggle. In a factious political climate, people could not come together to sustain libraries.

(3) In both periods, libraries were unostentatious, but prior to independence this aspect of libraries was an advantage for revolutionary politics. In the post-independence period, in an era of mass demonstrations and strikes, libraries provided a less fiery and dramatic prescription for change.

(4) In the period before independence, the political power in the city was in the hands of the upper middle class Bengali bhadralok, the vanguard of the library movement. The political climate was imbued with their characteristic liberal cosmopolitanism (Chaudhuri, 1990). In the second half of the 20th century, political power had transferred into the hands of labor unions and laboring classes who sought to bring change by revolution. Patronage of libraries in the midst of a class struggle may not have been paramount.

(5) By the time of independence, the Bengali bhadralok were replaced by a
    new set of elites. These elites were not Bengalis but represented com-
    munities that had migrated from different parts of India and were now
    at the helm of the most important industries in the eastern region – coal,
    iron and steel, and tea. They lacked the intellectual culture and aspi-
    rations of the Bengali elites. Their philanthropic role in the city was
    often limited to needs within their own communities.
(6) The political and civic culture following the frenzied political struggles
    of the 1960s and 1970s was one of negativism and disillusionment and
    lacked the idealism and optimism of the pre-independence times (Bane-
    rjee, 1987). The youth displayed neither the zeal nor the enthusiasm for
    the social activism that had resulted in the founding of many libraries.

Thus, the public library enterprise grounded in and spurred by community level participation and social networks of the neighborhoods suffered as
a result of the general decline in political climate in spite of the involvement
of the state since the early 1980s.

In the past couple of decades during the 1980s and 1990s, change has been
the keynote of Calcutta. Change is evident in the city's skyline, marked by
skyscrapers and multistoried apartment blocks replacing old-style houses.
The influx of luxury goods and a consumerist life-style have created new
patterns of life and leisure, generating new needs. For instance, the introduction and promotion of new modes of entertainment such as television in
the 1980s and satellite and cable TV in the 1990s has eroded the membership
base for libraries (conversation with librarians and managing committees).
Expensive housing is pushing the under-privileged out of the city or into the
slums while more and more land on the outskirts of the city is being developed (Roy, 2003). Previously neglected areas now have expensive apartment developments, marginalizing the traditional middle class inhabitants
and the slum-dwellers.

On the economic front, foreign direct investment and multinational corporations made their entry into the Indian economy. The consequence has
been immense competition among job seekers to secure lucrative positions
with them. Social and cultural ties in neighborhoods have been disintegrat-
ing. People's interrelationships and interactions with their immediate neighborhoods are less frequent. Greater mobility has meant that people seek
friendships and companionships outside their old neighborhoods. In the
past, communal events (pujas) would draw young and old in a neighborhood to come together, but these communal events are increasingly being
organized and attended by the more nefarious elements of the locality. In

this context, the corporatization of the Indian mind, proliferation of bureaucratic power, mindless consumerism, and greater emphasis on quest for power, privilege, and status attained by being associated with a MNC have had negative implications for the success of libraries, which called for cooperation, group effort, and "reform mindedness."

SPATIAL AND TEMPORAL GROWTH OF LIBRARIES

An analysis of the spatiotemporal growth and distribution of libraries is discussed in three phases: 1850–1900, 1900–1960, and 1960–1991. The spatial distribution of public libraries may indicate the extent to which the libraries serve the information needs of the population and the extent to which areas are under-served, well-served, or over-served. In a western context, mapping the spatial distribution of public libraries may serve to reinforce findings of earlier studies of public amenities (parks, fire protection, health services) that highlight disproportionate accessibility by race, income, and ethnic characteristics (Knox, 1978; Talen, 1997; McLafferty, 1982). To enable a better understanding of the current pattern of library service distribution, a historical perspective is taken. It is important to draw out the evolution of a public service and its generative processes in a non-western setting as it may differ from those in western countries. Furthermore, such information of service development provides a basis for cross-cultural comparisons.

Temporal Trends in the Growth and Distribution of Libraries

The data for number of libraries established in Calcutta can be subdivided into three stages, which follows a bell-shaped curve. The first stage, from 1870 to 1910, was characterized by an upward trend (Fig. 5). This trend is attributable to the effect of western education, the advent of the printing press, and initial participation and patronage of elites in the cause for libraries. The earliest public libraries began to make their appearance and at least 20 libraries were established between 1881 and 1900. The second stage, from 1910 to 1940, marked a period of rapid rise particularly between the decades 1920 and 1940. The distinctive features of this period are the establishment of the All Bengal Library Association, the rise of nationalism, and the role of libraries in social and religious reform. Altogether, 265 libraries were established during this period. The highest number of libraries established was in the pre-independence period. Fig. 5 shows that the peak occurred between 1930 and 1939 when new libraries established reached a total of 94 libraries. In the third stage, from 1940 to 1990, the rate of establishment of new libraries began to decline. This trend showed a slower rate between 1940 and 1960 but was relatively rapid after 1960 and has since leveled off. An average of 6.975 libraries were established every year during this period.

Spatial Patterns in the Growth and Distribution of Libraries

Library Growth and Spatial Distribution, 1850–1900
In the early phase (1850–1900), libraries were primarily established in north and central Calcutta. The small community-based public libraries' early concentration in the "native" sections of the city, the seat of the bhadralok community, and the newly emerging educational center is not unexpected. The European town to the south witnessed few libraries.

Library Growth and Spatial Distribution, 1901–1960
The broad nature of the spatial distribution and spread of libraries in Calcutta between 1901 and 1960 is shown in Figs 6–12. In the first decade of the 20th century new libraries were still predominantly in the north and central parts of the city. Beginning in the 1920s, more libraries are seen in the south, which was undergoing expansion to provide living space for the growing number of native elite. By the 1930s, the expansion of the railways led to further growth of the city and more libraries are seen scattered all over the city. Fewer libraries are seen on the eastern periphery of Calcutta, a vast low-lying industrial tract.

By 1960, both sections of the city had a vast number of small libraries distributed across its expanse. The highest number of libraries coincided with the areas of highest population densities in north and south Calcutta. As Calcutta expanded southwards, many libraries are seen in the southern most areas of the city.

Areas of the city that show notably fewer libraries are central east and west Calcutta (except Kidderpore). Factors affecting the growth of libraries in these areas are related to land use (Fig. 3) (industrial and manufacturing in the east and northeast, docks and port areas in the west and administrative and commercial areas in the west central sections of the city). These areas are not uninhabited. Population numbers in these areas are high as is the population density. However, the socioeconomic characteristics of the people may differ (literacy and education levels, occupation and organizational power), leading to insufficient support for library establishment.

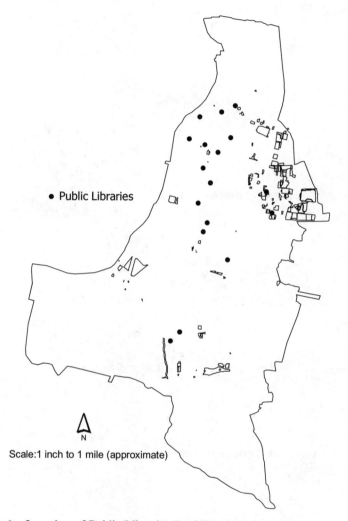

Fig. 6. Location of Public Libraries Established Between 1881 and 1900.

Aside from large-scale urban processes of physical expansion and population increase operating over the city, three concurrently occurring processes at the neighborhood scale have operated in the distribution and diffusion of public libraries over the decades. These are a *copycat effect, proximity, infilling, and spread.*

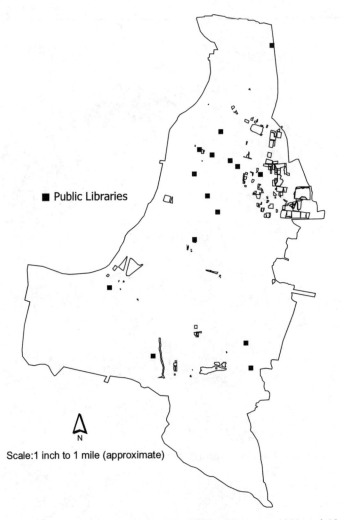

Fig. 7. Location of Public Libraries Established Between 1901 and 1910.

Copycat effect (or temporal clustering) and proximity have worked simultaneously whereby new libraries open close to one that has recently
appeared in a neighborhood. New libraries have very often appeared within
a couple of miles of ones previously established. An early example of this
phenomenon is noted in the western part of the city when the Michael
Madhusudan Library (1915) was established close to the Hemchandra

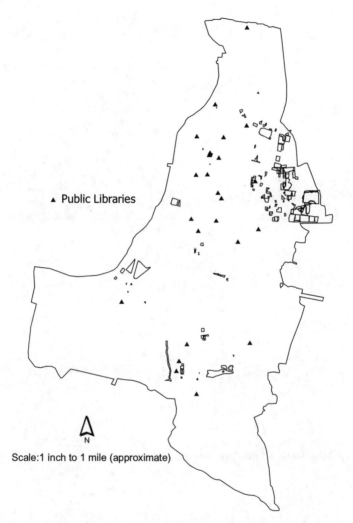

Fig. 8. Location of Public Libraries Established Between 1911 and 1920.

Library which was established in 1906. Similarly, the Kasba Uttarpara Club Library (1920) is in close proximity to the Kasba Library (1904). Voluntary organizations and altruistic workers with an innovative spirit easily come forth to set up small neighborhood libraries as the requirements are not insurmountable. A small ground-level room, some second-hand shelves, a few hundred books, journals and newspapers, and three or four score

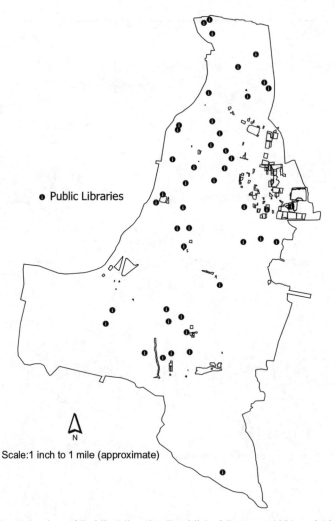

○ Public Libraries

Scale:1 inch to 1 mile (approximate)

Fig. 9.   Location of Public Libraries Established Between 1921 and 1930.

members and a new library is born. The process of infilling allows areas of the city previously not served by libraries to have library services. Examples of this are found in north and south Calcutta in the years between 1931 and 1950. As many of the libraries of the late 19th century have gained institutional character, smaller libraries have appeared in and around them along major roads, lanes, and bylanes. Libraries also spread spatially as

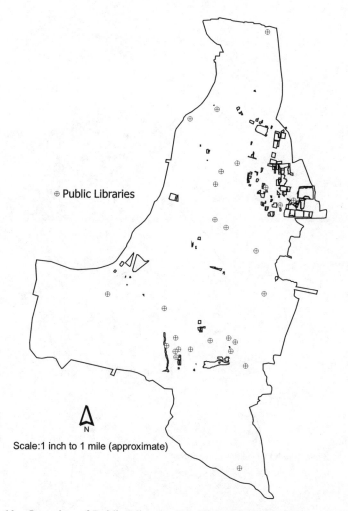

⊕ Public Libraries

N

Scale:1 inch to 1 mile (approximate)

Fig. 10. Location of Public Libraries Established Between 1931 and 1940.

population moved to the south and east and the political boundaries of Calcutta extended.

Table 1 shows that by 1961 the largest percentage of libraries, comprising nearly 59% of all libraries in the city, were in the small category with a book stock of less than 10,000. Large and very large libraries are fewer, together making up less than 3% of all libraries. Almost one quarter of the city's libraries had less than 1,000 books.

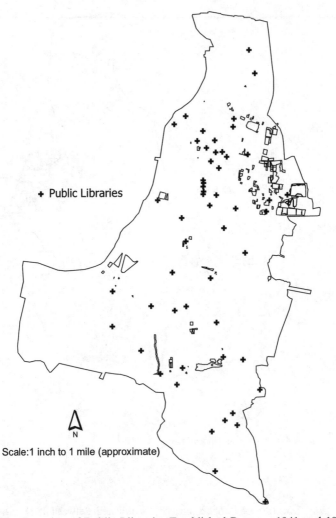

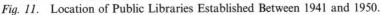

Fig. 11. Location of Public Libraries Established Between 1941 and 1950.

Library Growth and Spatial Distribution, 1960–1991
The period between 1960 and 1991 witnessed two new phenomena. First, after 1960 a sharply declining trend in library growth and development (Fig. 5) was an indication of the eroding political, economic, and social climate in the city. Second, the Libraries Act of 1979 established a much needed library board at the state legislature that would promote the

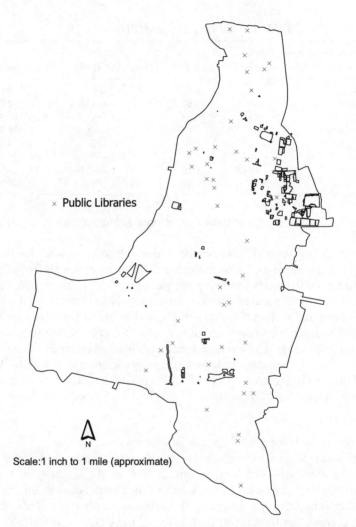

Fig. 12. Location of Public Libraries Established Between 1951 and 1960.

establishment of government-sponsored public libraries. Thus, by the early 1980s a large number of existing libraries came under state sponsorship within a relatively short period of time.

In this period, public libraries can be divided into two broad categories – government-sponsored libraries and non-government-sponsored libraries.

Table 1. Library Size and Structure 1961.

Total Volume of Books in 1961 Library Book Stock	Number	Percentage	Number of Books	Percentage of Books
<500	19	6.60	7,394	0.59
501–1,000	48	16.67	34,484	2.73
1,001–10,000	169	58.68	605,393	47.99
10,001–20,000	25	8.68	333,336	26.42
20,001–30,000	4	1.39	105,522	8.36
>30,001	4	1.39	175,459	13.91
Unknown	19	6.60	0	0.00
Total	288	100.00	1,261,588	100.00

Government-Sponsored Libraries

Government-sponsored libraries are public libraries funded by the State Library department and whose employees' salaries is drawn from the state exchequer. In the years following the passage of the Library Act, the State government proceeded to convert existing (private) libraries into government-sponsored ones. Of the 110 libraries that are government-sponsored, 88 (89.9%) have been converted and 11 (10.1%) are new libraries set up by the administration. The average membership of government-sponsored libraries was 401 persons, and the average book collection was 6,739. The membership ranges from a high of 1,720 members to a low of 31 members, while the range for book stock is 65,000 and 1,957, respectively.

Distribution of Government-Sponsored Libraries

Distribution of government-sponsored libraries does not deviate greatly from the distribution of libraries up to 1960 as the majority of these are preexisting ones (Fig. 13). Thus, in north Calcutta the distribution shows an axis that runs from northwest to the southeast with most of the libraries being clustered in the central east sector of the city. In south Calcutta another axis of government-sponsored libraries may be found extending from the southwest to the southeast.

Areas of south and west Calcutta have received a favorable number of new libraries under the Library Act of 1979 (Table 2). New government-sponsored libraries are located in areas previously underserved. Such location decisions are usually made by the District library officer after a "tour" of the area to determine whether a library is "required" or not. This is most striking in west Calcutta, an area dominated by docks and port facilities

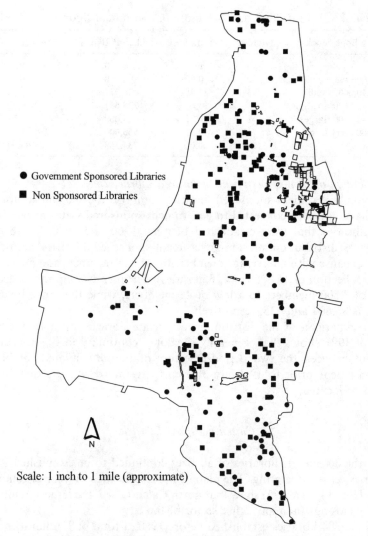

Government Sponsored Libraries

Non Sponsored Libraries

N

Scale: 1 inch to 1 mile (approximate)

Fig. 13. Distribution of Public Libraries, 1991.

where government libraries have spread into areas not previously served. Subscription lending libraries remain elusive in Alipore where the National Library (formerly the Imperial Library) is located. Historically, Alipore is an elite residential area of affluent industrialists and businessmen, and the need or demand for lending libraries may not have been so great.

Table 2. Library Size and Structure (Government-Sponsored, 1991).

Library Book Stock	Number	Percentage	Number of Books	Percentage of Books
< 500	0	0	0	0
501–1,000 (very small)	0	0.00	0	0
1,001–10,000 (small)	93	84.55	420,937	57.30
10,001–20,000 (medium)	15	13.64	225,631	30.72
20,001–30,000 (large)	1	0.91	23,000	3.13
> 30,000 (very large)	1	0.91	65,000	8.85
Total	110	100.00	734,568	100.00

Distribution of Non-Government-Sponsored Libraries
The non-government-sponsored libraries comprise the old public libraries that have not been converted to government-sponsored status as well as 83 new libraries that were established between 1960 and 2000. There is an extensive distribution of non-government-sponsored libraries across the city's expanse with an average membership of 321 members and an average book collection of 15,865 ($n = 26$ libraries). The membership ranges from a high of 2,500 members to a low of 25 members, while the range for book stock is 86,604 and 935, respectively.

A comparison of the distribution of private libraries prior to 1960 and that of 1991 shows that, generally speaking, continuity in site selection is evident between the two periods. Sectors of the city favored for library establishment prior to 1960 are also currently areas where a new library could be located.

Closed and New Libraries

Over the decades as libraries of all sizes continued to be established, many libraries ceased operating. The map of library closings by year of establishment (Fig. 14) (Table 3) show that north Calcutta saw the largest number of library closings than any other sector of the city.

Of the 284 libraries established before 1960, a total of 126 libraries have closed. The highest number of closures occurred in the small (53%) and very small (34%) categories of libraries (Table 4) leading to the conclusion that small libraries, prey to perennial problems of low membership and small size of book stock, find it most difficult to survive. Two features of the period between 1960 and 1991 are (a) a declining trend in the establishment of new libraries (Fig. 5) and (b) libraries established prior to 1960 closing at a faster rate than new libraries being established.

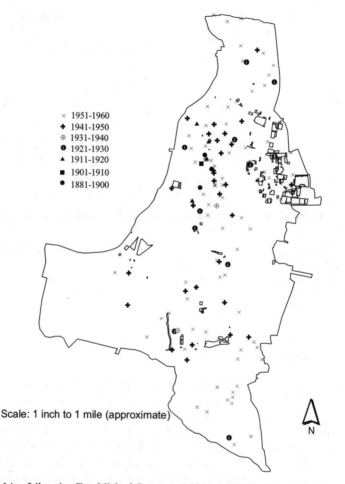

Fig. 14. Libraries Established Between 1881 and 1960, Closed by 1991.

Libraries established prior to 1920 outlasted those established after. The highest number of libraries closures were those established between 1940 and 1960. Two possible explanations are (1) founding fathers of older libraries and (2) time. Many of the older libraries were established by leading figures of the Bengal Renaissance. For example, the Taltala Public Library (1882) was established by Surendranath Banerji, a leading revolutionary of the time. Shashipada Banerji established the Shashipada Institute (1876) while the Chaitanya Library (1889) has stalwarts such as Bankimchandra

Table 3.   Library Closure By Year of Establishment.

By Year	Total	Closure	Percentage of Total (142)
1870–1899	16	3	2.4
1900–1909	11	1	0.8
1910–1919	23	4	3.12
1920–1929	49	10	8.0
1930–1939	28	2	1.6
1940–1949	49	28	22.2
1950–1959	49	28	22.2
Prior 1960	59	50	39.7
Total	284	126	100

Table 4.   Library Closure by Size of Library Book Stock.

Book Stock	Closure	Total	Percentage of 142
> 30,000 (very large)	0	4	0
20,001–30,000 (large)	0	4	0
10,001–20,000 (medium)	5	25	4.0
1,001–10,000 (small)	67	169	53.2
501–1,000 (very small)	43	66	34.1
Unknown (not available)	11		8.7
Total	126		100

Chatterji and Rabindranath Tagore associated with its history. Some of Rabindranath Tagore's famous articles and speeches were first read here. Similarly, Baghbazar Reading Room is associated with Iswarchandra Vidyasagar, Debendranath Tagore, Girish Chandra Ghosh, and R.G. Kar. Because of their historical association with luminous figures of an illustrious era these libraries hold a special place of pride in the community. The library's history is inseparable from the social and political history of the city and indeed the nation [a common saying of the time was – what Bengal (meaning Calcutta) thinks today, India thinks tomorrow]. These libraries were also important institutions in their localities providing night schools, study circles, sessions for discussion and debate of topics of economic and political significance as well as being meeting halls for the literati. Those managing the libraries presently strive to maintain the traditions and aspirations inherited from their predecessors. Secondly, the passage of time itself has helped the older libraries cement their presence in the community by building on previous experience and skills. This has helped them survive turbulent political and economic times than libraries with a shorter history.

Population and Libraries

The overall growth of public libraries is examined by looking at the relationship between number of libraries and population and the number of libraries and population density (Table 5). There is a strong positive correlation between population and number of libraries, borne out by the correlation coefficient with a value of $r = 0.93$. The relationship between population density and number of libraries is less strong with a value of $r = 0.77$.

The total for number of libraries in 1971 represents all known libraries and is therefore high as no information is available about when and how many libraries had ceased to operate. Similarly, in 1981 and 1991 the number of libraries remained the same as no reliable estimates are available for those decades. The total number of libraries has remained unchanged between 1960 and 1991 though population growth is evident. Growth within libraries is evidenced from increased book collections of those libraries that were part of the 1961 BLA survey as well as the postal survey of 1999/2002.

SPATIAL VARIABILITY AND SPATIAL EQUITY

To study spatial variability in the provision of library services the specific question asked was: what are the site-location strategies of public libraries?

Table 5. Population, Growth, and Libraries.

Year	Area (Square Mile)	Population	Population Growth	Population Density	Total Number of Libraries	Population/ Library (1,000s)
1881	7.87	433,219		55,062.32	2	217
1891	20.51	468,552		22,840.88	13	36
1901	18.67	847,796		45,404.31	24	35
1911	18.67	896,067	8.86	47,989.50	45	20
1921	18.67	1,156,753	3.63	61,950.72	84	14
1931	31.40	1,163,771	15.94	37,065.41	164	7
1941	28.31	2,070,619	77.49	73,153.82	181	11
1951	28.33	2,698,000	24.5	95,240.00	230	12
1961	36.92	2,914,412	8.48	78,938.57	287	10
1971	38.14	3,136,391	7.57	82,227.56	292	11
1981	38.14	3,288,148	4.54	86,206.21	279	12
1991	63.48	4,385,176	33.66	69,076.86	279	16

1901 and 1951 population figures are inflated as they include fort and port areas.

For instance, do public libraries locate primarily in wards with higher literacy and lower poverty rates? Spatial equity in the distribution of public libraries is explored by examining differential access of different subgroups in society.

General Overview

Public libraries in Calcutta operate from a set of fixed locations. Books are the only material available and issued. New digital technologies such as computers and Internet access that enable other types of tools and information – data, images, and sound – are absent. Neither there is reciprocity of service nor is there opportunity for interlibrary loan service between government-sponsored and non-government-sponsored libraries or within each of the two subgroups. The users are dependent on the library at which they are members. Many of the libraries have closed access so that members cannot browse shelves or handle the books but must fill a request form for the book required. The present distribution reflects not only specific historical factors but also more recent policy decisions.

Administratively, libraries in Calcutta are organized on an area basis. At present there is a large central library at the apex with 5 town libraries and 103 primary unit libraries forming an administrative hierarchy. Administrative status is mainly a function of library size and overall planning strategy.

Variation in Spatial Distribution of Public Libraries

Mapping the spatial distribution of public libraries provides a useful first step to begin to better understand the implications of the topography of information distribution and consumption on the urban landscape (Figs 6–13). A more rigorous method of assessing the significance of the spatial variation in the distribution of public libraries can be achieved by use of difference of means test. The characteristics (as represented by literacy and poverty distributions) of those wards with no public libraries can be compared with wards with public libraries so that an analysis of their location strategies can be undertaken. This test is designed to test two hypotheses. The basic hypothesis is that if public libraries are randomly located (because of constraints of space and resources) then there will be no statistically significant difference between the mean literacy and poverty (using surrogate variables – percentage of schedule caste and schedule tribe – (SC/ST) and percentage of slum population in 1961) compositions of wards with public libraries and the wards without public libraries. Another hypothesis holds that statistical differences between the data groups will be increasingly evident as the population (as represented by population density and number of occupied residential houses) of the study area increases over time.

As a prelude to testing the hypothesis, the street addresses of public libraries from 1960 and 1999 lists were manually geo-coded with a GIS program. Once the addresses of public libraries were mapped, each ward containing any public library was extracted from the map. Collectively, these extracted wards form a subset of data hereafter referred to as "wards with libraries." The process was repeated for wards without libraries. Collectively, these wards form a second subset of data hereafter referred to as "wards without libraries." Literacy, population, and poverty variables for each time period were compared against the subsets of wards using a two-sample difference of means test.

This test was chosen for several reasons. First, the test is a relatively simple one, and its ease of use is valuable in longitudinal studies where use of census data is limited because of missing categories across time and/or changing definitions of categories. Second, it is capable of testing the fundamental questions issued by the test hypotheses. Similar tests have been successfully applied in other access studies albeit in a western context wherein income and ethnicity comparisons were sought (e.g., Talen, 1997; Graves, 2003). Third, the lack of data to undertake cluster analysis (the classical method) or gravity model analysis because of scale issues makes the use of competing accessibility measures difficult.

This test is designed to determine whether or not two samples were drawn from a single population. As the test value of t grows, the probability that differences between the two sample means are due to chance decreases. When the value of t exceeds ± 1.96, the probability that the two groups are statistically similar drops to 0 at the 95% confidence interval.

Results and Discussion, 1961

The results of the difference of means tests suggest that public libraries are located in wards that have higher concentrations of non-working populations and with higher numbers of occupied residential houses (Table 6). The tests reveal that there is no pattern of locational bias among public libraries, i.e., one that favors wards that are more literate or have fewer poor people (Table 7).

The lack of significant statistical differences for variables such as literacy, poverty, and population density can be directly attributed to the spatial distribution of wealth and poverty in Calcutta. Slums are ubiquitous and their presence is noted in every ward. Homeless populations too can be found in the CBD, north and central Calcutta as well as in high-income

Table 6. Income and Literacy Means for Wards (1961).

	Sample Size (n)	Percentage of Illiterates	Percentage of Slum Population	Percentage of Non-Working Population	Number of Occupied Residential Houses	Population Density	Percentage of SC/ST
Ward with library	74	39.53	21.64	58.84	7,510.57	148,106.09	4.18
Ward without library	6	41.59	20.81	46.78	4,520.67	147,646.50	4.01

Table 7. t-Test Scores for Comparison of Wards with Libraries Versus Wards without Libraries (1961).

Percentage of Illiterates	Percentage of Slum Population	Percentage of Non-Working Population	Number of Occupied Residential Houses	Population Density	Percentage of SC/ST
−0.55	0.11	3.09*	2.27*	0.01	0.14

*Significant at the 95% confidence interval.

areas of Park Street and Alipur. Site location strategies of public libraries are conditioned more by limitations on space and resources and less by income or ethnicity (class or caste). Inertia in location decision has played a strong role.

The reader should be mindful that the test used the number of libraries but variation among facilities in size, membership, service, and hours of operation were not included in the analysis.

Results and Discussion, 1991

The results of the difference of means tests for all libraries in 1991 suggest that there is a positive bias towards location in densely packed neighborhoods where there is a high number of residential houses (Table 8 and 9). Site location strategies are not conditioned by income or literacy. Illiteracy is higher in wards without libraries. This result is statistically significant at the 0.90% confidence interval. Hence, there is some indication that literacy plays a role in site selection of libraries. The density of population is also significant at the 0.90% confidence interval. Other variables do not add a significant understanding of the location strategies adopted by libraries. The underlying demographic and socioeconomic characteristics of the wards have undergone little or no change between 1960 and 1991.

Table 8. Income and Literacy Means for Wards (1991).

	Sample Size	Density/ Square Mile	Number of Residences	Percentage of SC/ST	Percentage of Illiterates	Percentage of Non-Workers
All libraries						
Wards with libraries	103.00	161,710.51	6,268.85	6.62	28.00	66.39
Wards without libraries	38.00	112,909.57	5,228.71	6.81	31.10	67.78
Government-sponsored libraries						
Wards with libraries	69.00	148,070.33	6,592.52	6.67	26.91	68.13
Wards without libraries	72.00	149,026.30	5,409.71	6.68	30.67	65.45
Non-government-sponsored libraries						
Wards with libraries	76.00	187,974.50	6,261.83	5.99	27.89	65.39
Wards without libraries	65.00	102,472.07	5,668.98	7.48	29.93	68.37

Table 9. *t*-Test Scores for Comparison of Wards (1991).

	Density/ Square Mile	Residential Houses	Percentage of SC/ST	Percentage of Illiterates	Percentage of Non-Workers
All libraries	1.90	3.31*	−0.11	−1.64	−1.49
Government-sponsored libraries	−0.03	3.33*	0.00	−2.26*	3.35*
Non-government-sponsored libraries	3.13*	1.66	−1.05	1.21	−3.73*

*Significant at the 95% confidence interval.

Differential Access

The pattern of accessibility and its relationship with the sociospatial structure of the city is scrutinized to ascertain whether there is differential access for particular social groups? The differential access of particular social groups may be useful for planning purposes to identify such groups and to relate their spatial distribution to that of the libraries.

Correlation analysis was used to examine the relationship between the distribution of the number of libraries in a ward and socioeconomic cultural factors. Nine variables from the 1961 census data were examined as shown in Table 10.

Relatively high correlations are found for percentage of Bengali speaking population ($r = 0.44$) and percentage of non-working population ($r = 0.42$).

Table 10. Correlation Coefficients for Wards (1961).

Variables	Percentage of Hindus	Percentage of 60+	Percentage of Slum Population	Population/ Square Mile	Number of Occupied Residential Houses	Percentage of Bengali Speakers	Percentage of Total Illiteracy	Percentage of Non-Working Population	Percentage of SC/ST	Percentage of Libraries
Percentage of Hindus	1.00									
Percentage of 60+	0.32	1.00								
Percentage of slum population	−0.12	−0.12	1.00							
Population/square mile	0.00	0.06	−0.30	1.00						
Number of occupied residential houses	0.00	−0.16	0.36	−0.17	1.00					
Percentage of Bengali speakers	0.61	0.51	0.21	−0.17	0.23	1.00				
Percentage of total illiterates	−0.39	−0.57	0.63	−0.13	0.41	−0.30	1.00			
Percentage of non-working population	0.41	0.49	0.35	−0.02	0.38	0.75	0.00	1.00		
Percentage of SC/ST	0.00	−0.30	0.48	−0.48	0.26	0.07	0.55	0.06	1.00	
Percentage of libraries	0.32	0.21	0.01	−0.08	0.33*	0.44*	−0.15	0.42*	−0.04	1.00

*Significant at the 95% confidence interval.

The number of occupied residential houses ($r = 0.32$) and percentage of Hindu population (0.32) are weak but positively correlated. The multiple correlation coefficient R for 1961 is 0.55, suggesting a moderate linear relationship to explain the percentage of libraries found in a ward and the socioeconomic characteristics outlined above. The results of the correlation of percentage of libraries with select socioeconomic indicators are consistent with the results of the *t*-test of spatial variation. Libraries are more inclined to be located in wards with a higher presence of Bengali-speaking population who are more likely to be Hindu, a higher non-working population and a higher number of occupied residential houses. The location of libraries does not seem to be dependent on the population density within a ward or the presence or absence of slums or the percentage of SC/ST. These findings are not inconsistent with our understanding of the historical roots of library evolution in the city.

Correlation analysis was also employed to examine the relationship between the distribution of the number of libraries in a ward and socioeconomic cultural factors in 1991. Five variables from the 1991 census data were examined as shown in Table 11.

Correlations obtained for population density and schedule caste and schedule tribe mirrors those of 1961. The negative correlation with percentage of illiterates is higher in 1991, so that as number of libraries increases in a ward, the percentage of illiterates decreases. A regressive locational arrangement can be inferred from the results. The multiple correlation coefficient R for 1991 is 0.41. There is a weak-to-moderate linear relationship for explaining the percentage of libraries in a ward and the variables outline above.

Table 11. Correlation Coefficients for Wards (1991).

	Density/ Square Mile	Residential Houses	Percentage of SC/ST	Percentage of Illiterates	Percentage of Non-Workers	Total Libraries by Ward Number
Density/square mile	1.00					
Residential houses	−0.13	1.00				
Percentage of SC/ST	−0.24	0.06	1.00			
Percentage of illiterates	−0.06	0.16	0.29	1.00		
Percentage of non-workers	−0.12	0.16	0.19	0.10	1.00	
Total libraries by ward number	0.05	0.28	−0.12	−0.23	−0.05	1.00

Table 12.   Correlation for Two Subgroups 1961 and 1991.

	R	r^2
1961		
Illiterates	0.17	0.03
SC/ST	0.46	0.21
1991		
Illiterates	0.29	0.09
SC/ST	0.32	0.1

Two subgroups were identified for more detailed study of differential access. Such differential access is typically measured by the correlation between distance to nearest facility and income. A positive correlation implies a progressive locational arrangement. In the absence of income data, the number of illiterates in each ward and the number of scheduled tribe and scheduled castes are related to the distance to the nearest library, following the example of Lineberry (1977), and McLafferty and Ghosh (1982). Absolute numbers are used rather than percentages. Although wards vary in size, it seems appropriate to see how many potential users are within particular distances of their nearest library (Cole & Gatrell, 1986).

Based on the computed figures for r and r^2 it is seen that in 1961 there was a positive spatial arrangement between number of libraries and schedule caste and schedule tribes (Table 12). In 1991, this relationship was positive but weak. The regression r^2 in all cases yields very low positive coefficients, thus leading to the conclusion that the relationship between number of libraries and illiterates and number of libraries and SC/ST is random. These results indicate that there is no pattern of bias in location. Spatial equity and inequity are difficult to determine.

SPATIAL PATTERN OF LIBRARY USE

The spatial pattern of utilization is a product of the location of the service used and the frequency with which each patron uses it (Hays et al., 1990). The objectives of this section are

1. to characterize the spatial patterns of use of library services with regard to the location of libraries (and residence of patrons) and
2. to examine attributes of libraries and of a sample of users in an attempt to explain the pattern of use that emerged.

Two ideas have been influential in hypothesizing the patterns of attendance at libraries. These are distance decay and socioeconomic status of patrons as it relates to mobility. A study of the Port Harcourt Central Library revealed a distance decay relationship as there was a decline in the number of library users and in the number of times users visited the library with increasing distance of residential locations from the central library (Obokoh & Arokoyu, 1991). While distance from a library is a powerful explanatory variable, characteristics of the user are also important. In a Philadelphia study, library patronage declined with distance and the rates of distance decline were greater for higher socioeconomic groups than for less affluent groups (Coughlin, 1972).

The variables considered likely to influence use patterns in this analysis are (1) characteristics of the libraries – book stock, age, (2) demographic characteristics of users, (3) socioeconomic characteristics of users, (4) personal mobility of users, (5) criteria for selection, and (6) the frequency of visits by users.

This section focuses on location and frequency by analyzing survey data collected from library users during 1999 and 2002. The questionnaire was designed to determine the spatial distribution of library users, the distance, frequency, and mode of transportation to the library, as well as of socioeconomic characteristics of library users and their reading preferences (Appendix A). Libraries from each of the sectors of the city – north, south, east, west, and central were represented. In order to obtain a representative sample it was important that the library be a fully functioning institution with an established membership and with regular operating hours. A consequence of this is that a majority of the libraries surveyed are medium or larger ones in terms of their book collection. Smaller libraries often operate on an irregular basis or it was difficult to determine if they were operating at all. Less consideration was given to whether a library was a government-sponsored or not.

The selection of sampled individuals was based on those who volunteered or responded to the survey instrument. A total of 573 surveys spanning 30 libraries were completed. The statistical methods used in the study of library users include contingency analysis and correlation analysis techniques.

The Spatial Pattern of Use

The most striking feature of the spatial interaction pattern is the highly localized pattern of movement. However, the friction of distance acts strongly in reducing the likelihood of visits to those libraries which are not in close proximity to the homes of users. The median travel time to a library is 10 min, but due to distance outliers, the mean travel time is 16.67 min.

The most commonly cited reason for visiting the library surveyed was that it was closest to where the patron lived. Of the survey population, 75.39% attended the library closest to them. The nearest center hypothesis is therefore a strong predictor of spatial behavior. The major contributor to this attendance pattern is the location of the libraries themselves. Most libraries surveyed are located in residential neighborhoods within walking distance of where patrons lived.

Service area delineation to gain knowledge of patron distribution is another means of assessing the spatial delivery of public library services. Service areas were delineated by mapping the residential locations of patrons as provided in the survey instrument. Patrons were given the choice of providing a street intersection, locality of residence, or a street address. For most libraries the service areas are highly localized.

Influence of Library Characteristics

Given the influence of library location on the pattern of attendance, do other library characteristics affect use? A large book stock might be expected to have large trade areas, since the large size would attract greater numbers of users from further away. Furthermore in the case of Calcutta, the age of the library may also influence the size of its trade area. This is because an older functioning library will have a well-established reputation, is perceived as being more consistent in its daily operation and will be involved in the community and provide other functions such as drama and debating societies, programs related to various festivals and the like.

Support for the above observations was not provided by the sampled results. There was no significant correlation between size of book holdings and the median distance traveled to a library. The correlation coefficient obtained was 0.1 while the coefficient of determination was 0.005. When a log transformation was applied to the data, a slightly higher correlation coefficient was obtained: $r = 0.23$ and $r^2 = 0.05$. The median travel time for the largest and the smallest libraries in the sample were 10.5 and 15 and mean travel times were 23.5 and 15 min, respectively. There was no correlation between age of library and the median distance traveled. The correlation coefficient was 0.28, and the coefficient of determination was 0.08. The median travel times for the oldest and youngest libraries in the sample were 11 and 6 min and the mean travel times were 21.8 and 9.97 min, respectively.

Influence of Demographic Characteristics

To what extent do demographic characteristics affect use of public libraries? The following variables were examined further to study this question.

Age Distribution: The age distribution of library users shows variation with the highest percentage of users in the 20–24 years age group (21.60%) followed by those in the 60+ age group (15.82%). A possible explanation could be that a large number of undergraduate students and those who are studying for competitive exams frequent the library. Retired people also are drawn to using the library more frequently than other age groups. No children are represented in the surveys because most libraries do not cater to younger age groups.

Significant differences were identified between age groups in terms of the relative travel time. Differences in mean and median travel times emerged between age groups (Table 13). Given the relative rates of personal mobility, it would seem likely that older age groups would be more likely to attend local libraries while younger age groups would travel further afield.

Sex Distribution: Female attendance to libraries is 47% as opposed to 52% for males. Overall there is no significant difference in the percentages. No significant statistical difference emerged with mean and median travel times in reference to the sex of the users (Table 13).

Language Spoken at Home: The language spoken at home or mother tongue most frequently cited is Bangla (97.34%). Urdu speakers comprise 1.56% followed by Hindi speakers. One factor could be that the majority of the libraries (surveyed or other) are located in residential areas with large concentrations of Bengali Hindus.

Significant differences emerged when the language spoken at home and travel time were considered. Whether the respondent spoke Bangla, Hindi, or Urdu at home emerged highly significant for the travel time to a library. A comparison of the median and mean travel times shows Urdu speakers to be the least spatially constrained in attending a library. However, the higher mean travel time may be more an indication of the small numbers involved ($n = 9$) rather than consistent differences among language groups (Fig. 15).

Influence of Socioeconomic Characteristics

In a large urban setting in India do higher socioeconomic groups exhibit a more rapid decline in library usage over distance than would lower socioeconomic groups?

Table 13. Mean and Median Distances: User Characteristics.

Variables	N	Mean	Median	Standard Deviation
Age (years)				
0–17	40	8.14	5.00	6.62
18–59	433	18.62	10.00	30.12
60+	92	11.10	5.00	11.83
Sex				
Male	369	16.00	10.00	28.63
Female	193	16.68	10.00	17.82
Mother tongue				
Bengali	553	16.55	10.00	27.31
Hindi	5	15.00	12.50	14.07
Urdu	9	27.72	12.50	25.34
Income				
<3,000	54	23.17	10.00	44.17
3,000–5,000	78	18.75	10.00	30.28
5,000–7,000	73	13.15	10.00	13.19
7,000–10,000	67	11.08	8.00	9.37
10,000–15,000	64	27.31	15.00	42.10
>15,000	33	16.67	12.50	18.41
Transport				
Foot	424	9.94	7.00	11.03
Bus	88	46.44	30.00	53.00
Car	5	27.00	20.00	19.87
Combination	30	20.61	13.75	8.10
Cycle	10	11.25	7.50	19.43
Other		19.00	17.50	12.77
Education				
School	45	7.20	5.00	7.01
High school	68	12.11	7.75	13.50
In college	70	22.51	13.00	3.39
Undergraduate	231	19.02	10.00	33.25
Graduate degree	61	16.55	10.00	17.13

Based upon tabulated sample responses, correlation analysis was employed to measure the degree of association between patronage frequency and residence to library travel time (as a surrogate for distance) within various socioeconomic strata. Pearson's rank correlation was selected as the primary statistical technique.

The initial step was to determine if the service areas of the libraries surveyed are characterized by decreasing library patronage as travel time to the library increases (Fig. 16).

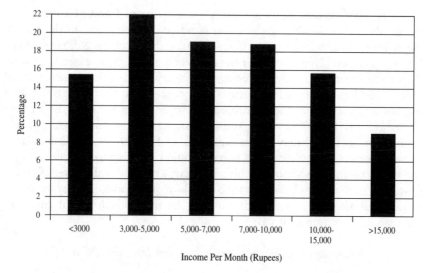

Fig. 15. Distribution of Library Users By Income.

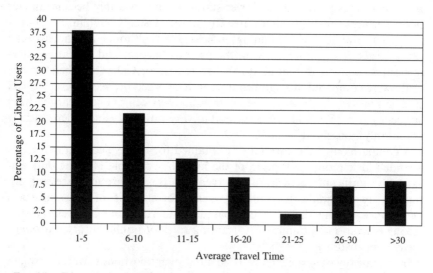

Fig. 16. Frequency of Library Users Based on Average Travel Time to Library.

Thirty-eight percent of library users spend between 1 and 5 min traveling to the library. A distance decay effect is noted as travel time to the library increases up to 25 min. As travel time increases, the percentage of users to the library declines. This effect is reversed when travel time exceeds 25 min. There is an increase in the percentage of library users with increased travel time beyond this point. This pattern of a decrease in library patrons with increased travel time and a subsequent rise beyond 25 min is seen in all sectors of the city – north, south, east, west, and central. A possible explanation is that it may indicate a break of bulk point – 20–25 min represents the maximum time that a person would be willing to walk (walking is the most common mode of reaching a library) or use local means of transportation such as a rickshaw or auto rickshaw. Beyond this other means of transportation such as a bus or car may be used which would cause an increase in the number of patrons.

Correlates of Library Patronage and Distance Decay

As a first test of the hypothesis, the relationship between visit frequency and residence to library travel time among various income and education strata was investigated. Findings on the influence of socioeconomic characteristics on library use has had mixed results. Some studies have found that library usage among higher socioeconomic groups declines more rapidly over distance than does patronage by lower status groups, possibly because higher income groups substitute alternatives for library visits (Coughlin, 1972). In a study of a rural library, the findings indicated that although a distance decay effect existed it was not related to the patrons' income and education characteristics (Bennett & Smith, 1975). In the case of Calcutta, when income strata were compared, no significant pattern emerged between average travel time and visiting frequency. The relationship between public library visiting frequency and time to library appeared to vary randomly and independently of monthly household income.

A comparison of the correlations obtained for the five educational levels provided little more verification of the hypothesis (Table 14). The only statistically significant correlation observed was for the group possessing education up to grade 10 (−0.46). Weak correlations of low statistical significance among the education-based strata ruled out any relationship linking educational attainment to varying rates of public library patronage decay over distance.

Economically heterogeneous residential neighborhoods would explain why no clear pattern has emerged between travel time and visit frequency.

Table 14. Pearson's Correlation Between Travel Time and Visiting
Frequency within Income and Education Subsamples.

Variable	Subsample	*r*	*p*-Value
Income	<3,000	0.02	0.18
	3,000–5,000	0.04	0.37
	5,000–7,000	−−0.16	−1.44
	7,000–10,000	−0.11	−0.90
	10,000–15,000	−0.16	−1.31
	>15,000	−0.09	−0.52
Education	School (grade 10)	−0.46	−3.42
	High school (grade 10–12)	−0.18	−1.47
	In college (1–3 years)	−0.08	−0.68
	Undergraduate (degree holder)	−0.03	−0.39
	Graduate (>4 years of college)	−0.26	−2.03

Alternatively, only patrons at the libraries were surveyed which would automatically filter out those who did not attend at all – presumably the very low income and the very high income groups.

The Influence of Personal Mobility
Access to some mode of transportation is an important factor in personal mobility. The less mobile are spatially constrained in their interaction with libraries. Almost 74% of library patrons walk to the library with a mean travel time of 9.9 min. Libraries are located in residential neighborhoods and their proximity to residences makes them attractive to use. The next frequent mode of transportation is the bus, followed by combinations of the two, or cycles and other methods. The automobile is the least frequent mode of transportation used (Fig. 17).

Reason for Library Selection
A number of factors can be involved in the selection of a library. Proximity to home or work accounted for 75.39% of library selection criteria. The next important selection criteria was that the library attended had the books needed by the patron (67.71%). Third in importance was the fact that the library had an easy access to books (57.59%).

Frequency of Visits
Forty-seven percent of library users visit the library between 1 and 5 times in a month. The percentage declines steadily up to 21–25 visits per month. Thereafter a rise in visits is seen again where visits between 26 and 30 times is 7.2%.

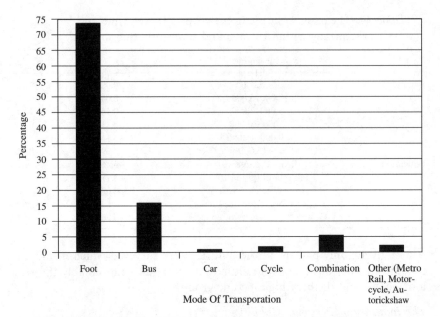

Fig. 17. Distribution of Library Patrons By Mode of Transportation.

SUMMARY AND CONCLUSIONS

An empirical investigation of the growth and distribution of public libraries in Calcutta and the spatiotemporal changes in patterns of information provision and accessibility formed the investigative core of this research.

The study shows that the historic sociospatial structure of a colonial city exerts a strong influence on the distribution of libraries currently. The earliest libraries grew in north Calcutta, the seat of the bhadralok community and the epicenter of Bengali culture and tradition – an area inseparable from social and political movements of the 19th and 20th centuries and from major developments in education, the arts, theater, and literature. In the analysis of the distribution of public libraries, north Calcutta is prominent with the highest number of libraries and forms the central core of high accessibility and use. The spatial distribution of libraries has remained unaltered for nearly 150 years, surviving both colonial and post-colonial periods.

Secondly, the study finds that there is no locational bias in the distribution of libraries. Both correlation analysis and an investigation of spatial variability using *t*-tests show no association between socioeconomic variables and libraries. The geography of wealth and poverty in the city suggests a complex sociospatial structure, and cleavages in income, education, and the like are not manifest spatially. In other words, there is lack of economic clustering and residential location does not reflect economic status. Slums are distributed almost ubiquitously over the city. The history of prominent libraries reveals that they emerged as a result of philanthropy, social, or political activism. Thus, no progressive or regressive spatial arrangement based on socioeconomic indicators is suggested.

Factors that aided the establishment of libraries are (1) age of neighborhoods, (2) role of elites, (3) role of youth, (4) cohesiveness of neighborhoods, and (5) homogeneous neighborhoods in terms of religion, language, and ethnicity.

SUGGESTIONS FOR FUTURE RESEARCH

Some suggestions and thoughts for future research are outlined in this section and fall into three categories: (1) suggestions that pertain to questions that arise from the findings of this research; (2) suggestions on research on library systems in general; and (3) the broader questions of urban service delivery in developing countries.

Some questions that could inform future research include an investigation of the factors that account for variation in library service delivery.

A look at the social history of Calcutta and its various neighborhoods would provide explanatory insight into the processes of libraries establishment and location strategies. The social structures, social practices, and the role of individual agents in their contextual relationship to each other would be important. The individual neighborhood as the spatial unit of study would be more appropriate level of spatial aggregation than census wards.

A deeper probing of the economic and political power of the bhadralok and their role in library establishment could be reconstructed to inform the causal relationships of library evolution, formation, and location.

Adoption of an intensive research strategy of a sample of libraries established at the height of the British rule would provide explanation of the causal mechanisms of library establishment and location strategy. Many of these libraries are important institutions in their communities today and an examination of their role in the community, what sustains them, why and how they function in the present socioeconomic climate would provide insight into patterns of growth of libraries and their survival strategies. In the context of current history, a study of individual agents and their role in managing and operating a library (chiefly voluntary) would enhance understanding of these institutions.

The concepts of accessibility and spatial equity may be examined by use of different measures as well as an examination of other types of data such as road networks and transportation, car ownership, income, and the like. Access to a library is dependent upon an individual's access to available transportation as libraries are an "immobile" service.

Future studies can examine the decision-making process of citizens of Calcutta in their use or reluctance to use library services as they exist, rather than a (self-selected) subgroup comprising library users. This could throw light on who uses the library and why. Spatial equity can be reexamined in light of the findings of such research.

Factors that may throw light on variation in service delivery may include perception of users about the libraries. The attractiveness factor of a library may play an important role in the selection process. In the questionnaire survey and in informal talks with library visitors clean and quiet surroundings, friendly staff, quality of book collections, regular hours of operation, open rather than close access, and lending practices were some of the reasons cited that attracted people to a particular library.

Questions and suggestions pertaining to public library distribution include a geographical study of library distribution and use at different spatial scales namely, urban, regional, and national and different settings, i.e., urban versus rural. International comparisons between western and non-western settings or within cities with a colonial past would provide insight not only into library growth and establishment but into patterns and processes as well.

Libraries ought to be studied in conjunction with other services such as schools, neo literacy programs, etc. as a service bundle to gain a full picture of services in the city. Research on urban service delivery can be broadened from its present focus on basic services to include non-basic services in developing countries so as to examine the geographical distribution of schools, libraries, parks and playgrounds and the like in order to understand "who gets what and why."

Non-basic services such as public libraries, parks and playgrounds, recreational centers, and schools have a huge impact on the quality of life for millions of people in cities and also contribute to the social, economic, and cultural development of its citizens. In large urban centers such as Calcutta hundreds of thousands of people are affected by the availability and accessibility to such services. This study, using the case of Calcutta, sought to demonstrate the provision of information services and accessibility and spatial equity thereof. It presents an investigation of the relationship between public library accessibility and socioeconomic variables, which together form the basis of an understanding of social/spatial equity in urban service distribution. It is hoped that this study offers a methodological as well as an empirical contribution to the analysis of spatial equity in the distribution of urban public services in a non-western setting.

In the information age, the public library is a vital player in fostering economic development of a region. The lack of electronic resources and digital capabilities at public libraries in Calcutta profoundly affect accessibility to information as well as social and economic development. However, the task is not a simple one. Some preconditions to the introduction of electronic resources to libraries are necessary. Library services are fragmented and the lack of interlibrary loans among libraries makes them isolated entities operating within small spheres of influence. The interlibrary loan provision would breathe new life into a system that is struggling with outdated and limited collections, financial problems, capital improvement, and falling membership. Libraries could expand their collections, share expertise, and strengthen their membership base. For library patrons, it would throw open vast possibilities in accessing information. Moreover, interlibrary loan services with universities and research institutions would also profoundly affect the reader's ability to access information. But the small public libraries of Calcutta are small cogs and system-wide changes of a fundamental nature are required. For instance, the National Library (akin to the Library of Congress) despite its vast and rich collection lacks open access to both material and electronic resources. Lack of open access is present at state-level libraries and those sponsored by the government. Most of these libraries including the non-sponsored public libraries have the unenviable task of updating and modernizing their collections, incorporating reference sections, and providing a trained and knowledgeable staff to usher in an information revolution.

However, the vast network of small libraries serving particular neighborhoods, embedded in their communities with a long history of association with the area, intimately knowledgeable about the needs of its clientele, provide an established infrastructure and are in a uniquely advantageous position to fundamentally alter the notion of accessibility to information and knowledge. Public libraries in Calcutta grew as a cooperative enterprise and have a history of social reform and political activism. Their role in these spheres can again revitalize these institutions and make them a pivotal figure in the social, economic, and cultural development of Calcutta's society.

REFERENCES

Antunes, G. E., & Plumlee, J. P. (1978). The distribution of an urban public service: Ethnicity, socioeconomic status and bureaucracy as determinants of the quality of neighborhood streets. In: R. L. Lineberry (Ed.), *The politics and economics of urban services* (pp. 51–70). London: Sage Publications.

Banerjee, A. (1987). Calcutta: Political culture. In: *The urban experience: Calcutta* (pp. 113–121). Riddhi-India Ohdedar; Calcutta-World-Press.

Bennett, W. D., & Smith, B. W. (1975). The correlates of library patronage distance decay. *East Lakes Geographer, 10*, 33–44.

Bhatt, R. K. (1995). *History and development of libraries in India*. New Delhi: Mittal Publications.

Bose, N. K. (1968). *Calcutta: 1964 – A social survey*. Calcutta: Lalvani Publishing House.

Burgess, E. W. (1925). The growth of the city. In: R. E. Park, E. W. Burgess & R. McKenzie (Eds), *The city* (pp. 47–62). Chicago: University of Chicago Press.

Chakravorty, S. (2005). From colonial city to global city? The far-from-complete transformation of Calcutta. In: N. R. Fyfe & J. T. Kenny (Eds), *The urban geography reader* (pp. 84–92). London and New York: Routledge.

Chaudhuri, S. (Ed.) (1990). *A living city, volume I and II*. New Delhi: Oxford University Press.

Cingranelli, D. L. (1981). Race, politics and elites: Testing alternative models of municipal service distribution. *American Journal of Political Science, 25*, 665–692.

Cole, K. J., & Gatrell, A. C. (1986). Public libraries in Salford: A geographical analysis of provision and access. *Environment and Planning A, 18*, 253–268.

Coughlin, R. E. (1972). *Urban analysis for branch library system planning*. Connecticut: Greenwood Publishing Co.

Cox, K. R. (1973). *Conflict, power and politics in the city: A geographic view*. New York: McGraw-Hill.

Crompton, J. L., & Lue, C. C. (1992). Patterns of equity preference among Californians for allocating park and recreational resources. *Leisure Sciences, 14*, 227–246.

Dear, M. J. (1974). A paradigm for public facility location theory. *Antipode, 6*(3), 46–50.

Dutt, A. K. (1983). Cities of South Asian. In: S. D. Brunn & J. F. Williams (Eds), *Cities of the world: World regional urban development* (pp. 326–368). New York: Harper and Row.

Dutt, A. K. (1993). Cities of South Asian. In: S. D. Brunn & J. F. Williams (Eds), *Cities of the world: World regional urban development* (pp. 351–388). New York: Harper and Collins.

Dutt, A. K. (2003). Cities of South Asia. In: S. D. Brunn, J. F. Williams and Zeigler (Eds), *Cities of the World: World Regional Urban Development* (pp. 331–372). Third Edition. Lanham Boulder, New York: Rowman and Littlefield Publishers, INC.

Dutt, B. K., & Ghosh, R. (1934). The library movement in Calcutta: Some constructive suggestions. *The Calcutta Municipal Gazette, pp*, 12–13.

Getz, M. (1978, October). *The efficient level of public library services*. Working Paper no. 55. The Joint Center for Urban Studies of M.I.T and Harvard University.

Gould, W. T. S. (1993). *People and education in the Third World*. UK: Longman Scientific and Technical.

Graves, S. M. (2003). Landscapes of predation, landscapes of neglect: A location analysis of payday lenders and banks. *The Professional Geographer, 55*(3), 303–317.

Harris, C., & Ullman, E. (1945). The nature of cities. *Annals of the American Academy of Political and Social Science, 242*, 7–17.

Harvey, D. (1973). *Social justice and the city*. Maryland: The Johns Hopkins University Press.

Hay, A. M. (1995). Concepts of equity, fairness and justice in geographical studies. *Transactions of the Institute of British Geographers, 20*, 500–508.

Hays, S. M., Kearns, R. A., & Moran, W. (1990). Spatial Patterns of Attendance at General Practitioner Services. *Social Science and Medicine, 31*(7), 773–781.

Hepworth, M. E. (1987). Information technology as spatial systems. *Progress in Human Geography, 11*, 157–177.

Hero, R. E. (1986). The urban service delivery literature: Some questions and considerations. *Polity, 18*, 659–677.

Herskovitz, S., Metzer, D., & Shoham, S. (1991). Development of Spatial structure of libraries: The case of Tel Aviv. *Libri, 41*(2), 121–131.

Hodgart, R. L. (1978). Optimizing access to public services. *Progress in Human Geography, 2*, 17–48.

Hodge, D., & Gatrell, A. (1976). Spatial constraint and the location of urban public facilities. *Environment and Planning A, 8*, 215–230.

Hornsby, S. J. (1997). Discovering the mercantile city in South Asia: The example of early nineteenth-century Calcutta. *Journal of Historical Geography, 23*(2), 135–150.

Hoyt, H. (1939). *The structure and growth of residential neighborhoods in American cities*. Washington, DC: Federal Housing Administration. Publish info [Washington, U.S. Govt. print. off. 1939].

Joardar, S. D. (1993). Perception and use of residential parks in Calcutta. *Ekistics, 362–363*, 276–282.

Kabir, A. M. F. (1987). *The libraries of Bengal 1700–1947*. London: Mansell Publishing Limited.

Kellerman, A. (1984). Telecommunications and the geography of metropolitan areas. *Progress in Human Geography, 8*(2), 222–246.

Kirby, A., Knox, P., & Pinch, S. (Eds) (1984). *Public service provision and urban development*. London: Croom Helm.

Knox, P., & Pinch, S. (2000). *Urban social geography: An introduction*. Pearson Education Limited, England.

Knox, P. L. (1978). The intraurban ecology of primary medical care: Patterns of accessibility and their policy implications. *Environment and Planning A, 10*, 415–435.

Koontz, C. M. (1997). *Library facility siting and location handbook*. Westport: Greenwood.

Kosambi, M., & Brush, J. E. (1988). Three colonial port cities in India. *Geographical Review, 78*, 32–47.

Kronus, C. L. (1973). Patterns of adult library use: A regression and path analysis. *Adult Education, 23*, 115–131.

Lineberry, R. (1977). *Equality and urban policy: The distribution of municipal public services*. Beverly Hills, London: Sage Publications.

Lucy, W. (1981). Equity and planning for local services. *Journal of the American Planning Association, 47*, 447–457.

Marsh, M. T., & Schilling, D. A. (1994). Equity measurement in facility location analysis: A review and framework. *European Journal of Operational Research, 74*, 1–17.

Mcguire, J. (1983). *Making of a colonial mind. A quantitative study of the Bhadralok in Calcutta 1857–1885*. Canberra: Australia National University.

McLafferty, S. (1982). Urban structure and geographical access to public services. *Annals of the Association of American Geographers, 72*(3), 347–354.

McLafferty, S. L., & Ghosh, A. (1982). Issues in measuring differential access to public services. *Urban Studies, 19*, 383–389.

Meier, K. J., Stewart, J., & England, R. E. (1991). The politics of bureaucratic discretion: Educational access as an urban service. *American Journal of Political Science, 35*, 155–177.

Miranda, R. A., & Tunyavong, I. (1994). Patterned inequality? Reexamining the role of race and politics. *Urban Affairs Quarterly, 29*, 509–534.

Mladenka, K. R. (1980). The urban bureaucracy and the Chicago political machine – who gets what and the limits to political control. *American Political Science Review, 74*, 991–998.

Mladenka, K. R. (1989). The distribution of an urban public service: The changing role of race and politics. *Urban Affairs Quarterly, 24*(4), 556–583.

Mladenka, K. R., & Hill, K. Q. (1977). The distribution of benefits in an urban environment. *Urban Affairs Quarterly, 13*, 73–94.

Mukherjee, S. K. (1969). *Development of libraries and library science in India.* Calcutta: World Press.

Munshi, S. K. (1981). Genesis of the metropolis. In: J. Racine (Ed.), *Calcutta 1981. The city, its crisis and the debate on urban planning and development* (pp. 29–49). New Delhi: Concept Publishing Company.

Murphey, R. (1964). The city in the swamp: Aspects of the site and early growth of Calcutta. *Geographical Journal, 130*(2), 241–256.

Noble, A. G. (1998). Using descriptive models to understand south asian cities. *Education About Asia, 3*(3), 24–29.

Obokoh, N. P., & Arokoyu, S. B. (1991, March). The influence of geographical location on public library use: A case study from a developing country. *SLA Geography and Map Division, 163*, 30–42

Ohdedar, A. K. (1966). The growth of the library in modern India 1498–1836.

Pacione, M. (1989). Access to urban services – The case of secondary schools in Glasgow. *Scottish Geographical Magazine, 105*, 12–18.

Ray, N. R. (1938). A municipal library scheme for Calcutta. *The Calcutta Municipal Gazette*, pp. 329–331.

Rich, R. C. (Ed.) (1982). *Analyzing urban service distribution.* Lexington, MA: Lexington Books.

Roy, A. (2003). *City requiem, Calcutta. Gender and the politics of poverty.* Minneapolis: University of Minneapolis Press.

Shaughnessy, T. W. (1970). *The influence of distance and travel time on central library use.* Unpublished Doctoral Dissertation, Rutgers University, New Brunswick, NJ.

Shaw, G. (1981). *Printing in Calcutta to 1800. A description of printing in late 18th century Calcutta.* London: The Bibliographical Society.

Talen, E. (1997). The social equity of urban service distribution: An exploration of park access in Pueblo, Colorado, and Macon, Georgia. *Urban Geography, 18*(6), 521–541.

Talen, E., & Anselin, L. (1998). Assessing spatial equity: An evaluation of measures of accessibility to public playgrounds. *Environment and Planning A, 30*, 595–613.

Toregas, C., & ReVelle, C. (1972). Optimal location under time or distance constraints. *Papers of the Regional Science Association, 28*, 133–143.

Truelove, M. (1993). Measurement of spatial equity. *Environment and Planning C: Government and Policy, 11*, 19–34.

Wicks, B. E., & Backman, K. F. (1994). Measuring equity preferences: A longitudinal analysis. *Journal of Leisure Research, 26*, 386–401.

Wordsworth, W. C. (1937), Libraries and the age: A plea for a municipal library Calcutta. *The Calcutta Municipal Gazette*, p. 7.

Zweizig, D. L. (1973). Predicting the role of library use: An empirical study of the role of the public library in the life of the adult public. Unpublished Doctoral Dissertation, Syracuse University, New York.

APPENDIX A. QUESTIONNAIRE SURVEY

Date: _____   Time: _____ a.m/p.m.   Name of the library: _____

Age: _____ years   Sex: M/F

Are you a ( ) Student; ( ) Employed; ( ) Seeking Employment or preparing for exam; ( ) Retired; ( ) Research Scholar; ( ) Teacher.

Mother Tongue: _____

Please list all languages spoken/read, in descending order of fluency.

Language Fluency _____

1. Please state your place of residence. Provide an address/street crossing or locality/para (Example New Alipore, Garia, Baghbazar) so that it can be placed on a map.

2. How many times in a month, on average, do you visit this library?

3. What is your primary mode of transportation to the library? If combination of transportation modes, please indicate all applicable.

( ) Bus
( ) Metro Rail
( ) By foot
( ) Car
( ) Other (please specify)

4. Please provide an estimate of how much time, on average, it takes you to travel to the library?

5. What is your level of education?

( ) School (class 1–10)
( ) High School (class 10–12)
( ) In college

( ) Finished College
( ) Doing M.A./M.Sc. or equivalent degree
( ) Finished M.A./M.Sc. or equivalent degree
( ) Doctoral Degree
( ) Post-Doctorate

The next question is of a more personal nature, dealing with family income. This information is necessary for the study as it will provide a better understanding of who uses the library. You may choose not to answer it. If you do answer it, please be assured that the information will be strictly confidential.

6. Please provide an estimate of your monthly family income?

( ) Less than Rs 3,000
( ) Rs 3,000 to Rs 5,000
( ) Rs 5,000 to Rs 7,000
( ) Rs 7,000 to Rs 10,000
( ) Rs 10,000 to Rs 15,000
( ) More than 15,000

7. What is your occupation?

( ) Housewife
( ) Retired Person
( ) Teaching
( ) Research
Self-Employed Professional
  ( ) Lawyer
  ( ) Chartered Accountant
  ( ) Doctor
  ( ) Other
Employed Professional
  ( ) Engineer
  ( ) Private Company Employee

() Other
() Government Employee
() Student
() Person preparing for competitive exams for jobs/entrance exams

8. If employed with the government, please indicate one of the following:
() Govt. Official—Retired
() Govt. Grade I Officer
() Govt. Grade II Officer
() Any other
() Not applicable

9. What sector of the economy would you categorize your job to fall under?
() Private for profit
() Government
() National level
() State level
() District level
() Municipal
() Other
() Private, not for profit
() Not applicable

10. Please provide an estimate (a date) of when you or a member of your family last purchased a book.

11. How many magazines does your household obtain through purchase or subscription each month?

12. To how many different daily newspapers do you subscribe (or purchase regularly)?

13. What language(s) are these newspapers published in? Please indicate all languages applicable.

() Bengali   () Chinese
() Hindi   () Oriya

( ) Urdu
( ) English
( ) Other

( ) Gujarati
( ) Gurumukhi

14. Please list other libraries in the city that you are aware of. Of these which libraries are you a member of? These could be lending libraries, college or university libraries, reading rooms, or other.

15. List the three subjects whose books you borrow most frequently. Some examples include but not restricted to engineering, law, fine arts, cooking, medicine, English literature, literature in a regional language, etc.

16. Please describe the major **reasons** why you patronize this library. Some reasons include but are not restricted to

( ) Close to where to live or work
( ) Library has most of the books I need/use
( ) Computer facilities
( ) Because my friends come here

( ) Easy access to books
( ) Only library I know of
( ) Air conditioned environs
( ) Other

17. Finally, which two of the above reasons do you consider most important.

APPENDIX B. LIBRARY POSTAL SURVEY

Please provide information on the following items and return this sheet in the self-addressed stamped envelope enclosed with this package. Thank you.

Name of Library: _____

Hours Open: _____

Year of Establishment: _____

Total Book Stock: _____

Total Male Members (Readers): _____

Total Female Members (Readers): _____

Total Children Members: _____

ABOUT THE AUTHORS

Dana W. R. Boden is an associate professor, and has been a subject specialist liaison librarian for the College of Agricultural Sciences and Natural Resources and the Research and Extension Centers at the University of Nebraska-Lincoln for over 20 years. As liaison to five departments in the College of Agricultural Sciences and Natural Resources, she received her B.S. from Western Kentucky University; M.S.L.S. from the University of Kentucky; and Ph.D. in Educational Administration from the University of Nebraska-Lincoln.

Deonie Botha is a full-time lecturer in both the pre and postgraduate programs of the Department of Information Science at the University of Pretoria, specializing in Information and Knowledge Management. She graduated from the University of Stellenbosch and obtained a Masters in Information Science and a Diploma in Human Resource Management, for which she received the Merit Award for Outstanding Achievement, from the Centre for Business Management at the University of South Africa (UNISA). Currently, she is enrolled in a Ph.D. program at the University of Pretoria. The topic of her thesis is: *The strategic training needs of managers in a selection of large South African companies.* Botha also maintains a strong interest in competitive intelligence, decision making, and organizational sensemaking.

Zohra Calcuttawala received her Ph.D. from the Department of Geography of the University of Cincinnati in 2004. Her research interests span urban and medical geography, feminist critiques, and environmental sustainability with a regional interest in South Asia. At present she is taking a break from her academic career to raise her family.

Marvin J. Dainoff received his Ph.D. in psychology from the University of Rochester in 1969. He is currently Professor Emeritus of Psychology at Miami University and President of the Human Factors and Ergonomics Society.

Paula R. Dempsey has held positions managing instruction, reference, access services, and document delivery for the DePaul University Libraries since

1992. She earned the M.A.L.I.S. from Rosary College in 1992, an M.A. in sociology from Loyola University Chicago in 2002, and anticipates the Ph.D. in sociology from Loyola in May 2006. She has written articles for Reference Services Review (2002), Library Trends (1998), Current Research on Occupations and Professions (1998), and Research Strategies (1996) and coedited Designs for Active Learning (ALA, 1998).

Rich Gazan is an assistant professor in the University of Denver Library & Information Science Program. He holds a Ph.D. from UCLA and his research interests center around the many challenges of integrating knowledge from diverse systems, collections, and people.

K. Brock Enger is social sciences librarian at North Dakota State University, teaches graduate courses in Education at Minnesota State University, Moorhead, and is associate professor of Leadership in Higher Education and General Studies at Northcentral University. She received her MLIS from The University of Iowa, and doctorate in Educational Leadership, Higher Education from The University of North Dakota.

Anna Maria Guerra, Ph.D., MLIS has dedicated her academic career to studying patterns regarding the Hispanic population. She has researched health habits and information literacy in the Hispanic population, as well as utilization of public services such as mental health centers and public libraries.

Leonard S. Mark received his Ph.D. in psychology from the University of Connecticut in 1979. He is currently a professor of Psychology at Miami University where he conducts human factors research in physical and cognitive ergonomics.

Charles B. Osburn is dean and professor emeritus of University Libraries at the University of Alabama, where he teaches part time in the School of Library and Information Studies. He is author or editor of several books and a number of articles, primarily in the field of library management.

Kevin J. Simons received his Ph.D. in psychology from Miami University in 2005. He is currently a senior human factors engineer at LexisNexis in Miamisburg, OH.

Delmus E. Williams is a Professor of Bibliography at the University of Akron in Akron, Ohio, USA.

AUTHOR INDEX

SUBJECT INDEX